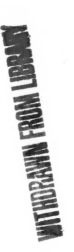

# Medicating Children

# Medicating Children

 ADHD AND PEDIATRIC MENTAL HEALTH

RICK MAYES

CATHERINE BAGWELL

JENNIFER ERKULWATER

HARVARD UNIVERSITY PRESS

Cambridge, Massachusetts, and London, England   2009

Copyright © 2009 by the President and Fellows of Harvard College
All rights reserved
Printed in the United States of America

Library of Congress Cataloging-in-Publication Data

Mayes, Rick, 1969–
    Medicating children : ADHD and pediatric mental health / Rick Mayes,
Catherine Bagwell, Jennifer Erkulwater.
        p. ; cm.
    Includes bibliographical references and index.
    ISBN-13: 978-0-674-03163-0 (alk. paper)
1. Attention-deficit hyperactivity disorder—Chemotherapy—United States—
History.  I. Bagwell, Catherine.  II. Erkulwater, Jennifer L.  III. Title.
    [DNLM:   1. Attention Deficit Disorder with Hyperactivity—drug therapy.
2. Central Nervous System Stimulants—adverse effects.  3. Child.  4. Drug
Therapy—ethics.  5. Health Policy.  6. Mental Health Services.
WS 350.8.A8 M468m 2009]
    RJ506.H9M4234   2009
    362.198'928589—dc22        2008007899

# Contents

# Acknowledgments

We wrote this book primarily for a diverse professional audience, which, among others, would include educators, policy analysts, legal experts, allied health professionals, physicians—in primary care, psychiatry, pediatrics, and neurology—and consumer leadership organizations such as Children and Adults with Attention Deficit/Hyperactivity Disorder (CHADD). We also tried to write for a more general audience of parents and adults with a strong personal interest in the clinical, policy, and historical issues surrounding childhood mental disorders in general and ADHD in particular, and stimulants such as Ritalin, Adderall, Dexedrine, and Concerta.

Most of the voluminous clinical literature on ADHD and stimulant pharmacotherapy involves "large n" research studies that focus primarily on diagnostic and treatment issues and the impairments associated with ADHD. In the social sciences, "n" refers to the number of individuals studied, which means that these "large n" studies examine the clinical outcomes of a large group of individuals. Yet this literature often ignores how the disorder and drug treatment for it both affect and are affected by the pharmaceutical industry, health insurers, the law, and a host of different public policies (educational, disability, and health care). In many cases, it also largely misses the real-world experiences of children and families coping with ADHD. Conversely, most of the popular literature on ADHD and stimulants seems more polemical or advisory/self-help in nature. Our book is unique in that it attempts to pull together different research traditions and academic disciplines to produce a single study of how and why ADHD and stimulants have evolved over time to become the most commonly diagnosed disorder and form of pharmacotherapy among children and adolescents, as well as one of the most controversial.

We are very grateful to Ann Abramowitz, Russell Barkley, Elizabeth Bromley, William Carey, C. Keith Conners, Peter Conrad, Lawrence Diller, Leon Eisenberg, Lydia Furman, Myron Genel, Stephen Hooper, Kelly Kelleher, Rachel Klein, Laurel Leslie, Christopher Nicholls, Gina Pera, Adam Rafalovich, Judith Rapoport, Jerry Rushton, Russell Searight, Ilina Singh, Gerald Solomons, Sydney Spiesel, Paul Wender, and Julie Zito for their insightful comments, suggestions, and constructive criticism on individual chapters or entire drafts (ultimate or penultimate) of this manuscript. Any errors that remain, particularly given this impressive group of scholars and researchers, are solely our fault. We are also grateful to Richard Scheffler, Agnes Rupp, Jill Duerr Berrick, the National Institute of Mental Health, and the Center for Child and Youth Policy at the University of California, Berkeley, which provided financial support to Rick Mayes to begin collecting statistical data and archival materials for this book back in 2001–2002. Catherine Bagwell's work was supported by a summer research fellowship from the University of Richmond in 2007. We have all benefited greatly from the support of colleagues and administrators at the University of Richmond who have encouraged and helped make possible our interdisciplinary collaboration, and we are appreciative of that support.

Portions of Chapter 4 appeared in the *Journal of the History of the Behavioral Sciences* (2005) in an article entitled "DSM-III and the Revolution in the Classification of Mental Illness." A shorter version of Chapter 3 appeared in the *History of Psychiatry* (2007) in an article entitled "Suffer the Restless Children: The Evolution of ADHD and Pediatric Stimulant Use." Parts of Chapter 5 appeared in the *Journal of Policy History* (2008) in an article entitled "Medicating Kids: Pediatric Mental Health and the Tipping Point for ADHD and Stimulants." Portions of Chapters 1, 2, and 8 appeared in the *Harvard Review of Psychiatry* (2008) in an article entitled "ADHD and the Rise in Stimulant Use among Children." We appreciate the generosity of these journals' editors in allowing us to use our scholarship from their publications in the present volume.

We wish to thank Harvard University Press, Vanessa Hayes, and especially Ann Downer-Hazell for supporting our work and helping us through the rigorous and lengthy review process. Without their excellent guidance and encouragement, it is unlikely we would have managed to complete this project given how controversial the subject is. We are indebted to the four anonymous reviewers whose extensive comments on the first draft of our manuscript helped us significantly sharpen our central arguments and improve our book's narrative flow. Gerry Lynn Shipe did her usual outstanding work in creating the index, which was financed by a grant from the University of Richmond. Eileen Chetti and Susan Rescigno were invaluable in helping us navigate our book through the editing and production process. And we are grateful to Leanne Anderson at Lynne Rienner Publishers, who initially encouraged us to start this project many years ago.

Finally, this book is dedicated to our families. Back when we started our research, we had one child among the three of us. Today we have six children, with more on the way. Since we began this project, we have all become much more knowledgeable about how intensely personal the issues surrounding childhood mental disorders, diagnostic processes, and treatment decisions are for millions of children and their families. As is the case for most parents, our children—Tim, Ben, Noah, Ada, Will, and Nat—are the focus of much of our time and thoughts. More and more of their lives involve longer and longer periods of the weekday interfacing with teachers, other school personnel, caregivers, and their peers. The less well they are able to manage these interactions, the more we need to become involved. This is the central dilemma that all parents face when they navigate the complicated clinical, educational, and personal aspects of their children's lives. We have not resolved the pressures and controversies that stem from this dilemma, but we do understand them better, and we hope readers will too when they finish this book.

# CHAPTER ONE

# Introduction

It is obvious that overdiagnosis and overmedication
exist . . . And I do think that a certain portion of what
is sometimes labeled as pathology in children can be attributed to poor parenting, poor schools, and the
pathological levels of stress and pressure that kids (and
adults) now experience . . . But there's a difference between people who exhibit these signs of distress under
certain conditions and those who show consistent signs
of disorder under all conditions. Overdiagnosis is
surely happening within the former group. But the
latter group, in many communities, actually remains
underdiagnosed.

—JUDITH WARNER, *NEW YORK TIMES*, MARCH 1, 2007

Attention deficit/hyperactivity disorder (ADHD) holds the distinction
of being both the most extensively studied pediatric mental disorder
and one of the most controversial,[1] due in part to the fact that it is also
the most commonly diagnosed mental disorder among minors.[2] On average, 1 in every 10 to 15 school-age children in the United States has
been diagnosed with the disorder, and 1 in every 20 to 25 uses a stimulant medication—often Ritalin, Adderall, or Concerta—as treatment.[3]
These figures, however, mask significant geographic, racial, gender,
age, and socioeconomic variation across the United States in per capita
use of the drugs,[4] for which to date it has been difficult to provide a satisfactory empirical explanation. The largest increase in the number of
youths diagnosed with ADHD and prescribed a stimulant drug occurred during the 1990s, when the prevalence of physician visits for
stimulant pharmacotherapy increased fivefold.[5] This unprecedented
growth in the number of U.S. children using psychotropic medication
triggered an intense public debate.[6]

Ironically, neither the debate nor ADHD and stimulants were new.
Methylphenidate, more commonly known by the trade name Ritalin,
was first introduced in the United States in 1955 and was approved by
the Food and Drug Administration in 1961.[7] Prior to Ritalin, another

stimulant (Benzedrine) had been tested and used by small numbers of children as early as 1937.[8] As for ADHD, the basic symptoms of the disorder have gone by several different diagnostic labels since the early 1930s: "organic drivenness," "minimal brain damage," "hyperkinetic impulse disorder," "minimal brain dysfunction," "hyperkinesis," "hyperactive child syndrome," and "attention deficit disorder."[9] Even the core of the controversy, children using physician-prescribed psychoactive drugs, dates back almost four decades. Nevertheless, negative publicity over the "drugging of problematic children" in the early 1970s—together with another negative media blitz and a wave of lawsuits against physicians, school personnel, and the American Psychiatric Association in the late 1980s—greatly reduced the prevalence of ADHD diagnoses and pharmacotherapy compared with current levels. When the 1990s began, there were around 900,000 youths in the United States diagnosed with ADHD, and most schools across the country had only a handful of children (if any) diagnosed with ADHD and using stimulants.[10] By 2000, there were upwards of 3 to 4 million children diagnosed with the disorder.[11] Currently, almost 8% of youths from 4 to 17 years of age have a diagnosis of ADHD, and between 4% and 5% of this group both have the diagnosis and are taking medication for the disorder.[12] If one includes the adult population using physician-prescribed stimulants for ADHD, the prevalence of drug treatment in the United States has continued to increase by almost 12% per year since 2000.[13]

This book seeks to answer a number of questions. Given the fact that ADHD has been present under different diagnostic labels in the United States for roughly 70 years, what accounts for the rapid growth in diagnoses, stimulant treatment, and the disorder's popular acceptance within the past 20 years? To what extent has the evolution of ADHD and stimulants been unique compared to other mental disorders and forms of pharmacotherapy? And why did stimulant use by American youths become so controversial yet commonplace?

As we attempt to explain, the massive increase in the number of U.S. children diagnosed with ADHD and using stimulants stemmed from a convergence in the first half of the 1990s of a confluence of *trends* (clinical, economic, educational, political), an alignment of *incentives* (among clinicians, educators, policy makers, health insurers, the pharmaceutical industry), and the sizable growth in *knowledge* about ADHD and stimulants. Growing political movements advocating for children's welfare and mental health consumers,[14] along with the decreasing stigma associated with mental disorders, led to three seemingly minor policy changes in the early 1990s that helped trigger the surge in ADHD diagnoses and related stimulant use.[15]

First, in 1990, a Supreme Court ruling led to a modification of the Supplemental Security Income (SSI) program—which provides financial assistance for individuals with disabilities—to include low-income children diagnosed with mental disorders such as ADHD. Congress later rescinded this expansion, and many children with ADHD were cut from the SSI program in the latter half of the 1990s, but in the first half of that decade, rates of new children enrolling in the program with a qualifying diagnosis of ADHD increased almost threefold.[16] Second, due largely to lobbying pressure from parents of children with ADHD, Congress in 1991 urged the Department of Education to clarify that ADHD was a protected disability under the Individuals with Disabilities Education Act (IDEA).[17] As a result, more children diagnosed with the disorder became eligible for special accommodations on tests (including the SAT), homework, and other school-related activities. Low-income children with ADHD could receive the same benefits in school, plus cash assistance for their families from SSI. These changes made many parents and educators more aware of ADHD and the services and benefits available to children with learning and behavioral problems who received a medical diagnosis.[18] Third, beginning in the early 1990s, policy makers expanded tremendously the number of individuals, especially children, eligible for Medicaid.[19] As a result, between 1988 and 1993, the total number of children receiving Medicaid services grew by 53%, as the proportion of U.S. youths eligible for Medicaid increased from 19% to 31%.[20] These expansions fueled massive increases in Medicaid spending on psychotropic drugs in general—from $0.6 billion in 1991 to $6.7 billion in 2001—and particularly on stimulants: between 1991 and 2001 real (inflation-adjusted) spending per child on stimulants grew almost ninefold, as the number of prescriptions increased sixfold.[21]

These policy changes reflected a shift that occurred over the course of the 1980s and 1990s in much of the public's view of mental disorders and their optimal treatment.[22] Back in the 1970s, a growing number of leaders in psychiatry and psychology sought to change the definitions of mental disorders.[23] Their efforts eventually led to the "biological" view of mental health—which stresses the neurosciences, brain chemistry, and psychotropic medications—eclipsing the "psychodynamic" or "psychosocial" view, which had dominated for decades and which sees mental disorders as largely influenced by individuals' personalities and relationship development, as well as life's social problems and personal stresses (poverty, bad parenting, broken families).[24] Clinicians usually subscribe to a combination of both mental health perspectives, psychosocial and biological, and encourage treatment regimens that weave the two together.[25] Yet when it comes to what third-party payers—employers, health insurers, government health plans—are willing to pay to treat mental disorders, the two approaches are very different.[26] Thus, it is of major political and clinical importance which approach dominates, as the ramifications for health insurance, education policy, and disability eligibility are extensive.[27]

ADHD and stimulant use have been and remain controversial, partly because most children are diagnosed and medicated as the result of decisions made by their parents and clinicians.[28] In short, the treatment is ordinarily decided *for* them instead of *by* them, a scenario that invites criticism that a patient's autonomy is being compromised to some extent.[29] Yet many medical decisions involving children are made this way and are not controversial. Mental disorders such as ADHD, however, are different.[30] They are regularly diagnosed based mainly, if not solely, on the presence of behavioral symptoms—inattentiveness, hyperactivity, and impulsiveness—that are common and thus not unique to ADHD (despite the fact that the fourth revised edition of the American Psychiatric Association's *Diagnostic and Statistical Manual of Mental Disorders,* the DSM-IV-TR, outlines a much more rigorous—albeit still subjective—approach to making a proper diagnosis of ADHD than relying exclusively on rating an individual's symptoms). The key difference is one of degree. Children with ADHD are *significantly* more inattentive, impulsive, distractible, and/or fidgety than their peers, such that their symptoms cause major personal impairment and interfere with daily human functioning.[31]

At the same time, mental disorders usually involve matters of degree, so why has ADHD been more controversial than other mental disorders? One of the main reasons has to due with the disorder's dominant educational aspect.[32] The majority of ADHD diagnoses originate with the observations of a child's teacher,[33] and many of the disorder's symptoms—rated on behavioral scales—require teacher reports to make a diagnosis (that is, the child "often fails to give close attention to details or makes careless mistakes in schoolwork, work, or other activities," "often does not follow through on instructions and fails to finish schoolwork, chores, or duties in the workplace," "often avoids, dislikes, or is reluctant to engage in tasks that require sustained mental effort [such as schoolwork or homework]," "often leaves seat in classroom or in other situations in which remaining seated is expected," "often blurts out answers before questions have been completed").[34] With ADHD, teachers are typically the primary source of diagnostic information.[35] Only a minority of children with the disorder exhibit symptoms during a physician's office visit,[36] and, as is the case with all mental disorders, there is no definitive medical (blood, urine, radiological) test to verify an ADHD diagnosis. Therefore, the diagnosis contains a large element of unavoidable subjectivity, which leaves it open to competing definitions of what is considered "normal" childhood behavior.[37] In addition, it is not clear why the fourth edition of the *Diagnostic and Statistical Manual of Mental Disorders* (DSM-IV), the official diagnostic manual that categorizes and defines mental disorders, emphasizes the symptoms of ADHD more than impairment criteria.[38]

For these and other reasons, people debate the sources of the ADHD and stimulant phenomenon in the United States. On the one hand, it can be ascribed to medical science making progress on a long-misunderstood disorder. On the other hand, it is claimed that ADHD has largely been "socially constructed,"[39] under the biological vision of mental health, as a response to nonmedical problems such as underperforming schools, increased academic demands and expectations, and higher poverty and divorce rates than existed before the 1970s.[40] What makes this question so contentious is that the debate is as much political and philosophical in nature as it is clinical and scientific.[41] Meanwhile, teachers, parents, clinicians, health plans, and policy makers are all trying to determine—within their separate but overlapping spheres of influence—what is in the best interests of literally millions of children.

This book is designed to try to explain how and why ADHD and stimulant use have evolved over time. As a case study, it is also intended to illustrate the larger changes associated with how mental disorders have been defined and treated over the past three decades, ADHD and stimulants being one of the more striking and controversial examples. Chapter 2 provides an overview of ADHD. Drawing from scientific studies of ADHD, it focuses on the disorder's symptoms and diagnostic criteria, prevalence and developmental course, relationship with other disorders, effects on individuals' daily functioning, possible underlying causes, and effective treatment interventions. The chapter concludes with a discussion of where future research efforts on the disorder are principally aimed. We start our book on a clinical note with a description of the state of scientific knowledge about ADHD because the general public often misunderstands what is and is not known about ADHD.[42] This understanding of the disorder and review of scientific research on its identification, causes, and consequences provide a context for evaluating the changes in public policy and resulting controversies we review in subsequent chapters.

The next two chapters (3 and 4) survey how ADHD as a diagnosis and stimulants as a form of treatment evolved from the early 1900s to the late 1980s. In synthesizing the vast literature on ADHD and the drugs, the chapters explain why, over time, the neurobiological view of the disorder—along with that of most mental disorders—came to dominate and thus strongly influence mental health, insurance, disability, and education policies. The chapters demonstrate that ADHD did not arise as a new diagnosis in the 1990s. What changed, beginning in the early 1980s, was how clinicians formally diagnosed the disorder and the extent to which stimulants became the dominant form of treatment.[43]

Chapter 3 provides a historical survey of both ADHD and the use of stimulants from the beginning of the twentieth century to the late 1970s. It traces the origins of the diagnosis in London by an English pediatrician, Sir George Frederick Still,[44] to the first official listing of "Attention Deficit Disorder" as a mental disorder in 1980 in the third edition of the *Diagnostic and Statistical Manual of Mental Disorders* (DSM-III). During this long period of time, the diagnostic terms used to describe excessively hyperactive and inattentive children changed frequently, as did the claims for what caused the disorder. What remained relatively consistent over the seven decades were the symptoms the children exhibited. Yet even as clinicians and researchers from different eras reached similar conclusions that the disorder was biological in nature, they often reached very different conclusions as to what caused the disorder and how exactly its biological basis operated on a child.[45]

Chapter 4 serves as a bridge connecting the older history of ADHD and stimulants to the larger changes in the field of mental health that transpired from the late 1970s to the early 1990s. One of the main goals of the chapter is to step back and examine the broader trends in mental health during that period. It is necessary to understand these trends in order to make sense of how ADHD and psychopharmacology have evolved over the past three decades. The chapter examines one of the most consequential postwar developments in the area of mental health: the publication in 1980 of the American Psychiatric Association's third edition of its *Diagnostic and Statistical Manual of Mental Disorders*.[46] Developed primarily by academic researchers—rather than the tens of thousands of rank-and-file clinicians—the DSM-III transformed the way in which all mental disorders, including ADHD, were defined, diagnosed, and, as a result, treated.[47] In so doing, the DSM-III also radically expanded the opportunities and funding for research.[48]

The critical change associated with the DSM-III was that diagnoses were defined more as categories of disorder (a person has or does not have ADHD) and less as dimensions of disorder (a person has more or less depression, ADHD, anxiety, and so on).[49] This predominantly categorical—rather than dimensional—approach to diagnosing mental disorders led to many improvements in clinicians' understanding and treatment of mental disorders.[50] But it also gave rise to heated debates over where diagnostic lines should be drawn between, for example, introverted and depressed, shy and phobic, active and hyper, scattered and dysfunctionally inattentive.[51] Consequently, even as the new DSM increased the level of reliability in diagnosing mental disorders, it did not—and could not—resolve debates over the validity of several mental diagnoses (are there really hundreds of qualitatively different and distinct mental disorders?).[52] Additionally, the DSM-III provided much more specific diagnoses for drug companies to target their products at, which over time has led to a disconcerting level of financial interconnectedness among clinical researchers, physicians, and the pharmaceutical industry.[53] For example, 13 of the 21 individuals who created the most recent version of the DSM criteria for ADHD had financial ties to the pharmaceutical companies that market stimulants.[54] More than one-third of all U.S. physicians receive reimbursement for costs associated with professional meetings or continuing medical education. And more than a quarter receive payments for consulting, giving lectures, or enrolling patients in trials.[55] "There's an irony that psychiatrists ask patients to have insights into themselves, but we don't connect the wires in our own lives about how money is affecting our profession," noted Steven Hyman, provost of Harvard University and former director of the National Institute of Mental Health.[56] To many observers, drug companies' direct-to-consumer marketing fosters problems by, among other things, making serious mental illnesses seem banal and creating an easy, overeager and underscrutinized market for psychotropic drugs.

Chapter 4 also analyzes the convergence in the latter half of the 1980s of several major clinical and policy developments related to

ADHD and stimulants. This convergence contributed significantly to the huge increase in the number of children diagnosed with the disorder and prescribed stimulant medication in the following decade. During the 1980s, spending on mental health services and treatment increased markedly, with a huge expansion of inpatient psychiatric facilities for adolescents and those with substance-abuse problems.[57] The dramatic increase in spending on mental health gave rise to employers' and insurers' cost-control response: managed care. Managed behavioral health companies emerged in the late 1980s and focused on finding less expensive ways of treating mental disorders, with decreased hospitalizations, shorter lengths of stay, greater use of primary-care physicians, limited psychotherapy, and the increased use of psychotropic drugs.[58] These new trends coincided with major changes in the pharmaceutical industry, the introduction of Prozac, and the rise of a new mental health advocacy organization: Children and Adults with Attention Deficit/Hyperactivity Disorder (CHADD).

Chapter 5 outlines the large and rapid increase in ADHD diagnoses and stimulant use in the early 1990s. The chapter highlights the linkages among minor changes in federal disability, education, and public health insurance policy in 1990 and 1991 that contributed to this rapid increase. The changes in public policy were partly the result of years of lobbying efforts by a broad coalition of medical professionals, antipoverty activists, and disability and children's health and welfare advocates.[59] The coalition had been pushing for more generous and expansive interpretations of how children qualified for programs designed to aid those with disabilities.[60] Their efforts—alongside changes in public perceptions of mental disorders—inadvertently provided the spark that resulted in a huge surge in ADHD diagnoses and stimulant pharmacotherapy, as well as growing public debates over their appropriateness.[61]

Chapter 6 examines the backlash that arose in the latter half of the 1990s. In tone, it was similar to the controversies over pediatric stimulant use in the early 1970s and late 1980s.[62] In size, though, it was far more widespread.[63] The mid- to late 1990s, therefore, is the period when most Americans first became familiar with ADHD and stimulants.[64] Old allegations that children were being diagnosed improperly and for nonmedical reasons—poorly performing schools, family problems, pharmaceutical greed—resurfaced in newspapers, books, television reports, school board hearings, and other venues.[65]

Chapter 6 also analyzes the Food and Drug Administration (FDA) Modernization Act of 1997, which provided new financial incentives to pharmaceutical companies for developing and testing drugs on children by extending their patent exclusivity.[66] As a result, pediatric psychopharmacology research underwent a major expansion,[67] which led to the development of new once-a-day or "long-acting" stimulants. These new drugs represented an important clinical event and one that, while not solving them, did address many complaints about children's embarrassment taking the drugs during the school day, as well as the drugs' diversion in school settings for illicit use.[68] By both avoiding the need for school personnel—particularly the dwindling number of school nurses in the United States[69]—to administer the drugs to children at midday and increasing confidentiality for families, the long-acting drugs made stimulant treatment an easier choice for many parents and youths.[70] The introduction of slow-release forms of stimulant medications played an especially important role in increasing the attractiveness of this form of treatment because children with ADHD are often sensitive to a change in their internal states.[71] The rapid fluctuations in the effects that result from short-acting medications made many of the children using the short-acting stimulants uncomfortable and thus more likely to reject the treatment.[72] The introduction of long-acting (or extended-release) forms of stimulant medication led to a smoother, less disturbing response, which many children found more attractive.[73] Nevertheless, even as benefits and services for disabled children expanded and ADHD became more widely recognized among educators, many parents of children with ADHD still harbored doubts about their children's diagnosis and treatment, doubts stoked by the polarizing popular debate about the disorder.[74]

Chapter 7 addresses three current issues and questions resulting from the marked increase in ADHD diagnoses and stimulant consumption. First, as the number of minors diagnosed with the disorder grew significantly in the 1990s, so too did the amount of stimulants in circulation.[75] This increased availability—most children and adolescents know someone who has a prescription for stimulants—has raised questions about illicit diversion of the drugs and fostered new controversies over illegal use of stimulants for academic and competitive advantage.[76] In Chapter 7 we review the literature on illicit use of stimulants by adolescents and college students and discuss the degree to which this is a significant concern.[77] Second, a common concern for many parents when making decisions about the use of medication to manage their children's ADHD is whether taking a stimulant will make their children more susceptible to drug use and abuse in the future.[78] We discuss the research on the relationship between the use of stimulants and abuse of other drugs in Chapter 7. Third, the number of adults diagnosed with ADHD and using stimulant medication is growing.[79] Chapter 7 concludes with a discussion of the diagnosis of ADHD in adulthood and the effectiveness of stimulants as a treatment for adults diagnosed with the disorder.

The conclusion (Chapter 8) summarizes our findings, compares ADHD and stimulants to other mental disorders and treatments, and highlights the growing use of protocols and guidelines for clinicians' diagnosis of the disorder. It also explains how and why similar rates of increase in antidepressant and antipsychotic medication use by children lagged a few years behind the significant increase in stimulant use.[80] The differences in timing are due in part to the fact that stimulants—unlike the newer generation of SSRI antidepressants and antipsychotics—are older drugs that have been used to treat a disorder (ADHD) that has traditionally been seen as one that affects children. Thus, while the rate of increase in children's and adolescents' use of antidepressants and antipsychotic drugs has been greater than that of adults over the past decade,[81] the rate of increase in stimulant use has been greater in adults than in children over the same period. Nevertheless, the *overall* use of psychotropic drugs by children, adolescents, and adults has increased by several orders of magnitude over the past two decades.[82]

This book grew out of our separate teaching, training, and research experiences. Rick Mayes is a public policy analyst and former National Institute of Mental Health postdoctoral fellow specializing in healthcare policy and mental health; Catherine Bagwell is trained in child clinical psychology and has worked in clinics for children with disruptive behavior disorders, including aggression and ADHD; and Jennifer Erkulwater is a political scientist whose research has focused on disability, education, and social welfare policy. The book is unique in that it attempts to pull together different research traditions and academic disciplines to produce a single study of how and why ADHD and stimulants have evolved over time to become the most commonly diagnosed disorder and form of pharmacotherapy among children and adolescents, as well as one of the most controversial.

Occasionally the book shifts in tone and literary style due to the fact that our professional backgrounds vary and our respective fields employ different analytical approaches for answering questions about subjects such as ADHD and stimulants. Clinical discussions are followed and preceded by social science analyses of the historical, political, economic, and sociological aspects of the disorder and the drugs. We allow these shifts in tone and style to remain because they reflect the reality that mental disorders and treatments for them are strongly influenced by their cultural and environmental contexts.[83] In other words, ADHD and stimulants do not exist in a clinical vacuum.[84] Like all mental disorders and mental health care, noted medical anthropologist Byron Good, they are "social, psychological and cultural to the core," powerfully influenced by public opinion and varying expectations of what is considered normal and abnormal behavior by girls and boys of different ages and stages of development.[85] So it is not surprising or unusual that ADHD and stimulants have become intensely politicized issues for debate, a debate that sometimes seems to border on being religious in nature.[86]

One of our main goals was to write a book that fills the large gap in the literature on ADHD and stimulants. The majority of publications on the disorder and the drugs are either scientific in nature—and thus aimed more narrowly at research and clinical audiences—or polemics from skeptics who directly or indirectly question the existence of ADHD. The reality is that there *is* an abundance of research findings from the past 3 decades that strongly suggests that ADHD is a real disorder and that stimulants are a generally safe and effective treatment for it when used properly.[87] At the same time, the disorder is often diagnosed, and the drugs prescribed, in a less than thorough manner due to a number of intense pressures experienced by parents, children, teachers, and clinicians.[88] In everyday clinical settings, ADHD is often seen as a somewhat messy, ambiguous, and even residual diagnosis,[89] which leaves many clinicians with a great deal of uncertainty and questions about the extent to which a child's complex of ADHD behaviors—or symptoms, when the behaviors are medicalized—are more a form of developmental delay[90] than a single condition (with three unstable subtypes: predominantly hyperactive-impulsive, predominantly inattentive, combined)[91] connected to a single etiology (cause).[92] One of the many reasons that ADHD is such a controversial mental disorder has to do with the fact that the symptom complex of inattentiveness, hyperactivity, and impulsiveness can reflect not ADHD but some other mental disorder or a learning disorder, or it could simply reflect a child's maturational lag, differences in temperament, or rigid or age-inappropriate parental or societal expectations.[93]

In addition, while decades of research support the position that ADHD is a valid disorder with neurobiological underpinnings, most children are on something of a continuum in terms of their vulnerability (as is now the dominant conceptualization of autism spectrum disorders).[94] And although the standard diagnostic conceptualization of ADHD is that a child either does or does not have the disorder, the reality is that children diagnosed with ADHD vary considerably in terms of the severity and number of symptoms they exhibit.[95] Furthermore, psychosocial and environmental factors—such as more demanding school environments[96] and busier home settings, along with different forms and rates of cognitive development—play very important roles in the complex interaction with biological vulnerabilities to the disorder. These factors cannot be disaggregated[97] and are more influential for children on the high-functioning end of the spectrum.[98] For example, "[a] disproportionate number of children labeled 'ADHD without hyperactivity' are exceptionally bright and creative children," noted Sydney Spiesel, a pediatrician at Yale University School of Medicine who has treated children for many years. "I've often thought that these kids find their own inner theater much richer and more interesting than the outer theater of the classroom and, so, naturally, focus on it at the expense of classroom attention . . . The proper fix for this problem would be done at the school level, a place where I am unlikely to have any significant effect. I can, however, help these children concentrate and return their attention to the classroom."[99] Arguably the most important thing for many clinicians and parents regarding an ADHD diagnosis is that it provides the basis for financial reimbursement by health insurance companies and access to a variety of therapies and educational accommodations.[100] In other words, for many the diagnosis is essentially a bureaucratic necessity to get a struggling child treated and helped.[101]

By integrating our analyses of the clinical, political, historical, medical, educational, cultural, economic, and legal aspects of ADHD and stimulants, we hope that readers will gain a better understanding of the immense challenges of taking scientific progress in research laboratories and flawlessly translating these findings into both public policy and such unscientific settings as schools, families, and clinicians' offices.[102] Given that none of the authors receives any funding from pharmaceutical companies, as many clinical researchers do who publish their findings on ADHD and stimulants in academic journals,[103] we have what we believe is a unique and valuable vantage point from which to analyze the story of ADHD and pediatric stimulant use. Essentially, we have no vested interest in either ignoring or overemphasizing any aspect of the history, current practice, or controversy surrounding the disorder.

Our desire is that this book will increase the public's understanding of the enormous difficulties that exist when it comes to accurately and consistently defining, diagnosing, and treating mental disorders in children. We also hope to shed light on how these difficulties contribute to the ongoing controversies over how mental disorders should best be addressed in terms of crafting and interpreting a number of important health, educational, disability, and welfare policies. As previously mentioned, the dominant diagnostic and public policy models in the United States are built primarily on categorical frameworks (that is, the child does or does not have ADHD and thus does or does not qualify for treatment and special accommodations).[104] Yet, as this book demonstrates, most children in question do not fit this typology well.[105] Thus, much of the controversy surrounding ADHD and stimulants is not over the comparatively smaller number of children with clear and extreme cases of ADHD, which often coexist with other problems such as depression, learning disabilities, and conduct disorders (and who constitute the majority of subjects in clinical research studies).[106] The controversy centers, instead, on the much larger number of children with less clear behavioral symptomology—or those with a shadow of ADHD in the form of mild-to-moderate behavioral difficulties—using stimulants where there is legitimate disagreement over how best to treat them.[107] Consequently, one of our main objectives has been to add a large dose of reason and thought to a debate that has sometimes lacked both.

# CHAPTER TWO

# An Introduction to ADHD

Advances in genetics or neuroscience related to ADHD can be especially difficult to evaluate, and their clinical relevance may not always be apparent . . . This leads to a complex state of affairs. Even as scientists are refining theories of neurobiology in ADHD, clinicians and other professionals are reading arguments that ADHD is not a valid disorder, is overdiagnosed, is excessively treated with medication, or represents a dangerous reductionism that mistakenly views all behavioral and adjustment problems merely in terms of biology.

—JOEL NIGG, *WHAT CAUSES ADHD?* 2006

To publish stories that ADHD is a fictitious disorder or merely a conflict between today's Huckleberry Finns and their caregivers is tantamount to declaring the earth flat, the laws of gravity debatable, and the periodic table in chemistry a fraud. ADHD should be depicted in the media as realistically and accurately as it is depicted in science—as a valid disorder having varied and substantial adverse impact on those who may suffer from it through no fault of their own or their parents and teachers.

—RUSSELL BARKLEY AND COLLEAGUES, INTERNATIONAL CONSENSUS STATEMENT ON ADHD, 2002

The bad news: Attention deficit/hyperactivity disorder (ADHD) is one of the most prevalent disorders in childhood and adolescence. As many as 50% of children seen in child psychiatry clinics suffer from ADHD. Also, ADHD is persistent. Approximately 50%–80% of children with ADHD will continue to meet diagnostic criteria for the disorder into adolescence and adulthood. Perhaps most important, ADHD has a significant impact on children's academic, social, and emotional development and interferes with functioning in important life domains, such as school, family, and peer groups. The good news: ADHD is also one of the most well-researched psychiatric disorders in children, and as a result, we know much about its features, developmental course, etiologies (causes), and management and treatment. The goal of this chapter is to provide a clinical perspective by reviewing the current state of knowledge about ADHD with special focus on symptoms and diagnosis, prevalence and developmental course, co-occurrence with other disorders, other associated impairments, etiology, and effective treatment interventions. Because this book examines ADHD from a variety of perspectives and disciplines—mental health, politics, economics, health care—and because there is misinformation and misunderstanding about what we actually know about ADHD, we begin the book with an overview of what we know about ADHD from scientific research. This review will provide a solid foundation with which to evaluate the arguments in the chapters that follow.

## What Are the Symptoms of ADHD, and How Is It Diagnosed?

Current conceptualizations of ADHD focus on two behavioral dimensions that underlie the core symptoms of ADHD—inattention and hyperactivity/impulsivity. The diagnostic criteria in the fourth edition of the *Diagnostic and Statistical Manual of Mental Disorders* (DSM-IV)[1] include 18 specific symptoms. The 9 symptoms that reflect impaired attention indicate that children with ADHD are unable to sustain attention and follow through on instructions and that they are easily distracted. The hyperactivity/impulsivity dimension of ADHD is also captured in 9 specific symptoms, with 6 for hyperactivity and 3 for impulsivity. These behavioral symptoms involve an inability to inhibit responses. Children with these symptoms of ADHD have an excessively high level of activity—including fidgetiness, running and climbing, and failing to sit still—and act impulsively by blurting out responses, interrupting others, and having trouble waiting for a turn. Three subtypes of ADHD are based on an individual's pattern of symptoms. ADHD, combined type, is diagnosed when children display at least 6 symptoms of inattention and at least 6 symptoms of hyperactivity/impulsivity. The predominately inattentive and predominately hyperactive/impulsive subtypes are reserved for youths with at least 6 symptoms in one dimension and fewer than 6 in the other.

One reason that the diagnosis of ADHD has been criticized is that many, if not most, children can display behavioral characteristics of inattention and hyperactivity/impulsivity. Take toddlers and preschoolers, for example. It is rare that preschoolers are *not* easily distracted by things around them, *not* impatient and challenged by having to wait their turn, and *not* described by their parents as "on the go." Thus, if one naively focuses only on these 18 concrete behavioral symptoms, it is easy to see why there has been public concern about overdiagnosis of ADHD. A correct diagnosis of ADHD, however, depends on much more than this checklist of behaviors. There are five criteria for a diagnosis. The first defines the specific symptoms (described above) and indicates that these behaviors must occur at a level that is developmentally inappropriate and must have persisted for at least 6 months. In other words, the child must display levels of inattention and hyperactivity that are significantly higher than those that are expected for children at his or her age or developmental level, and these symptoms must be persistent and chronic. Second, at least some of the symptoms of ADHD must have an onset before the age of 7 years. This criterion of onset age has been questioned because it may exclude at least two groups—children whose symptoms (particularly of inattention) are not readily apparent until school-related demands increase and adults who do not have clear records of their developmental history.[2] The third criterion requires that the symptoms cause significant difficulty for the child in at least two different settings, such as at home and at school. Meeting this criterion assures that the symptoms are pervasive and do not occur only in specific situations. Fourth, the symptoms of ADHD must cause significant impairments in the child's functioning in salient life domains. These can include impairments in family and peer relationships and in educational and academic settings. Finally, the symptoms and impairment must not be better explained by another disorder. Consequently, the criteria for diagnosing ADHD are not lax or vague (as they are sometimes presented in the media). They are detailed and specific.

Youths with ADHD often show considerable variability in their symptoms depending on the situational context.[3] For example, children with ADHD often function better in play settings than in settings that require persistence in work (such as completing homework) or that place limits on activity levels (such as in restaurants or in the library). Teachers may also see variability in symptoms throughout the school day, with more problem behavior in the classroom than at lunch or at recess, where less work-related persistence is necessary.[4] This situational variability reflects the interaction between a child's vulnerabilities and the demands of the particular environment he or she is in at the moment. Such an interaction is not unique to ADHD but explains variability in many mental disorders. Although symptoms of ADHD may be most likely to emerge in situations that are boring or repetitive, they also manifest in play settings. A common complaint of parents is that their child with ADHD starts an activity and then moves from one toy or game to the next, eventually pulling all the toys off the shelves and leaving them strewn on the floor around them. Similarly, when school-age children play on organized sports teams, parents and coaches often note that a child with ADHD has trouble focusing on his or her own activity and instead is too often distracted by the game on the next field, the dog walking by, or the bees on the clover in right field. In addition to this situational variability, the behavior and task performance of a child with ADHD is often inconsistent, with good performance (completing homework, getting a high test score, finishing chores at home) one day and poor performance the next.[5]

As with other psychiatric disorders, there is no blood test, X-ray, or other laboratory test that can identify ADHD. A careful clinical diagnosis of ADHD is made based on the collection of a detailed history of the child's symptoms and their developmental course, including the child's medical, neurological, and social history.[6] Variability in diagnoses is thus in part due to variability in assessment and in how strictly DSM-IV criteria are applied.[7] Most thorough assessment batteries rely on a combination of clinical interviews, behavior-rating scales, and various other tests and observations, including IQ and achievement tests, computerized continuous performance tests, and/or medical tests to rule out alternative explanations. In addition, information is gathered from multiple sources, including parents, teachers, the child, and others who might have knowledge about the child's functioning. This multimethod approach is important for ensuring that all DSM-IV criteria are met. For example, the assessment of developmental inappropriateness of symptoms is better accomplished with rating scales that have well-established norms than with clinical interviews that require a parent's, educator's, or clinician's subjective assessment of where a child's behavior fits with other children of the same age.[8]

## How Common Is ADHD, and How Does It Change over the Life Span?

In U.S. samples, the prevalence of ADHD is approximately 4% to 6% of school-age children,[9] and DSM-IV reports an estimated prevalence between 3% and 5%. However, not surprisingly, prevalence rates differ substantially depending on the characteristics of the sample (such as age, sex composition, clinic versus community based) and how ADHD is assessed (based on a comprehensive clinical assessment versus based on a rating-scale cutoff). For example, if teacher ratings are used alone, prevalence rates soar as high as 15%.[10] Using parent reports and complete DSM-IV criteria as opposed to simple cutoffs on behavior-rating scales brings the prevalence rates down. This variability highlights the importance of the DSM-IV criteria of developmental deviance, functional impairment, persistence, and pervasiveness of symptoms. In one study that rigorously applied DSM-IV criteria using a representative population sample and annual assessments over a number of years, the 3-month prevalence rate of ADHD was approximately 1% among 9- to 16-year-old children and adolescents.[11] In the same study, it was estimated that just over 4% of children would meet the criteria for a diagnosis of ADHD at some point before the age of 16 years.[12]

In clinic and community or epidemiological samples, ADHD is much more common in boys than in girls. These differential rates vary considerably, with an average ratio of approximately 3 to 1 across epidemiological samples.[13] Sex differences are much higher in clinic samples, which likely is a reflection of a referral bias. Specifically, girls tend to have fewer symptoms of aggression and other conduct problems than boys, and these are the symptoms that often precipitate referral. In addition, relying on teacher reports also accentuates gender differences in rates of ADHD.[14] Russell Barkley has argued that the uneven male-to-female ratio may be due in part to the fact that the symptom threshold in DSM-IV (at least 6 of 9 symptoms of inattention or hyperactivity/impulsivity) is less appropriate for girls than for boys.[15] Specifically, boys display more of the behaviors reflected in the DSM-IV ADHD symptom list than do girls, and the majority of participants in the DSM-IV field trial were boys.[16] Thus, in order to meet criteria for an ADHD diagnosis, girls must be more deviant relative to other girls than boys have to be relative to other boys. Nevertheless, there is some evidence that girls are more likely to be diagnosed with the inattentive subtype of ADHD[17] and that although girls with ADHD are less likely to show conduct problems than boys with ADHD, other academic and social impairments are similar for both boys and girls with ADHD. In addition, two recent follow-up studies of girls with ADHD demonstrate clearly that girls with ADHD show significant impairments 5 years later, even if their symptoms of ADHD improve. These impairments include much higher levels of mood and anxiety disorders, disruptive behavior, and substance abuse and dependence, and much lower levels of social skills and academic achievement than non-ADHD comparison girls.[18]

ADHD typically emerges in the preschool period, often around age 3 or 4 years.[19] A number of studies demonstrate that particular ADHD symptoms have different ages of onset and developmental courses. Hyperactive and impulsive behavior has the earliest onset, and inattentive behaviors often emerge after school entry.[20] Although some cross-sectional studies show declining rates of ADHD with increasing age,[21] this finding is likely due in part to the fact that the symptom list in DSM-IV is based on children between the ages of 4 and 16, and the behavioral symptoms of hyperactivity decline with development.[22]

Long-term studies indicate that many children do not "outgrow" ADHD, yet ADHD in adulthood has been a controversial diagnosis given that it has, until fairly recently, been described as a disorder of childhood.[23] Findings from a handful of studies that follow children with ADHD into adolescence and adulthood emphasize the persistence and pervasive impairment associated with ADHD symptoms. In two cohorts of approximately 100 children, 31% to 43% continued to be diagnosed with ADHD at a mean age of 18.5 years.[24] In another study, 50% of the sample of adolescents with a history of childhood ADHD had a current diagnosis of ADHD in late adolescence (approximately age 19).[25] With parent reports of ADHD symptoms, Barkley and colleagues found that ADHD persisted for 46% to 66% of the probands (the follow-up group who had an ADHD diagnosis in childhood) at age 21 and for 44% of the probands at age 27 (by self-report).[26] These rates are even higher in mid-adolescence. At an average age of 15, 70% of adolescents with a diagnosis of ADHD in childhood continued to meet DSM criteria for the disorder.[27] Likewise, Joseph Biederman and colleagues found that by age 14, only 15% of the probands no longer had a diagnosis of ADHD.[28] Severity of ADHD in childhood appears to be one of the best predictors of persistence of symptoms into adulthood.[29]

Follow-up studies show that not only do adolescents and adults with a history of ADHD in childhood often continue to have the disorder, but they also experience a host of other psychiatric, cognitive, and psychosocial impairments. By mid-adolescence, youths with a childhood history of ADHD have higher rates of conduct disorders and substance use;[30] greater impairment in academic functioning, including reading and math achievement and failing a grade;[31] and more problems with parents, siblings, and peers compared to control groups.[32] Findings have been inconsistent with regard to whether children with ADHD have an elevated risk for anxiety and depression in adolescence and adulthood. Biederman and colleagues identified a higher rate of both disorders for boys and girls with ADHD in mid-adolescence, and Russell Barkley,

Mariellen Fischer, and colleagues reported an increased risk for depression at age 21 and for anxiety disorders at age 27.[33] However, other studies have shown no differences between adolescents and adults with a history of childhood ADHD and control groups in rates of anxiety and depressive disorders.[34] There is some indication that increased risk for these disorders is limited to youths who also have serious aggression and disruptive behavior.[35]

## Does ADHD Occur with Other Disorders?

The diagnosis and treatment of ADHD can be complicated by its comorbidity—the co-occurrence of ADHD and other disorders. In particular, comorbidity raises a number of questions. Which symptoms should be the primary focus in treatment? Is there a causal relationship between the disorders such that ADHD can cause or be caused by another disorder? Is comorbidity simply due to an overlap in symptoms as defined by DSM-IV, or does the individual indeed suffer from two or more distinct disorders? Rates of comorbidity vary, but most epidemiological studies find that nearly half of children who are diagnosed with ADHD also meet diagnostic criteria for another disorder.[36] In clinic samples, these rates are higher, in part due to the fact that children with a greater number and severity of symptoms are more likely to be referred for treatment.

In the DSM-IV, ADHD is grouped with oppositional defiant disorder (ODD) and conduct disorder (CD) in the category of disruptive behavior disorders, and ODD and CD are the most common comorbid conditions with ADHD. ODD is characterized by a pattern of noncompliant and oppositional behaviors (for example, arguing, defying adults, losing temper). CD describes a constellation of serious aggressive and rule-breaking behaviors (for example, fighting, truancy, lying, stealing, destroying property) that typically develop later than ODD. In their compilation of results across many epidemiological studies, Adrian Angold and colleagues found that having ADHD results in a more than tenfold increase in the likelihood of having ODD or CD.[37] By adulthood, as many as 12% to 21% of youths with ADHD will be diagnosed with antisocial personality disorder, which is a persistent pattern of illegal, deceitful, impulsive, and aggressive behaviors that violate the rights of others.[38]

In addition to comorbid disruptive behavior disorders, anxiety and depression show considerable overlap with ADHD. Peter Jensen and colleagues reviewed many studies and reported that rates of comorbidity between ADHD and anxiety and depression vary from 13% to as high as 50%.[39] In clinic-referred and epidemiological samples, as many as one-third of children identified with ADHD also have anxiety disorders.[40] Some evidence suggests that the link between ADHD and depression may be even stronger than that between ADHD and anxiety. Angold and colleagues found a greater than fivefold increase in the likelihood of depression given a diagnosis of ADHD.[41] This association between ADHD and depression may be mediated by CD or ODD.[42] In one study of boys with ADHD who were followed into adulthood, levels of aggression in childhood predicted major depression in adulthood.[43] Similarly, in a follow-up study, childhood conduct problems, severity of CD in adolescence, and antisocial personality disorder in adulthood were related, and antisocial personality disorder predicted increased rates of major depression.[44] Thus, the association between ADHD and depressive disorders may be explained at least in part by links between ADHD and conduct problems, showing that ADHD without conduct problems may not be associated with increased rates of depressive disorders.

A question that arises when comorbidity is considered is whether co-occurring conditions represent distinct and meaningful subtypes of ADHD. If there are unique causes and outcomes for ADHD depending on the presence or absence of comorbid disorders, there may also be different responses to the typical treatment approaches. Jensen and colleagues reviewed evidence for the co-occurrence of ADHD and CD, mood disorders such as depression, anxiety disorders, learning disabilities, and Tourette's syndrome.[45] Using a number of criteria to examine whether patterns of comorbidity represent distinct subcategories, they determined that ADHD with CD and ADHD with anxiety can be considered unique subtypes of ADHD. In a later study directly comparing four groups of youths with ADHD—ADHD with comorbid anxiety; ADHD with comorbid CD or ODD; ADHD with comorbid anxiety and CD or ODD; and "pure" ADHD, without comorbid anxiety, CD, or ODD—Jensen and colleagues found evidence for three distinct subtypes with different demographic characteristics, outcomes, and responses to treatment.[46] Specifically, the ADHD with CD or ODD and the ADHD with anxiety groups differed on multiple variables: the comorbid anxiety group had fewer hyperactive-impulsive symptoms and lower overall impairment, more diagnoses of learning disability, lower math and spelling achievement scores, and more positive indicators of family functioning than the comorbid CD or ODD group. In addition, anxiety and CD or ODD exerted their effects on different variables, which is an indication of different symptom profiles for these two groups. An interesting finding of this study is that youths with ADHD and anxiety had a better response to treatment and often showed better functioning than youth without anxiety, regardless of whether or not they had comorbid CD or ODD. Furthermore, the ADHD group with anxiety responded well to behavioral interventions, but the ADHD group with both CD or ODD and anxiety responded best to combined treatment that included medication management and psychosocial interventions.

Taken together, these studies indicate that ADHD is often complicated by comorbid conditions. As discussed below, youths with various patterns of symptoms may respond differently to particular treatment approaches. In addition, long-term outcomes associated with ADHD vary for children with different comorbid conditions. This suggests that careful attention not only to the recognized subtypes of ADHD in DSM-IV but also to patterns of comorbidity is essential in predicting current and future functioning and responses to treatment.

## How Else Does ADHD Affect Children, Adolescents, and Adults?

In addition to the risk for these and other psychiatric problems associated with ADHD, youths with ADHD encounter numerous cognitive, emotional, and social challenges and are likely to experience impaired functioning in all of these domains. Concluding that children and adolescents with ADHD face significant and long-lasting impairment across numerous domains of life, Stephen Hinshaw describes why understanding impairment is important: "This impairment magnifies the need to develop viable and durable intervention strategies; it provides validation of the disorder from a scientific and nosologic perspective; it illustrates the need for ecological research on the interplay between afflicted individuals and their social contexts; and it underscores the need for coordinated social policy related to preventing and accommodating ADHD."[47] Cataloging the myriad risks and impairments associated with ADHD is beyond the scope of this chapter, but we briefly review research in two particular areas—academic functioning and social functioning—to highlight the ways in which core ADHD symptoms have both direct and indirect effects on important areas of children's lives. In addition, the impairments associated with ADHD suggest particular domains that might be targets of treatment interventions and that might indicate treatment effectiveness above and beyond improvements in core symptoms of ADHD.

For many children with ADHD, the school setting is where their behavioral symptoms are most apparent and cause considerable difficulty. Sitting still, following directions, sustaining attention, completing difficult tasks, organizing materials, inhibiting responses, and delaying gratification are all demands placed on children throughout the school day, and they are all behaviors that are particularly challenging to children with ADHD. A significant number of children with ADHD experience learning disabilities or disorders in language and communication that adversely impact academic achievement and performance in school. Estimating the prevalence of learning disabilities in children with ADHD depends in large part on the definition of learning disability that is used. Using a fairly conservative definition—delay in reading, math, or spelling relative to IQ and achievement below the seventh percentile in that area—Barkley found that between 20% and 25% of children with ADHD have a single learning disability.[48] A more relaxed criterion—performing at two grade levels below actual grade level—results in prevalence rates of learning disabilities as high as 80% of children with ADHD.[49]

Even youths with ADHD who do not have a learning disability frequently struggle in school. Numerous studies have documented lower IQ scores for children with ADHD versus control groups, and these IQ differences are especially common in verbal intelligence.[50] In addition, youths with ADHD typically score lower than children without ADHD on standardized achievement tests.[51] According to a dual-pathway model proposed by Mark Rapport and colleagues, underachievement in school is associated with ADHD in two ways—one cognitive and one behavioral.[52] First, ADHD has an effect on school performance through its association with behavior problems. Specifically, as discussed above, ADHD increases risk for conduct problems that interfere with classroom behavior. As a result, academic performance and school functioning are poor. Second, ADHD is associated with deficits in IQ, working memory, vigilance, and other cognitive processes; these deficits interfere with school performance and academic achievement. Both of these trajectories explaining the link between ADHD and academic underachievement may be important targets for intervention. As discussed below, school-based interventions targeting classroom behavior as well as academic performance are frequently part of a comprehensive treatment plan for ADHD.

Some of the most important developmental tasks of middle childhood are in the social realm—getting along in the peer group and establishing and maintaining close friendships. The impulsive, disruptive, and often aggressive behavior displayed by youths with ADHD interferes with these developmental tasks in multiple ways. In their peer interactions, children with ADHD are often characterized not by the absence of positive or prosocial behaviors but by the presence of disruptive, emotional, and intense behavior that is often inappropriate for the particular play setting.[53] Children with ADHD may yell and run around at inappropriate times, and their intrusive behavior often interrupts and interferes with ongoing play interactions. Thus, they do not show the sensitivity to the rate, balance, and coordination of play activities that their peers expect from playmates.

Children with ADHD are overwhelmingly disliked by their peers. In studies that have observed children with ADHD in groups of unfamiliar peers, youths with ADHD are often rejected after even brief interactions, such as at the end of the first day.[54] For children with ADHD, this peer rejection has been shown to be fairly constant.[55] Peers perceive children with ADHD as disruptive, immature, bossy, intrusive, mean, and aggressive.[56] Thus, it is not surprising that they are highly disliked.

There is evidence that aggression and hyperactivity independently contribute to peer rejection.[57] Indeed, it appears to be the combination of ADHD with aggression that is associated with the highest levels of peer rejection.[58] In one study, a group of aggressive children with ADHD received on average approximately one negative nomination (as someone one would least want to be friends with) for every four peers. The nonaggressive ADHD group received one negative nomination for every 10 to 11 peers, and the non-ADHD comparison group received one nomination for every 20 classmates.[59] Nevertheless, irritable and inattentive behavior also predicts peer rejection apart from hyperactivity and aggression.[60] Inattention is often associated with immature behavior and results in "goofy" and insensitive behavior. This socially dysregulated behavior is not rewarding for peers, who find it difficult to predict and coordinate their partners' play behaviors and who find children with ADHD self-centered and unable to follow social cues and expectations.[61] Hinshaw found that among girls with ADHD, those with the combined subtype were more rejected than girls with the primarily inattentive type, yet the latter group experienced greater social isolation.[62]

Peer rejection in childhood has been associated with a host of negative outcomes in adolescence and adulthood, including psychiatric disorders, delinquency and criminality, and school-related problems, such as early school dropout.[63] This list of maladjusted outcomes contains some of the negative outcomes associated with ADHD. Thus, if poor peer relations contribute directly to these outcomes, children with

ADHD may be at increased risk due to the combination of poor peer relations and ADHD psychopathology.[64]

Peer rejection is an index of a child's poor acceptance or likability in the larger peer group. A second dimension of peer relationships that becomes increasingly important in middle childhood and early adolescence is the establishment of friendships—close relationships between two children based on mutual affection and reciprocity. Children with ADHD have fewer friends than children without ADHD, and some evidence suggests that they choose others with ADHD as their preferred play partners.[65] They have trouble sustaining associative play interactions, and the reciprocity that is a hallmark of friendships is often missing from their interactions.[66] In a study of friendship among girls with ADHD, friendship stability varied as a function of ADHD subtype.[67] Specifically, from the beginning to the middle of a 5-week summer camp, girls with the combined subtype had unstable relationships, but from the middle to the end of the camp, the inattentive subgroup had trouble with the maintenance of friendships. Consistent with the findings about peer behavior in general (discussed above), girls with ADHD had high levels of negative features (such as conflict) in their friendships but did not differ from girls without ADHD in the number of positive friendship features (such as companionship and support).

The problems in peer relations associated with ADHD are not fleeting. In a follow-up study with adolescents who had a history of ADHD in childhood, there was evidence of impairment in multiple domains of peer relationships. Youths with a childhood history of ADHD had fewer friends and were more rejected by peers, according to their parents, and they had friends who were involved in fewer conventional activities such as athletics and other extracurricular activities than were friends of the group without an ADHD history.[68] These differences were greater for youths with ADHD who had comorbid CD or ODD or persistent ADHD.

The evidence shows that ADHD is associated with a host of current and future adjustment difficulties and appears to have both direct and indirect effects on maladjustment. For example, symptoms of inattention interfere with appropriate classroom behavior directly, resulting in lower school performance, and symptoms of hyperactivity-impulsivity may lead to early school dropout indirectly, because of their association with peer rejection. When examining the effectiveness of treatments for ADHD, it is thus important to consider the improvements in specific symptoms as well as the effect on associated impairments, including school performance, peer relations, and the many other domains of functioning affected by symptoms of ADHD.

## What Causes ADHD?

One reason that critics have been quick to criticize the categorization of ADHD as a "real" disorder is that the causes of ADHD are not completely clear. Research in the past decade has contributed significantly to our understanding of potential pathways leading to ADHD, yet there continue to be questions about what specific factors cause ADHD for specific children. The search for etiologies is further complicated by the fact that researchers are not likely to find just one cause of ADHD. Rather, there appear to be multiple developmental trajectories that involve various combinations of neurological, genetic, cognitive, and other factors that lead to ADHD.[69] Nevertheless, as described in more detail below, at the level of heredity, genetics, and neurology, we are becoming increasingly knowledgeable about ADHD's etiologies.[70]

Our understanding of the biological factors that contribute to or cause ADHD has progressed substantially as the technologies available for studying neuroanatomy and neurological functioning have improved. Even so, research tends to be correlational in nature, and speculations about biological causes of ADHD rely on converging evidence from neuropsychology, neuroimaging, genetic, and psychopharmacological studies. Nevertheless, Barkley contends that this is true for all psychiatric disorders and that we know much more about the etiology of ADHD than about other childhood disorders.[71]

As early as 1963, Keith Conners and Leon Eisenberg proposed a dual mechanism underlying ADHD.[72] Based on the findings of their early methylphenidate trial, Conners and Eisenberg proposed that both inhibition and arousal or alerting are involved in ADHD. Specifically, deficits in inhibitory controlling symptoms are involved in the impulsivity symptoms of ADHD. A second mechanism, however, involves problems with arousal and may underlie symptoms of inattention. With regard to stimulant medication, Conners and Eisenberg suggested that methylphenidate both enhances the systems that control inhibition and increases alerting.[73]

Barkley's more recently developed model of ADHD[74] attributes ADHD symptoms to deficits in behavioral inhibition. Specifically, behavioral inhibition involves delaying responses that are likely to be reinforced and protecting this delay so that other self-regulatory functions (called executive functions) can occur and control responses. Behavioral inhibition deficits make it difficult to delay immediate reactions and also to stop behavior once it is begun. The executive functions that are disrupted by problems with behavioral inhibition involve processes such as holding events in mind and using hindsight (such as remembering a prior plan), reflecting to oneself ("Now, where did I leave my keys?" or "What should I do next?"), controlling emotions (such as managing frustration), and breaking down and synthesizing behaviors (such as coming up with multiple solutions to a problem).

Barkley presumes that the underlying dysfunction in behavioral inhibition is biologically based. Specifically, executive function deficits imply neurophysiological problems in the prefrontal cortex and projections of the cortex to other parts of the brain. Considerable research has documented deficits in frontal lobe functions on a variety of neuropsychological tests that assess motor inhibition, interference control, and cognitive inhibition, and the evidence suggests that the inhibition deficits associated with ADHD are better explained as executive inhibition (which is deliberate inhibition of a response so that a later goal can be achieved) as opposed to motivational inhibition (which is inhibition driven by anxiety or fear, such as awareness of impending punishment).[75] Although Barkley's theory is not the first to suggest behavioral inhibition as a core deficit with ADHD,[76] it goes further in explaining how problems with inhibition result in the particular constellation of symptoms and impairments associated with ADHD. In addition, the theory makes specific predictions and hypotheses that can be tested, and although there is considerable support for the theory, additional research is needed to test and clarify it. Nevertheless, Barkley concluded that "the totality of findings in the neuropsychology of ADHD is impressive in further suggesting that some dysfunction of the prefrontal lobes (inhibition and executive function deficits) is involved in this disorder."[77]

Neurological studies have compared cerebral blood flow and cerebral glucose metabolism (using positron emission tomography, PET) between ADHD and control groups. These studies have shown decreases in blood flow in the prefrontal areas of the brain and also in the connections between these regions and the limbic system in the ADHD group.[78] With PET studies there is some evidence of reduced glucose metabolism, but these findings have not been consistent.[79] Finally, with the availability of newer neuroimaging technologies such as magnetic resonance imaging, researchers have found differences in particular regions of the brain in ADHD and control samples. The brain regions that have been implicated in these studies (though not with complete consistency) include, among others, regions of the temporal lobes that control auditory detection; the corpus callosum, which is involved in transferring information between the two hemispheres; the caudate nucleus, which is involved in motor control; and areas of the cerebellum that might be involved in executive functioning.[80] In general, the findings of neuroimaging studies converge to suggest that the inhibition problems associated with ADHD may be the result of impairments in several frontostriatal regions of the brain,[81] and functional magnetic resonance imaging (fMRI) studies show correlations between activation of these areas and ADHD severity.[82]

As this research continues, particularly with fMRI studies, which can examine activity in particular regions of the brain while neuropsychological tests and other tasks of attention and inhibition are being completed, it will be critical to confirm that ADHD symptoms and executive function deficits are associated with differences in brain structures and functioning. Only then can we attribute a role in the etiology of ADHD to these brain abnormalities. In addition, it is important to recognize that studies using these types of scanning technologies are relatively new and still somewhat small in number. Thus, conclusions based on these studies need to be made somewhat tentatively and with attention to the fact that ADHD often co-occurs with other disorders, and it is important to question whether brain differences that emerge are associated specifically with ADHD (and not comorbid disorders). In addition, studies that are based on comparisons of scans of children's brains—children who have ADHD versus those who do not—need appropriate comparison groups. Specifically, children's brains are still developing, and developing at different rates, so we need to be sure that differences attributed to ADHD are not better explained by normal developmental phenomena.

Likewise, there is some debate about whether ADHD results from brain structure and functioning that deviates from typical development—an "abnormal" brain—or whether ADHD is due in part to a delay in maturation of the brain.[83] The studies reviewed above support the former perspective. Recent evidence, however, provides some support for the latter view. Evaluating brain scans over time of children diagnosed with ADHD and children without ADHD, Philip Shaw and colleagues compared the age at which children attained peak cortical thickness.[84] Typically, the cerebral cortex thickens during childhood and then begins a period of thinning as the brain matures. With repeated scans of children who were followed from childhood into adolescence, the researchers were able to compare the age of peak cortical thickness—the age at which increases in thickness cease and thickness begins to decrease—for children with and without ADHD. The findings showed that the median age at which half of the cortical points assessed reached their peak thickness was 3 years later for the ADHD group than it was for the children without ADHD—10.5 years versus 7.5 years. The authors concluded that their findings best represent maturational delay rather than deviance, in part because the sequence of development was similar in the ADHD and non-ADHD groups. Interestingly, the maturational delay tended to be greatest in regions of the brain that have been associated with ADHD. Unfortunately, data were not available to assess whether differences in the age of peak cortical thickness among children with ADHD were associated with clinical outcomes or other behavioral markers of ADHD.

Even with the identification of differences in brain structures, differences in brain functioning, and delays in brain maturation such as those discussed above, the next question is, Where do these differences come from? Given that brain damage probably accounts for only a very small percentage of cases of ADHD (roughly 5%),[85] we turn to genetic factors. Indeed, there is considerable evidence that heredity plays a substantial etiological role in ADHD. It has long been observed that between 10% and 35% of family members of children with ADHD also have the disorder.[86] Looking at these data another way, Biederman and colleagues found in one sample that if a parent has ADHD, the chance that a child will have the disorder exceeds 50%.[87]

Studies of twins provide a valuable tool for specifying the genetic contribution to ADHD. Twin studies compare the rates of ADHD in pairs of monozygotic twins, who share 100% of their genetic material, to those in dizygotic twins, who are no more similar genetically than non-twin biological siblings. Rates of concordance (when both twins have the disorder) are dramatically higher for monozygotic twins—81% versus 29% in dizygotic twins in one study[88] and 82% versus 38% in another.[89] In a third study, correlations between mothers' reports of impulsivity-hyperactivity symptoms correlated .92 for monozygotic twins and only .32 for dizygotic twins.[90] The correlations were .70 and .30, respectively, for inattention. Heritability estimates provide another statistic for evaluating the role of genetics. They range from 0 to 1.0 and indicate the extent to which genetic factors are responsible for ADHD. A recent study with preschool twins found that heritability ranged from

.78 to .81 across the preschool period and further that 91% of stability in ADHD symptoms across this period was due to genetic factors.[91] Overall, average heritability estimates across dozens of studies hover around .80.[92] This value is at least as high as, if not higher than, the heritability of IQ (approximately .40 to .80)[93] and suggests a clear and substantial genetic contribution to ADHD.

Research investigating the role of various neurotransmitters in the etiology of ADHD is growing, but the findings are not yet conclusive and are inconsistent. The catecholamines have been implicated, with studies showing decreased availability of dopamine[94] and deficient activity in noradrenergic pathways.[95] In addition, other findings suggest that serotonin plays an important role in the etiology of ADHD, particularly the impulsive and hyperactive symptoms.[96] Given the complexity and variability in the expression of ADHD, the role of neurochemicals in many psychological disorders, and interactions among neurochemical systems, the hypothesis that one neurotransmitter would be implicated in ADHD is likely too simplistic.[97] One multistage model suggests that the norepinephrine, epinephrine, and dopamine systems are all involved, and that interactions among these systems are responsible for problems with both inattention and impulsivity. Similarly, comorbidity may relate to particular patterns of neurotransmitter activity. One group of researchers found that aggressive boys with ADHD who also had an aggressive parent had the lowest levels of serotonin function, followed by the nonaggressive ADHD group and the aggressive ADHD group without an aggressive parent.[98] In contrast, another group found no difference in serotonergic functioning for nonaggressive boys with ADHD, aggressive boys with ADHD, and aggressive boys without ADHD.[99] Research on neurotransmitters and ADHD is complicated by the fact that there are multiple indirect ways of measuring neurochemicals but no direct way to assess levels of brain chemicals, and different results may emerge from the variety of measurements used. As these and many other studies demonstrate, the jury is still out on the role of neurotransmitters in the etiology of ADHD.

What about the environment? As discussed above, twin studies reveal a small but not zero contribution of environmental factors to ADHD symptoms. These environmental factors include biological as well as psychosocial factors. Events that compromise the nervous system before, during, and after birth have been shown to contribute to inattention and hyperactivity/impulsivity. These include low birth weight,[100] prenatal exposure to alcohol and nicotine,[101] and exposure to high levels of lead.[102] Nevertheless, studies of lead exposure that control for confounding factors find a weak association between lead exposure and ADHD symptoms, and none have controlled for the presence of ADHD in parents.[103] Additional research on these environmental factors that carefully controls confounding variables (such as socioeconomic status) and that uses diagnoses of ADHD as an outcome (rather than measures of symptoms only) is needed.[104]

Current research indicates that psychosocial variables are not primary causal factors for ADHD. Etiological theories of ADHD that consider problematic family influences to be the primary causal agent have not received much support.[105] For example, twin studies have shown that shared environmental factors account for less than 5% of the variability in ADHD symptoms.[106] These studies have confirmed the limited etiological role of psychosocial factors in ADHD because they can directly compare estimates of contributions from genetics, shared environmental influences (similarities that arise because twins live in the same home environment), and nonshared environmental influences (environmental factors that affect only one twin, such as peer influences or school experiences that are not shared by the siblings). For example, after controlling for the contributions of parental smoking and drinking to ADHD, one research group reported that 86% of ADHD risk was due to genetic contributions and 14% to nonshared environmental influences.[107]

Even though psychosocial factors do not appear to *cause* ADHD, they can have a critical impact on the course of the disorder. Family, school, and other environmental influences may impact the severity of symptoms displayed, comorbid disorders that might develop, and long-term outcomes for children with ADHD.[108] Several avenues of research support this conclusion. First, findings of conflict-ridden parent-child interactions, chaotic environments, and other indicators of family dysfunction in children with ADHD are implicated in the development of co-occurring disruptive disorders (ODD and CD) rather than in the symptoms of ADHD.[109] As discussed above, comorbid ODD or CD forecasts more negative outcomes for children with ADHD. Second, the association between family variables such as harsh discipline, less positive engagement, marital disagreement, and family stress and ADHD appears to be bidirectional.[110] Research supports both the conclusion that poor parenting increases noncompliance and poor emotion regulation in children with behavior problems[111] and the reverse—that child behavior problems promote increasingly problematic parenting behavior and family stress.[112] Transactional views recognize that child problems exacerbate parental and family problems at the same time that parental and family problems promote escalations in children's behavior problems.[113] The impact of ADHD on the family is seen in increased demands on caregivers, lower satisfaction and sense of esteem about parenting, and increased distress for parents. In turn, these factors influence the emotional climate in the house, the well-being of other family members, and the quality of the parents' marital relationship—all important aspects of the child's social context.[114] Third, it is difficult to separate biological and environmental influences even to suggest how psychosocial factors, for example, affect the course of ADHD. For example, because of the heritability of ADHD, a child with ADHD may have a parent with ADHD (a genetic risk factor), and the parent's symptoms might interfere with his or her ability to provide the structure and consistency that could be helpful for promoting the child's adaptive functioning (a psychosocial risk factor).

In sum, recent research on the etiology of ADHD has resulted in greater understanding of the multiple trajectories leading to ADHD. The research to date clearly suggests strong genetic contributions and implicates the frontostriatal regions of the brain. Although psychosocial factors may influence the particular expression of ADHD and comorbid problems and are often an important target of intervention, there is little support for nonbiological factors serving the primary causal role.

## Can ADHD Be Treated Effectively?

A variety of treatments are commonly used to improve ADHD symptoms and manage the impairments associated with ADHD. In broad terms, the treatments fall into two categories—medication and psychosocial treatments—yet there are multiple treatment approaches within each of these categories. The most common medical treatments are central nervous system stimulant medications, and the most common psychosocial treatments involve some combination of parent management training, child-focused behavior therapy, and intervention in the school setting.

### Treatment with Medication

Stimulants are the most thoroughly studied and the most effective medical treatment for ADHD.[115] These drugs are named stimulants because of the effect they have on the central nervous system—increasing its activity, alertness, and arousal.[116] Across several hundred controlled trials of stimulants, 50% to 95% of children have shown improvements in the core ADHD symptoms as well as other areas of functioning, including academic, behavioral, and social.[117] That number is highest if different drugs are considered across multiple trials, given that some children have a better response to one stimulant than to another.[118] A number of different stimulant medications have been used to treat all three subtypes of ADHD. These include methylphenidate (Ritalin), dextroamphetamine (Dexedrine), and mixed amphetamine salts (Adderall). Pemoline (Cylert) is no longer a commonly used medication because of concerns about serious liver toxicity associated with its use in some children.[119] As a result of the seriousness of this side effect, pemoline was withdrawn from the UK market in 1997, the Canadian market in 1999, and the U.S. market in 2005.

Stimulants are available in a variety of formulations, including immediate release, intermediate release, and extended release.[120] Immediate-release preparations have a very fast onset of action (within about an hour), and because of their short half-life (a measure of the time it takes the substance to lose its effect), doses need to be repeated two to three times per day. Intermediate-release and extended-release preparations are designed to last longer so that they need to be taken only once or twice each day—a considerable advantage in that children do not need to take a dose during the school day. The onset of action is slower for these formulations. They have delivery systems that allow a pattern of release that is similar to immediate-release formulations given two or three times a day. For example, Adderall XR (an extended-release preparation) includes two types of beads. Half of the beads are immediate release, and the other half of the beads release medication 4 hours later. Concerta (an extended-release preparation of methylphenidate) uses a drug-delivery system that mimics three doses of immediate-release methylphenidate and lasts for 10 to 14 hours. In treating the core symptoms of ADHD, Concerta and thrice-daily immediate-release methylphenidate given at 4-hour intervals have been found to be similarly effective.[121]

Potential side effects differ for the various drugs from one child to another and also appear to differ with the age of the child. Among preschool-age children, the effectiveness of stimulant therapy is more variable than among school-age children, and side effects are reported more often among younger children. These include irritability, sadness, insomnia, emotional outbursts, and decreased appetite.[122] Perhaps more significant, there appears to be a risk for reduced growth rates in preschool-age children who are treated with stimulants.[123] Among school-age children, side effects of all of the stimulants may include trouble sleeping, decreased appetite, headaches or stomachaches, weight loss, irritability, and growth suppression.[124] In most cases, these side effects are mild, may be reduced over time, or can be managed by changing dosages.[125] Because of the nature of stimulant medications and effects they may have on the body, there has been some concern about their cardiovascular safety. In healthy children and adolescents, the effects on the cardiovascular system appear to be minimal and do not require special blood pressure or pulse checks.[126] In adults, however, monitoring of blood pressure and pulse rate may be indicated given the higher prevalence of hypertension in adults relative to children.[127] In addition, there has been recent concern about the use of Adderall XR (the extended-release preparation) when children have underlying heart anomalies (often silent). According to the FDA, there are 12 known cases of sudden death in children and adolescents treated with Adderall XR, and in Canada, the sale of Adderall XR has been suspended. Evaluation of these 12 cases did not result in suspension of Adderall XR sales in the United States, as it was concluded that the rate of sudden deaths associated with Adderall XR was not significantly higher than would be expected without treatment.[128] Chapter 6 discusses further the 2006 decision by the Food and Drug Administration (FDA) *not* to issue a "black box" label for stimulant medications.

In addition to the age of the child, the side effects profiles of the medications, and cardiac history, other factors to consider when evaluating the decision to use medication include the severity of the child's ADHD symptoms, the child's previous response to treatment, the presence of a family history of tics or Tourette's syndrome (which may be exacerbated with stimulants),[129] parents' attitudes toward medication treatment and ability to monitor use, and whether there are concerns about stimulant abuse in the family.[130] Despite the high rates of success with stimulants, researchers and clinicians caution that the response to stimulant medication may be very idiosyncratic. In addition to stimulants, various antidepressants, including tricyclic antidepressants, bupropion, and monoamine oxidase inhibitors, have also been used to treat ADHD symptoms with some success.[131] Atomoxetine (Strattera) is the first nonstimulant drug approved by the FDA for the treatment of ADHD in both children and adults. It is one of a new class of drugs called specific norepinephrine reuptake inhibitors (SNRIs) and has been shown to be effective in reducing core ADHD symptoms.[132]

*Psychosocial Treatments*

If medication, particularly stimulant medication, is so commonly used and has demonstrated success in managing ADHD symptoms, why are other treatments necessary? There are a number of theoretical and practical reasons for the use of psychosocial treatments. From a practical clinical perspective, not all children who take stimulant medication demonstrate significant improvement in their symptoms (perhaps 10%–20% do not),[133] and as noted above, side effects may make medication management undesirable for some children. For other children, parents may decide that medication is not a viable alternative, or there may be additional contraindications for the use of medication such as a history of drug abuse in the family or the presence of medical or other psychiatric conditions that preclude stimulant use. Thus, treatment with medication is simply not an option in some cases, and alternative therapies are necessary.

Additional justification for psychosocial treatments include the following. First, if Barkley's theory of ADHD as an underlying deficit in behavioral inhibition is correct, then behavioral treatments that increase awareness of and externalize the link between behavior and its consequences are expected to be effective.[134] Second, the success of psychosocial treatments, including parent management training, for common comorbid conditions such as ODD and CD[135] suggest that these treatments may be effective in improving functioning for children with ADHD and comorbid disruptive behavior problems. Finally, given the ADHD-related impairments across many domains of functioning and the likelihood (discussed above) that psychosocial factors may exacerbate these impairments, treatment interventions that address these factors may be effective in improving children's current and longer-term functioning, apart from their direct effect on core symptoms of ADHD.[136]

Several examples of psychosocial treatments that have been supported empirically include parent management training[137] and direct contingency management in intensive summer treatment programs[138] and in the school setting. Successful parent interventions include training parents to use contingency management such as positive reinforcement and time-out strategies. In addition, various programs might include sessions on anger management for parents, increasing parents' knowledge about ADHD, and promoting strategies for successful home-school coordination.[139] An additional benefit of parent training programs is that they may also result in decreased stress for the parents, increased parenting confidence, and other improvements in functioning within the family.[140]

School interventions include modifications in the classroom (some as simple as changing the classroom environment by moving the child's seat and increasing structure),[141] use of positive reinforcement to improve behavior and productivity as well as response cost and other punishments,[142] and, of course, academic interventions to target performance and achievement. One example of a commonly used intervention that requires collaboration between teachers and parents is the daily report card.[143] With this strategy, several target behaviors are selected (for example, following rules, completing assignments, remaining seated, cooperating with peers) and individually tailored to the needs of the child, and a rating system is used to indicate performance of the target behaviors. These ratings can include simple checkmarks indicating successful performance during particular periods of the day, frequency counts if the behavior is easily quantifiable (for example, number of interruptions), or a rating scale indicating degree of performance or compliance (for example, 1 for "poor" to 3 for "good"). Usually, the child is responsible for keeping the report card, and teachers provide feedback on a regular basis (such as during each period of the school day, or based on blocks of time). The child takes the report card home each day, and the teachers' reports are mapped onto a menu of rewards or negative consequences that all parties (child, parents, and teachers) clearly understand. For example, teachers' marks can be translated into points as part of a token economy system.

Finally, summer treatment programs (STPs), developed by William Pelham and colleagues,[144] have shown promising results.[145] These are intensive, manualized, full-day programs that take place over the course of 8 weeks in a camplike setting. Goals of the STP include improving peer relationships, academic performance, and self-efficacy.[146] In the STP, children participate in daily academic classroom instruction and in group-based recreation activities. An important part of the STP is training in sports skills, and several hours each day are spent in teaching and playing sports and games. In addition, social-skills training occurs, and the STP provides extensive opportunities for developing positive peer relations. A token economy system is employed throughout the STP and integrated into all activities throughout the day. Improvements have been documented in multiple domains as a result of participation in an STP—core ADHD symptoms, social skills, and academic performance.[147] There are now summer treatment programs based on the Pelham model throughout the United States.

## The MTA, New York/Montreal, and PATS Studies

The short-term benefits of stimulant medication, behavior modification, and the combination of the two have been established through many studies,[148] yet until recently, there was very limited evidence of the effectiveness of treatment beyond several months.[149] Thus, it is valuable to highlight in detail the Multimodal Treatment Study of Children with ADHD (MTA).[150] This collaborative project, involving six research teams and supported by the National Institute of Mental Health and the Department of Education, was a randomized clinical trial comparing the effectiveness of medication, behavioral treatments, the combination of the two, and standard community care over a 14-month treatment period. The 579 children recruited for the study were 7 to 9 years old and met criteria for a diagnosis of ADHD, combined type. Each family was randomly assigned to 1 of the 4 treatment strategies.

*Behavioral treatment* involved parent training (27 group sessions plus 8 individual sessions); an intensive 8-week STP for the child; and school interventions including biweekly teacher consultation, 12 weeks of assistance from a specially trained aide working directly with the child in school, and daily report cards to provide a link between parents and the school. *Medication management* involved a double-blind, daily-switch titration of methylphenidate for 28 days. The best dose was chosen based on reviews of parent and teacher ratings of the child's response. Monthly visits with pharmacotherapists were used for medication maintenance, such as to adjust doses if necessary. The *combined treatment* group received all of the treatments in the behavioral and medication management treatment arms, and the two were integrated so that the pharmacotherapists and teacher-consultants communicated about treatment decisions. Families in the *community care* group were provided a list of mental health resources and were able to seek services in their communities.

In terms of treatment with medication in the MTA, nearly 69% of children in the medication management and combined treatment groups responded well in the initial titration and were assigned to methylphenidate, and approximately 9% were titrated to dextroamphetamine because they did not respond well to methylphenidate. By the end of the study, 73% were successfully maintained on methylphenidate, 10% on dextroamphetamine, and 3% on other medications. In addition, 67% of children in the community care group received medication for their ADHD symptoms from their physicians.[151]

A comprehensive and thorough battery of assessments was completed with information gathered from parents, teachers, peers, and the children themselves; observations from trained staff; educational tests; and other methods indexing multiple domains of functioning. These measures assessed six primary domains: ADHD symptoms, oppositional/aggressive behavior, social skills, symptoms of anxiety and depression, parent-child interactions, and academic achievement. Overall, all four treatment conditions demonstrated a substantial reduction in ADHD symptoms over the 14-month period, but the improvements were not consistent across the four groups. Specifically, direct comparisons between the medication management and behavior treatment groups showed evidence of greater improvement in the medication management group for symptoms of inattention (rated by parents and teachers) and hyperactivity-impulsivity (rated by teachers) but not on any other measures of functioning. In addition, combined treatment resulted in greater improvements than behavioral treatment alone on particular measures in several domains (ADHD symptoms, parent ratings of aggression and internalizing distress, and reading achievement). Finally, ADHD symptoms showed greater improvements in the combined treatment and medication management groups (but not behavioral treatment) when compared with community care. Interestingly, only the combined treatment was also superior to community care on at least one measure in all of the other domains assessed (oppositional behavior, internalizing symptoms, social skills, parent-child relations, and achievement).

The comprehensiveness and complexity of the MTA study cannot be overemphasized, as it is arguably the most thorough and detailed study of treatment effectiveness, not only for ADHD, but for any psychiatric disorder of childhood.[152] As a result, the findings of the MTA have the potential to inform the standard of care for ADHD. For example, as noted above, a large percentage of children in the community care group received psychotropic medication, yet the treatment arms using medication in the MTA were more effective. The authors noted that their use of systematic feedback from parents and teachers, provision of educational material to parents, and use of higher doses (to maximize effectiveness and minimize side effects) given three times per day may be responsible for the improvements with MTA medication protocols over community care. Despite the success of the MTA intervention, several researchers have noted that the extensive 28-day medication titration with drug-placebo reversals and the expensive and intense behavioral treatments in the MTA may be unrealistic for clinical practice in most communities.[153]

Secondary analyses of the MTA data provide some evidence for concluding that the combined treatment was superior to treatment with medication alone.[154] Using a categorical outcome measure that indicated whether children were successfully treated or not, combined treatment yielded higher success rates (68%) than medication management alone (56%), behavioral treatment alone (34%), and community care treatment (25%). Using a composite outcome measure that incorporated a number of specific indicators of symptoms and behaviors rated by both parents and teachers, combined treatment was more effective than medication management alone, behavioral treatment alone, and community care treatment. Finally, the positive effects of combined treatment on children's functioning at school were most apparent in the families with the greatest decreases in negative and ineffective discipline, suggesting that changing parenting practices is an important process that explains the effectiveness of combined medication and psychosocial treatment for ADHD.

Several issues concerning behavioral treatments in the MTA are important. First, in further analyses of the MTA treatment outcome data, behavioral treatments were shown to be similar in their effectiveness to medication management and combined treatment for the subgroup of children with a comorbid anxiety disorder. For children without comorbid anxiety, behavioral treatments were similar to community care and less effective than the other MTA treatment strategies.[155] Second, parent satisfaction was highest for the two treatment strategies that included behavioral modification, and more than 75% of children who received behavioral treatment did not receive medication and were maintained successfully.[156] Third, children who received both medication and behavioral treatment used lower doses of medication than those who received only medication. These findings highlight the importance of considering comorbidity and other individual differences (such as the fact that some parents do not want their children to take medication) in designing comprehensive treatment plans for children with ADHD.

Fourth, Pelham and colleagues examined the value of medication above and beyond intensive behavioral treatment by comparing the behavioral and combined treatment groups *during* the STP (as opposed to once the behavioral treatment had been dramatically reduced in intensity but medication continued, which was the situation at the 14-month outcome assessment).[157] These comparisons revealed that across many measures, the incremental effects of medication during an intensive behavioral treatment were not substantial and thus supported the effectiveness of intensive behavioral treatments as an alternative to medication. One important exception to this conclusion is in the domain of peer relations, where children in the group that received behavioral treatment only (and who did not receive medication) were less liked by their peers and received more nominations from peers as someone who is not a friend than those in the combined group. This is despite the fact that the STP focused specifically on social skills and friendships.

Overall, then, the MTA suggests that both stimulants and intensive behavioral treatment are effective treatments for ADHD. Furthermore, to the extent that minimizing the amount of medication a child receives is a treatment goal, the MTA findings indicate that a combination of medication and behavioral treatments may be especially effective because the medication management and combined treatment groups showed similar outcomes at 14 months even though the combined group was maintained on significantly less medication.[158]

Although the randomly assigned treatment provided by the MTA ended after 14 months, the children involved in the study continue to be followed. The most recent reports examine outcomes at 3 years after the trial began.[159] By this time, the four treatment groups did not differ on the primary outcome measures—ADHD symptoms, ODD symptoms, social skills, reading achievement, and overall impairment. In addition, rates of ADHD diagnoses were similar at 36 months for all four treatment groups despite the fact that the combined treatment and medication management groups had shown substantial decreases in ADHD diagnoses at 14 and 24 months compared to baseline. Notably, for all four groups there were dramatic improvements in the primary outcome measures from baseline to 36 months,[160] even though ADHD symptoms remained much higher than for non-ADHD classmates of the MTA children who were assessed at follow-up.[161] Thus, ADHD symptoms were much improved, but the children's symptoms were not at normal levels.

Once the MTA intervention ended at 14 months, families managed treatment for ADHD on their own. Although at the end of the intervention more than 90% of children in the medication management and combined treatment groups took medication at least 50% of the time (defined as "high use"), this percentage dropped to 71% by 36 months. In contrast, 14% of children in the behavioral treatment group were in the high-medication-use category at 14 months, but by 36 months, 45% were. The percentage of children in the community care group in the high-medication-use category remained approximately 60% at both 14 and 36 months. Yet children who used medication during the 24- to 36-month follow-up period had increased symptoms compared to children not using medication.[162] These findings did not appear to be due to selection effects. Specifically, it was not the case that children with more severe problems would be more likely to have poor outcomes and thus be more likely to take medication, resulting in medication treatment for the most severely affected children.[163] Such effects might make it difficult to observe an overall positive effect of medication.

In other analyses, three groups of children were identified based on distinct trajectories of their symptoms over time—one group showed a linear trend of gradually decreasing symptoms over time from baseline to 36 months. Another group showed a large decrease in symptoms initially, and this improvement was maintained. The final group also showed a large initial decrease and then increasing symptoms that returned to baseline levels.[164] Interestingly, randomization to either medication management or combined treatment was associated with a greater likelihood of children being in the second group, with the most positive outcome. Perhaps, then, the MTA medication treatment had long-term benefits for some children with ADHD.[165] Clearly, continued follow-up assessments of the youths involved in the MTA will be important for understanding the long-term implications of treatment.

A second multisite trial comparing stimulant treatment, stimulant treatment plus a comprehensive psychosocial intervention, and stimulant treatment plus a control psychosocial intervention was conducted between 1990 and 1995 by research teams in New York and Montreal.[166] All children in the study received carefully titrated doses of methylphenidate for 2 years, and the psychosocial treatment interventions continued for 2 years as well. The study was designed specifically to examine whether the intensive psychosocial treatment resulted in significant improvements above and beyond medication alone, whether the hypothesized superiority of the combined treatment would have long-term effects, and whether children who received the combined treatment could be successfully withdrawn from medication after the first year of treatment. The psychosocial intervention included parent training, academic assistance and tutoring, individual psychotherapy, and social skills training, but it did not include a substantial school-based intervention as the MTA study did because the goal was to design an intervention that could be realistically implemented in community clinic settings.

The results of the study across a wide variety of outcome measures showed that children in all treatment groups improved significantly, and that these effects did not diminish over the 2 years of the study.[167] Parent and teacher reports and classroom observations showed decreases in

ADHD symptoms, and fewer children in all treatment groups were diagnosed with ODD at the end of the first year of treatment. Academic achievement improved, and homework problems decreased. Emotional well-being (better self-concept and fewer symptoms of depression) and social functioning with peers improved. Psychosocial treatment enhanced parents' knowledge of appropriate parenting practices but did not translate to improved parenting relative to the other treatments, as mothers' negative parenting behaviors were reduced across all treatment groups. Most notably, though, and contrary to the authors' hypotheses, the combined medication and psychosocial treatment yielded no substantial improvement over medication alone. Thus, in contrast to the MTA study, there were no apparent benefits from incorporating an intensive multimodal psychosocial intervention with treatment with stimulant medication.

Most studies of the efficacy of various treatments for ADHD have focused on school-age children. However, a recent NIMH-funded study at six sites across the United States examined the use of methylphenidate in preschool children.[168] The Preschool ADHD Treatment Study (PATS) included more than 180 children between 3 and 5 years of age who participated in a rigorous treatment study over the course of a year. Several conclusions of this study suggest clinically important differences between responses to methylphenidate in preschool- versus school-age children. First, children treated with methylphenidate (versus placebo) showed significant reductions in ADHD symptoms on all except the smallest dose of drug, yet the size of the difference between active treatment and placebo was not as large as differences generally reported for school-age children.[169] Second, a particular concern of the PATS investigation was the assessment of side effects (called "adverse events").[170] As compared to studies with school-age children, the study with preschool children showed higher rates of discontinuation of the medication due to adverse events—11% in PATS versus less than 1% in the MTA, for example. Thus, a number of the preschoolers did not tolerate methylphenidate as well as was expected. The pattern of adverse events spontaneously reported by parents of the preschoolers was not the same as in studies of school-age children. The most common adverse events included emotional outbursts, irritability, trouble falling asleep, repetitive behaviors, and decreased appetite. Importantly, no preschool children discontinued the study because of cardiovascular side effects. In addition, for some children, there appears to be a risk for reduced growth rates, which should be carefully monitored in young children taking methylphenidate.[171] Overall, the PATS study is an important step in examining the effectiveness of medication for treating ADHD outside the age-range typically studied and suggests that there may be important developmental differences in the effectiveness of stimulant treatment.

## Where Is Our Understanding of ADHD Headed?

Significant advances in our understanding of the development, course, and management of ADHD continue to be made each year. Despite the fact that ADHD is the most well-researched psychiatric disorder in childhood, there is much more to learn. Theories of ADHD, such as Barkley's theory of ADHD as a disorder of behavioral inhibition, provide very specific hypotheses to be tested.[172] Evidence is accumulating that the inattentive subtype of ADHD differs substantially from the combined subtype in its prevalence and patterns of impairment, associated features, and comorbidities.[173] Further research about this subtype and investigation of whether it is a separate disorder will be important. Most notably, perhaps, neuroimaging and genetic studies provide rich opportunities for enhancing our understanding of the etiology and impairments associated with ADHD. Finally, the MTA study and the New York/Montreal trial are by far the most comprehensive studies of treatment strategies for ADHD. As these researchers continue to follow their samples of children and as additional reports from the initial data appear, we will learn much more about longer-term outcomes of various treatments. There is certainly no shortage of questions to investigate, and with collaborations among researchers across various disciplines—psychology, neuroscience, biology, psychiatry, epidemiology, and education, to name a few—there is much promise that our understanding of ADHD will continue to increase dramatically in the near future.

# CHAPTER THREE

# A Survey of the Evolution of ADHD and Pediatric Stimulant Use, 1900–1980

In the 1950s, educators learned about [the] . . . psycho-pharmacological aspect of behavior modification, and began to encourage parents to seek such help from the child's physician. Soon it became evident that these drugs were being used indiscriminately—prescription would depend mostly upon a description of behavior by a teacher or parent. There was little awareness or use of the supporting information required to differen-tiate the hyperkinetic impulse disorder from other types of behavior disorders in which overactivity was also a predominant feature.

—ERIC DENHOFF, *JOURNAL OF LEARNING DISABILITIES*, 1971

To those who have seen the results of such treatment [stimulants] in minimal brain dysfunction children, many of whom had failed to improve or had worsened with traditional therapies, the present limited use of drug therapy is as upsetting as it is unbelievable . . . It would not be hard to argue that in many instances psychotherapy of children with this syndrome virtually constitutes malpractice—a harmful withholding of useful treatment from a child.

—PAUL WENDER, *MINIMAL BRAIN DYSFUNCTION IN CHILDREN*, 1971

If modern observers find the debate over ADHD and children's use of stimulants contentious and convoluted, they need only look at the history of the diagnosis and the drugs to better understand why. Extremely hy-peractive, restless, and inattentive children have been identified by clini-cians and medical researchers dating back to 1902. Since then, upwards of 20 different diagnostic labels have been used to categorize children who exhibit these problematic behaviors. The numerous terms used to describe these children have outlined behavioral symptoms similar to those that were first described in 1902. Yet while these children have remained recognizable in terms of their description decade after decade under different diagnostic labels, the explanations offered for their condition have varied dramatically. Even when researchers from different eras reached similar conclusions—that the disorder was partly biological in origin and the result of some damage to (or a deficiency in) a child's central nervous system—they often arrived at very different explanations for both the source of this damage or deficiency and how the disorder's biological basis operated on a child. In short, ADHD has been a recognized disorder—albeit under different diagnostic labels—for more than half a century, but that has not precluded controversy from developing over how best to accurately diagnose and treat it.

Another aspect of the controversy, and the one that principally drives it, has to do with children using psychotropic drugs. The discovery of the effectiveness of stimulants on hyperactive children was—like many psychiatric drug discoveries—accidental. It came in 1937, more than three decades after the first clinical description of inordinately hyperactive and inattentive children. Another three decades would elapse before the federal government made the first ever research grant to study the therapeutic effects of stimulants on children. During this period, most of the very few children in the United States who used psychiatric drugs were those with severe mental disorders and were hospitalized for either short or long durations. Sufficiently controversial was the issue of children using psychotropic drugs that pharmaceutical companies would not finance large-scale research in the area. The only substantial source of research funding for pediatric psychopharmacology in the 1960s and 1970s was the National Institute of Mental Health (NIMH).[1] Three years after the NIMH awarded the first grant for studying children's use of stimulants in 1967, the first in a long-running series of controversies erupted over the ethics of children using these drugs. As this chapter explains, the debate among clinicians and researchers and within the general public has always revolved around the same basic issue: the appropriateness of millions of children using stimulant drugs.

## A "Defect of Moral Control," Social Darwinism, and Sir George Fredrick Still

The diagnostic origins of ADHD lie in the clinical description of 20 behaviorally disturbed children by an English pediatrician, Sir George

Frederick Still, who practiced medicine at King's College Hospital in London. In a lecture series he gave before the Royal College of Physicians in March 1902,[2] Still observed that the children he studied were of normal intellect, but they "exhibited violent outbursts, wanton mischievousness, destructiveness and a lack of responsiveness to punishment."[3] Moreover, they were often restless and fidgety with a "quite abnormal incapacity for sustained attention, causing school failure even in the absence of intellectual retardation."[4] Unable to sit still, the children proved easily distractible, inattentive, and unable to focus for long on any one thing.[5] Still went on to state that "this pattern occurred more often in boys than in girls, became frequently apparent by early school years, was sometimes accompanied by peculiarities of physical appearance, generally showed little relationship to the child's training and home environment, and commonly shared a poor prognosis."[6] The resemblance of these children to modern-day boys and girls diagnosed with ADHD has been used both as a reference point for discussing the medical history of the disorder and as fodder for proponents on either side of the controversy.[7]

What separates Still's work, as well as the related observations of his contemporary Alfred Tredgold (examined in the following section), from virtually all subsequent research related to hyperactivity, inattentiveness, and stimulants is that neither Still nor Tredgold was primarily interested in the children's welfare or their prognosis per se. What they most cared about was the overall health of the British population and its future socioeconomic characteristics. Still and Tredgold were strongly influenced by the social prejudices and dominant scientific thinking that abounded in Britain during its Victorian era.[8]

In the nineteenth century, Britain experienced wrenching economic, political, and social transformations. The country's agrarian and land-based economy shifted to one based on industrialization and goods mass-produced in cities. Society became increasingly stratified by class, with the lower classes suffering the negative effects of a new degree of poverty.[9] Many of the men, women, and especially children who found employment at the lower end of the economic spectrum worked excessively long hours for absurdly low wages; they also lived in unspeakable and unsanitary conditions.[10] During this time the incidence of infant mortality, illness, and learning difficulties and delinquency in children rose dramatically. The leading medical and scientific thinkers of the day, however, tended to identify the moral and intellectual deficiencies of the lower classes as the *cause*, rather than the consequence, of the awful conditions associated with their physical environment.[11] As a result, the middle and upper classes became increasingly concerned with the character, conduct, and number of people from the lower class, who were seen as fundamentally "immoral."[12]

Still considered hyperactive children as suffering from a "defect of moral control."[13] Rather than a medical discovery, his work represented more of a plea to the medical community of his time for expanded research to better understand these children who were too intelligent to be considered "idiots" (defined medically as "extreme stupidity") and too young to be viewed as "criminal minds."[14] In his opening statement to the Royal College of Physicians, Still remarked, "For some years past I have been collecting observations with a view to investigating the occurrence of defective moral control as a morbid condition in children, a subject I cannot but think calls urgently for scientific investigation."[15]

His exhortation for more research reflected the public's growing enthusiasm for achieving social progress through the expansion of objective science. The theories of Charles Darwin's biological discoveries provided a scientific rationale for various kinds of social deviance, which Still found in abundance among the 20 hyperactive children he studied. They stole, lied, and were prone to violence and sexual "chicanery" (among other forms of immorality). He described the children's neurological deficit "as a severe lack of reserve signaled by persistent self-gratification, shamelessness, immodesty, and passionateness."[16] Still's central hypothesis was that this moral deficit represented "the manifestation of some morbid *physical* condition."[17] This integrated well with Darwin's larger picture of evolutionary development, in which he hypothesized that the environment provided a selective advantage to specific types of biological variation.[18] What Darwin initially proposed as one of several possible mechanisms accounting for evolution in animals and differentiation among species, noted Russell Schachar, was elevated to an "iron law" of the "survival of the fittest" in an attempt to explain not only biological but also *social* phenomena.[19] Evolutionary social science grew in popularity among intellectuals and social reformers, in large part because "social Darwinism" appeared to explain the key differences between "primitive races" and, say, refined Englishmen.

The children that Still identified, therefore, were painful reminders of the inferior and residual end of evolution's relentless process of natural selection. In an effort to explain the "defects of moral control" in the children he observed, he claimed that moral consciousness and moral control were essentially innate characteristics and "the highest and latest product of mental evolution" in both the individual and the human race. As such, Still argued, moral control showed "a special liability to loss or failure in development [that is] quite in accordance with the phenomenon of evolution."[20]

Still's observations were also informed by those of William James—arguably the leading nineteenth-century psychologist—whose seminal two-volume *Principles of Psychology* (published in 1890) noted that "effort of the attention is the essential phenomenon of will."[21] James's position was strongly influenced by Théodule Ribot, an experimental psychologist at the Collège de France. In Ribot's definitive treatise on the psychology of attention, he distinguished between "the faculty of spontaneous attention, an inborn trait, and voluntary or sustained attention, the product of education and training." While the former was present in children, animals, and savages, "the latter could be won only through civilization."[22] James's interpretation of "moral behavior" reflected the dominant concepts of mental illness in the nineteenth century, which held that "any stimuli affecting the sensorium can be a source of mental illness" because excess stimulation deflects an individual's will from making proper choices. Therefore, "moral" was an ability to make ethical choices, and a "moral defect" was rooted in the physiology of attention.[23]

Still believed that the "insufficiency of inhibitory volition" and the "morbid exaggeration of excitability," which characterized the morally defective children he studied, were caused by some form of brain damage. Meningitis, head injury, and tumors were likely suspects, but so too was prolonged or difficult labor and premature birth or ill health experienced by the child's mother.[24] Children with moral deficits, he believed, were most often the result of some physical disease acting *together* with a genetic defect. Still pointed to "disorders of intellect, epilepsy, or moral degeneracy of one kind or another" in 17 of the 20 families he observed as evidence for the high degree of heritability of moral deficiency.[25] Ultimately, the children's hyperactive, impulsive, and inattentive behavior, he proposed, "resulted from an interaction of inherited susceptibility and minimal brain dysfunction acting on a human faculty (moral control) that was essentially inherited, of late evolutionary acquisition and, therefore, susceptible to loss."[26]

## Alfred Tredgold, "Feeble-Mindedness," and the Epidemic of Encephalitis Lethargica

To substantiate Still's contention that the hyperactive behavior pattern found in morally defective children stemmed from actual brain damage, particularly when no such damage was clearly evident, Alfred F. Tredgold suggested that at least *some* form of mild damage had occurred—probably during birth—that went undetected until the formal demands of early education exposed it.[27] In the early twentieth century, Tredgold was widely considered to be Britain's leading expert on mental deficiency and, as such, was a senior member of the English Royal Commission on Mental Deficiency. "After the passing of the Education Act of 1876, making attendance at public elementary or other schools compulsory," wrote Tredgold, "it gradually became apparent that a group of children existed who were so far mentally defective that they could not be satisfactorily taught in the ordinary public schools, but who were not sufficiently defective to be certified as imbeciles or idiots under the Idiots Act of 1886."[28]

The Mental Deficiency Act of 1913, which was the outcome of the royal commission's work, "was intended to embrace all grades of defect."[29] It applied the term "feeble-mindedness" to the "mildest grade and divided individuals suffering from feeble-mindedness into two classes" (adults and children).[30] The term was not especially precise. "Mentally defective or feeble-minded children differ greatly in the degree of their deficiency. The lower members of the class closely approximate to, and cannot be distinctly separated from, the imbeciles. The higher members, on the other hand, are but little removed from the merely dull and backward of the normal population."[31] Tredgold noted that a number of the children exhibited a variety of slight physical "anomalies," or "the so-called stigmata of degeneracy," which included abnormal head shape and size (about half an inch less in diameter than that of a normal child), poor coordination, and "abnormalities of the palate."[32] Researchers many decades later found a similar relationship between minor physical anomalies and hyperactivity, which is now considered to be partly the result of intrauterine defects during the first trimester.[33] Yet to look at the pictures of the children Tredgold included in his textbook and identified as "Types of Mentally Defective School-Children" is to see virtually everyone's less-than-flattering elementary school photos.[34]

Not surprisingly, Tredgold was an enormously supportive proponent of the eugenics movement, which sought to "prevent the propagation" of mentally deficient individuals through forced sterilization, segregation "in suitable colonies," and the strict regulation—sometimes including the restriction—of marriage.[35] He was convinced that mentally, physically, and socially inferior individuals were "being produced at a rate which can only be described as alarming. This is due in part to the propagation by persons who are themselves mentally deficient, in part to the relatively increased fertility of persons who, whilst not actually aments [retarded], are of pronounced psychopathic inheritance."[36] Sensing apocalyptic outcomes, Tredgold argued, "the result is to bring about an increasing ratio of the mentally, physically, and socially unfit, which, if unchecked, must not only handicap social progress, but which may hurl the State into the abyss of degeneracy."[37] These quotes are drawn not from his book's first edition in 1908 or its second edition in 1914, but from its fourth edition in 1922, when evolutionary social science was conspicuous for its being in a state of rapid decline.[38] Although his opinions and enthusiasm for eugenics seem radical and bizarre today, at the time these views were widespread ways of thinking about urbanization and modernism. Tredgold essentially believed that misbehavior signified a threat to the health of the larger society, which was similar to what many of the progressive child welfare workers of the time believed.

Like Still's, Tredgold's continued notoriety is based largely on the fact that the children he described in the early years of the twentieth century bear a striking resemblance to modern-day children diagnosed with ADHD. After noting "a considerable preponderance of males" among the "feeble-minded," he estimated that they constituted approximately 1% of the entire childhood population and were disproportionately concentrated in towns as opposed to the country.[39] He concurred with Still that the moral deficiency was essentially a form of mental deficiency caused by some "organic abnormality on the higher levels of the brain" and argued that the areas of the brain where the sense of morality was located were also the product of the more recent development in the course of human evolution and thus were more susceptible to damage.[40] He also viewed environmental circumstances as "not the cause, but the *result*" of the condition's "pronounced morbid inheritance."[41] What stood out the most about these mentally defective children, noted Tredgold, was their profound inattentiveness:

> *Attention.*—The most trifling thing serves to distract these children from their occupation, so that even where the attention is readily gained, it is with difficulty held. Many of them become capable of pursuing a congenial task with a certain amount of patience, but the majority have neither sufficient power of concentration or will to be capable of sustained mental effort against inclination or interposed obstacles . . . School-teachers often complain of the lack of *memory* of these children . . . Control is very

feebly developed in these children, and action is always along the line of least resistance. Volition is by no means absent, but their behaviour is more often the result of sudden desires and impulses than of deliberate purpose.[42]

What made Tredgold unique from most other enthusiasts of "social Darwinism" at that time was that he did not consider "feeble-minded" children as disproportionately concentrated among the lower classes. Instead, they existed throughout society: "With regard to the social status of these children there is little to be said. The labouring classes have no monopoly of mental defect, and, although I am unable to give any actual figures, my general impression is that it is just as prevalent amongst the upper as the lower classes of this country."[43]

Tredgold firmly believed in a link between some form of brain damage and "feeble-mindedness," so anything that could cause brain damage on a wide scale would result in a vastly increased incidence of mental defectiveness in all social classes and geographic environments.[44] Beginning in 1922, the same year the fourth edition of Tredgold's *Mental Deficiency (Amentia)* was published, growing numbers of medical reports surfaced detailing the negative neurological and behavioral effects found in children who had survived a bout with *encephalitis lethargica*.[45] The epidemic killed upwards of 20 million people worldwide (approximately 500,000–600,000 in the United States) and infected roughly half of the earth's human population between 1917 and 1928.[46] An often fatal illness, encephalitis was "characterized by tremendous sluggishness, hallucinations, and fever, sometimes bringing with it periods of remission— something doctors viewed as a hopeful sign."[47]

After the influenza epidemic subsided, increasing numbers of clinicians began encountering children who had survived their infection but were exhibiting characteristics that would later be considered partially consistent with ADHD (albeit more severe), characteristics they had not exhibited prior to their illness.[48] The clinicians described symptoms of antisocial behavior, irritability, impulsiveness, severe emotional swings, and hyperactivity, but without significant cognitive damage.[49] Although only a few of the child survivors of the epidemic would perfectly fit modern descriptions of children with ADHD, "postencephalitic behavior disorder" (as it became known) seemed to buttress the notion that there was a link between both severe brain damage and severe behavioral disturbances and, by extension, mild brain damage and mild behavioral disturbances. The latter were the "feeble-minded" and mentally defective forerunners of children with ADHD.[50] Thus,

"the discussion of *encephalitis lethargica* was significant, not simply because it drew suspicion to the causal connection between behavior and
neurological impulse," noted sociologist Adam Rafalovich, "but because
it medicalized unconventional behavior specific to children. Many of
these symptoms would later be claimed by neurologists and placed under
the rubric of ADHD."[51]

## "Organic Drivenness," Amphetamines (Benzedrine), and Charles Bradley

In 1934, in a *New England Journal of Medicine* article, researchers Eu-
gene Kahn and Louis Cohen identified a number of patients whose clinical condition was marked by an inability to remain quiet, abruptness,
clumsiness, and explosiveness of voluntary activity.[52] They noted that
all the patients' symptoms were secondary to a primary behavioral abnormality, hyperactivity, which they argued was a result of "organic
drivenness" or "a surplus of inner impulsion."[53] Unlike the postencephalitic children or those described by Still and Tredgold, however,
most of these new children described by Kahn and Cohen did not have
a specific history of neurological trauma. To account for this, they suggested that a congenital defect in the brain-stem organization that controlled activity level could be responsible for this "organic drivenness."[54] They also revived hints of "social Darwinism" as a potential
causative factor, given "that the over- as well as the under-development
of certain brain areas serves as a sort of background of certain plus and
minus members of the species."[55] Essentially, Kahn and Cohen were
pointing to the existence of superior and inferior human genetic types
to buttress their belief in a biological—rather than an environmental—
basis for hyperactivity.

Kahn and Cohen's work did not garner widespread attention when it
was first published (it did later). But frequent reference to "organic drivenness" and Kahn and Cohen's article was made in a special "setting
known as the Bradley Home, which devoted itself to the emotional problems of children," according to Maurice Laufer, a medical researcher
who spent part of his residency there and who later went on to provide
the first specific name—"hyperkinetic impulse disorder"—for the cluster
of behavioral symptoms that characterized this "organic drivenness."[56]
The home's wealthy donors, Mr. and Mrs. George L. Bradley, had established it as a memorial to their only child, who had suffered from the se-

vere 1918 strain of influenza in her early childhood. It left her mentally retarded, cerebral-palsied, and epileptic.[57] Her parents, with all their wealth, found no resources available for her. In their wills they expressed the hope that their home in Rhode Island and their estate might be used so that from their suffering "might come comfort and hope for many."[58] Dr. Charles Bradley, a psychiatrist and the great-nephew of George Bradley,[59] headed the home's staff of pediatricians and psychiatrists, most of whom were imported from local adult private mental hospitals and Yale University's School of Medicine in New Haven, Connecticut.[60]

In the early days of the Bradley Home, noted Laufer, it was widely believed that abnormalities of the structure of the central nervous system were probably responsible for the children's difficult behavior and that neurosurgical remedies might be an effective treatment. Therefore, a procedure after the admission of some children to the home was to perform a pneumoencephalogram (a painful spinal tap) on them, which regularly resulted in complaints of severe headaches.[61] In response, Bradley began treating these children with a new amphetamine, Benzedrine. He reasoned that if he gave "it as a vasopressor [a medication that raises blood pressure], he could increase the production of cerebrospinal fluid and thereby shorten the duration of the children's headaches."[62]

Similar to the discovery of many new psychiatric drugs in the history of mental health, this one came entirely by accident.[63] The children's headaches were not particularly affected or relieved by the drug.[64] But "possibly the most striking change in behavior during the week of Benzedrine therapy occurred in the school activities of many of these patients," reported Bradley in 1937.[65] The behavior and school performance of many of the 30 children who received the drug underwent a dramatic change characterized by increased interest in schoolwork, better work habits, and a significant reduction in disruptive behavior. The drug calmed many of the children without dulling their attention span.[66] The effect was not limited to children with any particular behavioral disorder, but ranged from the child who had "specific educational disabilities, with secondary disturbed school behaviour, to the retiring schizoid child on the one hand and the aggressive, egocentric epileptic child on the other."[67]

Bradley prescribed the drug not only for children suffering from severe post-pneumoencephalogram headaches but also, as Elizabeth Bromley has noted, for children who had not recently undergone the spinal tap procedure.[68] As it turned out, Benzedrine had the same effect on both groups of children, who began to refer to the medication as their "arithmetic pills" and would often spontaneously remark, "I have joy in my stomach," "I feel fine and can't seem to do things fast enough today," and "I start to make my bed and before I know, it is done."[69] A month before Bradley's 1937 article on his patients appeared, two other researchers similarly found "improvement in the performance on IQ tests of subjects who were given amphetamines [Benzedrine]."[70]

Bradley acknowledged that "it appears paradoxical that a drug known to be a stimulant should produce subdued behavior in half of the children." He noted, however, "that portions of the higher levels of the central nervous system have inhibition as their function, and that stimulation of these portions might indeed produce the clinical picture of reduced activity through increased voluntary control."[71] Furthermore, on the first day that Benzedrine was discontinued, the effects of the drug disappeared and the children's behavior problems returned. "To see a single daily dose of Benzedrine produce a greater improvement in school performance than the combined efforts of a capable staff working in a most favorable setting, would have been all but demoralizing to the teachers, had not the improvement been so gratifying from a practical viewpoint," observed Bradley. Nevertheless, he concluded his article by cautioning that "any indiscriminate use of Benzedrine to produce symptomatic relief might well mask reactions of etiological significance [other physical, psychological, and/or educational factors that could be the underlying cause of the children's behavioral problems] which should in every case receive adequate attention."[72]

What ultimately proved critical from Bradley's accidental finding was that the first experimentation with amphetamines opened two avenues of research: the calming effect on children's behavior and activity and the stimulating effect on their academic performance.[73] In 1950, 13 years after his original article, Bradley summarized his treatment of 350 "individual maladjusted children" who were treated with amphetamines—this time Benzedrine and Dexedrine—and again found that they were effective in subduing extremely restless and fidgety children.[74] In his later reports, he concluded that "these drugs influence children's behavior by altering their emotional reactions to distressing situations."[75] In sum, Bradley came to believe that many hyperactive children were deeply unhappy and that their behavior problems were their way of conveying this. Administering amphetamines had a euphoric effect on them, which remedied their desire to convey unhappiness through deviant behavior.[76]

## Minimal Brain Damage and Hyperkinetic Impulse Disorder

In the 1940s and 1950s, the work of Alfred Strauss—an education specialist from Wisconsin and president of the Cove School for Brain-Injured Children in Racine, Wisconsin—seemed to provide additional support for the theory that "minimal brain damage" could be inferred from children's hyperactive and inattentive behavior even when scars or "lesions on the brain were not apparent."[77] Both Darwin and Kahn and Cohen's 1934 reference to an "organic drivenness" inspired Strauss's work.[78] In their 1947 book *Psychopathology and Education of the Brain-Injured Child*, Strauss and Laura Lehtinen argued that children who had been brain-injured—from causes such as anoxia (lack of oxygen) or head injury during the pre- or perinatal period—exhibited characteristics similar to children who were infected with the encephalitis epidemic following World War I and survived but with varying degrees of neurological damage.[79] In many respects, the pathological condition resulting from "epidemic encephalitis is similar to sequelae of brain injury, particularly in the general disturbances expressed in instability, lack of inhibition, impulsivity, hyperactivity, etc.," noted Strauss and Lehtinen.[80]

Strauss and his colleagues provided a scientific rationale for children's misbehavior and school failure in terms of unavoidable biological variation rather than genetic heritability or social and environmental factors. "In brain-injured children, disinhibition, hyperactivity, and distractibility should be regarded as manifestations of exaggerated responsiveness to stimuli and, in young brain-injured children, as behavior reactions beyond the reach of effective cortical control," they argued. "Such a child not only attends to the noise outside but is unable to inhibit the impulse to run to the window to find it."[81] In addition, Strauss and Lehtinen noted,

> Classmates sitting near-by or passing his desk are a constant source of excitation to which he responds by reaching out to hit or punch or push. Class games designed to motivate and interest the normal or familial mentally retarded child are overstimulating for the brain-injured child, with the result that a child who is hyperactive and disinhibited is driven to boisterous talking, shouts, uncontrolled laughter, running about the room, etc. This is the child whom the teacher describes as unresponsive to correction. Scoldings or deprivations, reasoning, subtle approaches by

precept or example are equally ineffectual, since the organic irritability and the situational irritating agents remain.[82]

The research by Strauss and his colleagues received a great deal of attention and became very popular among American educators, largely because they linked their findings directly to new educational policies for accommodating minimally brain-damaged children.[83] They even provided specific photographs of modified school settings for the "reduction of stimuli within the classroom."[84] The special education procedures that Strauss advocated were widely adopted by schools across the country and served to bolster the apparent link between brain damage and hyperactivity in the minds of many educators.[85] Subsequent research into the educational treatment programs and procedures advocated by Strauss and his colleagues, however, yielded minimal evidence for their effectiveness.[86] Additionally, their psychological findings could not be replicated.[87] But enthusiasm for their work continued in large part because there were so few special education procedures and programs available in the 1940s and 1950s for teachers of hyperactive children.[88] Trying something—anything—ordinarily seems better than doing nothing.

In the 1950s, the misbehavior and its treatment began to be described in ways that are more familiar to current observers. What later became known as ADHD was first officially named "hyperkinetic impulse disorder" by Maurice Laufer (a child psychiatrist and an electroencephalographer), Eric Denhoff (a child neurologist), and Gerald Solomons (a pediatrician) in 1957.[89] The three researchers worked at the same Bradley Home where Benzedrine was first found to be helpful to children with severe behavioral disorders 20 years before. Laufer became director of the Bradley Home after Charles Bradley.[90] In their article, they "acknowledged their indebtedness to Charles Bradley, M.D., whose pioneer observations provided the inspiration for these studies."[91] As a new and specific diagnostic category, noted Laufer and his colleagues, hyperkinetic impulse disorder is a behavior pattern that

> may be noted from early infancy on or not become prominent until five or six years of age . . . Hyperactivity is the most striking item . . . There are also a short attention span and poor powers of concentration, which are particularly noticeable under school conditions . . . The child is impulsive . . . irritable and explosive, with a low frustration tolerance. Poor school work is frequently quite prominent.[92]

Poor concentration was a second "cardinal symptom" of the disorder, which was observed as "more frequent in males than in females" and, peculiarly, more frequent "in first-born than in subsequent children."[93]

Similar to the nineteenth-century scientists who theorized about mental illness, Laufer and his colleagues suggested that hyperkinetic impulse disorder was the result of an "injury to or dysfunction of the diencephalon in early life."[94] The diencephalon, they explained, "is a small part of the brain that acts to sort, route and pattern impulses coming from sensory receptors before they become amplified at higher levels of the brain. In this capacity it functions as an inhibitor of irrelevant stimuli, keeping them from 'flooding' the cortex. If the diencephalon is not functioning properly, the cortex can become overwhelmed by more stimuli than it can adequately deal with."[95] The result, noted Laufer and Denhoff in a separate article, "is an undue sensitivity of the central nervous system to stimuli constantly pouring in from peripheral receptors . . . The resulting components of sensitivity and forced responsiveness to stimuli, inability to inhibit and delay responses, and visual-motor difficulties—all combine to produce the characteristics of the hyperkinetic syndrome."[96] Two decades later, researchers proposed a similar theory of "under arousal" of the cortex and brain stem in hyperkinetic children with minimal brain dysfunction.[97]

Laufer and his colleagues noted how the new diagnostic category was so welcome to many parents. "Often, the demonstration to the parents of an organic factor in the child's behavior leads to a great sense of relief concerning their own and the child's responsibility for the problem. They then are able to understand and accept the child's behavior more readily," they noted. "If the physician in turn shows the parents that he understands and is not critical of them, he can help greatly to bring about a *rapprochement* between parent and child."[98] At the same time, Laufer acknowledged decades later that he and his colleagues had "a nagging concern over the fact that so many children who presented the picture that we were coming to recognize and that we later characterized as 'hyperkinetic impulse disorder' presented no clear diagnostic evidence of involvement of the central nervous system and had nothing in their history that would provide an acceptable etiological statement."[99] In other words, many of the children they diagnosed with hyperkinetic impulse disorder did not have any evidence of brain injury, nor was there an obvious biological or physical explanation for their behavior (for example, retardation).

Regardless of what specifically caused hyperkinetic impulse disorder, Laufer and his colleagues confirmed that amphetamines were effective in counteracting its symptoms.[100] They suggested "that amphetamine may in some way, perhaps by raising the level of synaptic resistance, alter the functions of the diencephalon in such a way that it once more can keep the cortex from being flooded by streams of unmodulated impulses coming in through sensory receptors."[101] What is often overlooked in other historical accounts of Laufer and his colleagues' work is how they subordinated the importance of stimulant medications to psychotherapy and the Freudian views that dominated psychiatry at the time. Their articles are full of references to "associated ego disturbances" and "ego weaknesses," mothering issues, Freud, neurosis, and "the present permissive era of child management."[102] In the first article they published in 1957, Laufer and his colleagues wrote, "In other words the amphetamine did not interfere with the operation of the psychotherapeutic process and the fostering of a basic inner change."[103] They concluded their second article with the observation that "it would be unfortunate if, as a result of these observations, amphetamines were used indiscriminately for the treatment of behavior disturbance in children or if the need for specific psychotherapy were overlooked. Amphetamine has a specific role, but is no substitute for psychotherapy."[104] Laufer and his colleagues viewed misbehavior the way that most psychiatrists did in the 1950s and 1960s. They saw illness as psychodynamic in origin, yet treatable with medications that could facilitate psychotherapy. During this period, child psychiatrists rarely talked to one another in a professionally oriented sense—through academic journals and research conferences—and no large literature existed, so there was no single story of childhood misbehavior (a biological explanation did not become dominant until at least the late 1970s).

Laufer and his colleagues' work on hyperkinetic impulse disorder represented one of the very few research initiatives in the country at the time on children's use of psychiatric drugs. Fewer than a dozen clinical research papers were published between 1937 and the early 1950s on the use of stimulant drugs by children.[105] The general consensus among clinicians and medical researchers at the time, noted the NIMH's first director, Robert Felix, was that psychopharmacological drugs in children may be "tools of tremendous value but also may contain elements of danger."[106]

## Ritalin and the Rise of Psychopharmacology

At the same time, in the mid-1950s new psychiatric drugs became available for treating adults with severe mental illnesses. The whole field of psychopharmacology entered a phase of rapid acceleration, with experiments that showed the effectiveness of tranquilizers for adult psychiatric patients and antidepressants for severe mood problems.[107]

These developments led to a resurgence of interest in the use of drugs for hyperactive and emotionally disturbed children. A number of articles appeared in 1955 and 1956 that pointed to the effectiveness of chlorpromazine—a powerful and revolutionary psychiatric medication also known by its trade name Thorazine—in treating hyperactive children.[108] "At this point the question may justly be asked, 'Why use such a potent drug on these children instead of psychotherapy?'" wrote Herbert Freed and Charles Peifer in the *American Journal of Psychiatry* in 1956. "Fundamentally, the chief reason was the need to improve a situation, such as individual misbehavior in a school room where the authorities could use only limited controls in dealing with the student."[109] Besides, the authors noted, "Twenty of these children (80%) were either illegitimate or came from broken homes. Psychotherapy with the remaining parent was therefore, for economic or other reasons, impossible."[110] Most of all, they concluded, "Certainly the quieter child makes less demands on the environment, parental giving is more freely offered when placidity abounds, [and] learning is facilitated when teachers are not frustrated."[111]

Yet chlorpromazine was (and remains) a powerful psychiatric drug with some especially unpleasant side effects.[112] Its primary and most effective use was on adults in mental asylums suffering from psychosis.[113] Thus, it did not become a serious competitor to amphetamines, such as Benzedrine and Dexedrine (which had their own unpleasant side effects), for use by inordinately hyperactive and restless children. A Swiss pharmaceutical firm, Ciba-Geigy, had been working since the 1940s to develop a drug that would produce the same stimulant effects as amphetamines, but with fewer side effects and with less potential for abuse. In 1955, just as chlorpromazine was transforming the treatment of severely psychotic mental patients in many state mental asylums, Ciba-Geigy synthesized a drug called methylphenidate.[114] Given the brand name Ritalin, it was initially marketed as a treatment for narcolepsy in older patients.[115] Its first mention as a possible treatment for children with "hyperkinetic behavior syndrome" came in Laufer and Denhoff's 1957 article in the *Journal of Pediatrics*.[116] The authors noted, however, that their experience with Ritalin and a handful of other drugs was "too limited for any valid statement as to their usefulness."[117]

As part of an effort to build on the success of chlorpromazine and to aid in the development of new psychiatric drugs for treatment of depression such as imipramine (Tofranil), the NIMH created the Psychopharmacological Research Branch (PRB) in 1956.[118] In 1958, the

PRB sponsored the first ever conference "on the use of drugs in children with psychiatric problems."[119] One of the leading voices at the conference was a young psychiatrist from Johns Hopkins University's School of Medicine by the name of Leon Eisenberg. While noting how vitally important psychopharmacological research with children was, "we must, however, reckon with a host of unresolved methodological quandaries," explained Eisenberg. "Whereas the adult comes for treatment largely because of his own distress and at his own initiative, the child comes to our attention because of his family's or his community's initiative. Whom, then, are we to classify diagnostically: the child, the family, the community, or all three?"[120] Eisenberg was becoming something of an iconic and controversial figure in the field of psychiatry—which at the time was dominated by Freudian and psychodynamic theories—because he continually stressed to his colleagues the importance of empiricism, symptom-driven diagnostics, and the need for psychiatry to improve and advance public health. He became famous for, among other things, stating, "It's time to stop pulling drowning kids out of the river and start heading upstream to see who is pushing them in."[121]

The PRB conference on children's use of psychiatric drugs coincided with the federal government's first ever research grant on child psychopharmacology in 1958, which went to Eisenberg. The grant was for studying the use of tranquilizers on children, however, and did not include plans for the investigation of stimulants.[122] Eisenberg recruited a young instructor in pediatrics and medical psychology by the name of Keith Conners, and together they initiated a series of groundbreaking studies in pediatric psychopharmacology.[123] Conners, a former Rhodes Scholar who earned his doctoral degree with highest honors at Harvard University, and Eisenberg, who earned his MD at the University of Pennsylvania, interned at Mount Sinai Hospital in New York City, and served as a captain in the Army Medical Corps, brought a new level of scientific rigor and biomedical respectability to the study of using psychiatric medications on children.

Ritalin was eventually approved by the Food and Drug Administration in 1961 for use in children with behavioral problems.[124] In 1963, Conners and Eisenberg published the first article in a medical journal explicitly advocating the use of Ritalin for treatment of "disturbed" children.[125] In their study, they included 81 children who came from "two residential care institutions," one of which was a foster home for children "unsuitable for care in individual foster homes"; the other was a psychiatric treatment center.[126] Children who took Ritalin showed demonstrably and statistically significant improvement following their use of the drug.[127] Conners noted many years later that he was "struck by the size of the improvement effect in the children who received stimulants" because his "earlier experience treating similarly disturbed children with psychotherapy yielded virtually no improvement even after a year's worth of psychotherapy."[128] Key to Conners and Eisenberg's research was, first, the fact that parents and child-care workers, rather than physicians, rated the children's symptoms before and after treatment and, second, that the study was both double-blind (nobody knew which children received what treatment) and controlled (half of the children received a placebo).[129] "The only adverse side effect," noted Conners and Eisenberg, "was a high report (70%) of appetite loss in the drug group."[130]

With today's strict and demanding scientific requirements for "informed consent" by human research participants and other safety procedures, it is interesting to note how relaxed the research environment was back in the 1960s. "I would walk down the street in Baltimore to School 102, which served children with conduct disorders," recalled Conners, "and I'd tell the principal about the research I was interested in doing: using psychopharmacology to try to help the kinds of students he had. And the principal responded, 'If you could help us, that would be great!' The parents of the children were even more enthusiastic than the principal," he added. "I was able to conduct a safe, rigorous, double-blind, cross-over study within ten days."[131]

The composite picture of hyperactivity in the early 1960s, then, was that "of a brain damage syndrome to be treated with stimulant drugs, minimal stimulation classrooms, and possibly psychotherapy, and having a favorable prognosis for the adolescent years."[132]

## Minimal Brain Dysfunction, Stimulant Politics, and the Critical Role of the NIMH

By the mid-1960s, however, growing numbers of researchers were openly questioning the assumption that there was a definitive link between some degree of brain damage and hyperactivity.[133] Many children who were diagnosed with hyperkinetic impulse disorder showed no evidence of any brain damage.[134] The term "became recognized as vague, overinclusive, of little or no prescriptive value, and without much neurological evidence," noted Russell Barkley.[135] Consequently, the term "minimal brain damage" died a slow death and morphed into "minimal brain *dysfunction*," which still stressed some deficiency in the child's central nervous system but left vague what the underlying cause for this deficiency might be.[136] The new term's description of extremely hyperactive and inattentive children closely resembled many previous descriptions dating back to Still's famous 1902 lecture:

> The term "minimal brain dysfunction" refers . . . to children of near average, average, or above average general intelligence with certain learning or behavioral disabilities ranging from mild to severe, which are associated with deviations of function of the central nervous system. These deviations may manifest themselves by various combinations of impairment in perception, conceptualization, language, memory, and control of attention, impulse, or motor functions . . . These aberrations may arise from genetic variations, biochemical irregularities, perinatal brain insults or other illness or injuries sustained during the years which are critical for the development and maturation of the central nervous system, *or from unknown causes.*[137]

The new term's hedging on what caused minimal brain dysfunction partly reflected the reality that psychodynamic and Freudian-inspired psychotherapy still held sway within the field of psychiatry in the 1960s. Until Eisenberg replaced him in 1961, the chief of child psychiatry at Johns Hopkins was Leo Kanner, one of the first academic child psychiatrists in America.[138] While critical of psychoanalysis, Kanner espoused a "dynamic" approach to human personality that he learned from his profoundly influential mentor, Adolph Meyer.[139] Meyer's technique consisted of psychiatrists conducting "life-history" analyses that emphasized "the careful measurement of whole persons in the understanding of mental disorder."[140] According to Kanner, origins of present troubles were reactions to experiences of the past; mental illness was essentially the behavioral product of personal difficulties and sufferings stretching back to early childhood.[141] Thus, when the second edition of the American Psychiatric Association's *Diagnostic and Statistical Manual of Mental Disorders* (DSM-II) appeared in 1968, all childhood disorders were described as "reactions." "Hyperkinetic impulse disorder" or "hyperactive child syndrome" became "hyperkinetic reaction of childhood."[142] Parents and teachers were urged, among other things, to try to reduce the number of stimuli around children diagnosed with the disorder.[143]

As clinicians and researchers continued to debate the best diagnostic term for children with significant behavior disorders, the late 1960s marked the beginning of a turning point for research in pediatric psychopharmacology.[144] It was initiated almost exclusively by financial support from the federal government's NIMH. The pharmaceutical industry would supply researchers with psychotropic medications (a very small marginal cost) for their trials and place ads for their products in psychiatry journals.[145] Yet, as social psychologist Ilina Singh found, the industry would not depict children in advertisements for stimulants until the early to mid-1970s. Also, pharmaceutical companies would not provide major funding for research in the area of pediatric psychopharmacology, largely because administering psychoactive drugs to nonhospitalized children—except in the most extreme and extraordinary situations—was considered too controversial.[146] At the time, drug companies did not even envision that the pediatric market for psychiatric drugs would ever become big enough to be worth investing in.[147] They were focusing their efforts almost exclusively on the adult market.[148]

After the NIMH made the first two federal research grants for child psychopharmacology in 1958 and 1961, there was a temporary hiatus. Concerns arose in the mid-1960s over the indiscriminate use of phenothiazines (an antipsychotic drug group that includes chlorpromazine) in the treatment of people with mental retardation, many of whom, it turned out, had been receiving these powerful psychiatric drugs in state institutions on an "indefinite" basis.[149] In a 1966 report to the PRB's Clinical Review Committee documenting the abuse of patients with mental retardation, the authors stated, "The recent work of Eisenberg and Conners, much of which is still in press, has apparently not yet had an impact on the field."[150] With the scandal associated with the indiscriminate use of phenothiazines, the report added, many NIMH-funded researchers were turning "their attention toward the stimulants after negative experiences with the tranquilizers and with psychotherapy."[151]

The following year, in 1967, the NIMH made the first federal government research grant to study the effectiveness of stimulants on behaviorally disturbed children to Keith Conners, who had left Johns Hopkins for Harvard Medical School and Massachusetts General Hospital.[152] The PRB concluded that it "needed more quality studies comparing, in concurrent designs, the relative efficacy of drugs of different classes; stimulants, phenothiazines, antidepressants, and minor tranquilizers." It also wanted more long-term efficacy studies (e.g., longer than 8 weeks and hopefully as long as a few years).[153] Consequently, the NIMH made three additional grants in 1968 to researchers at the University of California, Davis; Hillside Hospital in New York; and the

District of Columbia's Department of Mental Health to study the "comparative drug effects in hyperkinetic children" and the "pharmacotherapy of hyperactive children."[154]

By the close of the 1960s, only an estimated 150,000 to 200,000 children in the United States were being treated with stimulants,[155] which represented roughly 0.002% of the entire childhood population.[156] Nevertheless, an event occurred in the summer of 1970 that permanently altered the field of pediatric psychopharmacology. It also served as a harbinger of the future debates and controversy over ADHD and stimulant use by children. On June 29, 1970, in an article entitled "Omaha Pupils Given 'Behavior Drugs,'" the *Washington Post* reported that 5% to 10% of schoolchildren in Omaha, Nebraska, were receiving behavior-controlling drugs (Ritalin), "that this was part of a directed program by the school system in which some parental coercion to submit to drug therapy was involved, and that drugs were being given without adequate medical supervision resulting in pill swapping in school."[157]

The *Post* article had several inaccuracies: the 5%–10% figure referred only to the percentage of special-education children using stimulants, not the entire student population. And parents were not being coerced into accepting drug therapy.[158] Yet the story generated considerable media attention.[159] It led to a congressional hearing,[160] a national conference on the subject ("The Use of Stimulant Drugs in the Treatment of Behaviorally Disturbed Young School Children"),[161] and an official report of the conference in 1971.[162] The 1970 congressional hearings, in particular, reveal the controversy's timelessness and its overarching philosophical orientation:

Representative John Wydler (R-NY): I would think that what you describe as a problem is practically almost the average child that goes to school. They all have these kinds of problems. All you are dealing with is the question of degree. Don't most children have a problem of attention span and things of this nature? This is almost natural. I would think that is a normal problem. I have that problem myself.

Dr. Ronald Lipman (NIMH): I think we all do . . . All I am saying is that hyperkinesis is frequently something that brings the child into conflict with his parents, peers, and teachers and that the teacher observes behavior and has a referral role to play, but, as you know, hyperkinesis is a medical syndrome. It should be properly diagnosed by a medical doctor . . .

Representative Cornelius Gallagher (D-NJ): At what age does the effect of amphetamines reverse itself?

Dr. Lipman: I would say after the age of 12 these drugs should be given with extreme caution, if at all.

Representative Gallagher: What happens to the hyperkinetic child when he is 12?

Dr. Lipman: Well, many hyperkinetic children, when they reach adolescence, outgrow the hyperactivity.[163]

The committee's hearing came amid mounting public and congressional concern over the abuse of all drugs, but particularly stimulants.[164] In 1970, Congress revised the nation's existing federal drug regulations with the passage of the Comprehensive Drug Abuse Prevention and Control Act.[165] The act placed amphetamines and methylphenidate (Ritalin) in the category of Schedule III, which put limits on the number of refills a patient could obtain and how long an individual prescription could run.[166] Recommending the use of stimulants for one purpose—treating children with minimal brain dysfunction—while trying to prevent their use for illicit purposes (for example, appetite suppression, performance enhancement in athletics, recreational use) was sometimes politically awkward.[167] As Representative Gallagher, who chaired the congressional hearing, stated at the hearing's conclusion, "The thing that really troubles me in this is a certain glibness about the experimentation on young children in this country, used as guinea pigs . . . Here we are acting in a way that rather assumes that the drug problem doesn't exist in America. I think the most tortuous problem in our country today is drug abuse. And the biggest part of drug abuse is amphetamines."[168]

With growing amphetamine abuse in the United States and a documented epidemic of Ritalin abuse in Sweden,[169] Congress instructed the Drug Enforcement Administration (DEA) in 1971 to reclassify amphetamines and methylphenidate as Schedule II drugs (along with opiates such as Demerol and morphine), which further tightened prescription regulations and created a production quota or limit for all stimulants.[170] This new classification had several important consequences. Henceforth, pharmaceutical companies had to make requests to the DEA for how much total amphetamines and other stimulants they were permitted to manufacture. The DEA reviewed these requests and then set an aggregate amount based on what it considered to be "appropriate." The DEA also began monitoring the distribution of these drugs nationwide, which has provided annual data on the amount of the drugs produced, and where they have been distributed, dating back to the early 1970s.[171]

At a symposium of NIMH officials and leading pediatric psychopharmacology researchers in March of 1972 in Key Biscayne, Florida, the opening speaker outlined the inherent difficulties and frustrations that he and his colleagues experienced in trying to explain their research efforts to Congress and the general public: "The area of pediatric psychopharmacology has been favored by having some old drugs of clear effectiveness such as *d*-amphetamine and methylphenidate and cursed by the fact that both these drugs can be abused," said Jonathan Cole. "It is also cursed by having a range of children who benefit from these drugs, which is hard to describe in terms other than those that encourage critics of all drug administration to all children to accuse doctors of drugging down the normal exuberance of childhood just to allow teachers to shirk arduous educational tasks."[172]

Growing concerns about the ethics of biomedical research in general led Congress to pass the National Research Act in the summer of 1974, which created the National Commission for the Protection of Human Subjects of Biomedical and Behavioral Research.[173] The commission made clear, noted Robert Sprague, that "research with children, particularly research that is considered *at risk*, defined as any increased possibility of harm above the probabilities ordinarily encountered in everyday life to the subjects, such as in psychotropic drug research," was going to be much more tightly controlled.[174] Meanwhile, the FDA established its own Pediatric Subcommittee to focus on "the many problems that have arisen in the area of psychotropic drug usage with children."[175]

The negative media blitz and increasing public and congressional interest in hyperactive children and stimulants culminated in 1975 with three major publications that found large audiences in both academia and the general public. The first, *The Myth of the Hyperactive Child and Other Means of Child Control*, by journalists Peter Schrag and Diane Divoky, argued that schoolchildren were being labeled with a dubious diagnosis and treated with unnecessary and dangerous medications, particularly Ritalin, by a conspiracy of authoritarian physicians, school administrators, and teachers.[176] The book was a classic screed. Stimulants were being used as "chemical straitjackets," the authors asserted, to control the natural exuberance and activity of children who came into conflict with teachers or other school personnel. The book was criticized for various inaccuracies, but it was widely read. A second book, Dr. Benjamin Feingold's *Why Your Child Is Hyperactive*, made an argument that has persisted off and on to this day, despite a continuing lack of evidence for it.[177] Hyperactivity in children, Feingold maintained, was the result of an allergic or toxic reaction to food additives (especially colorings and dyes). Remove these items from a child's diet, he claimed, and the hyperactivity would disappear.[178] Feingold's arguments became so widespread that Feingold Associates—part political organization, part public interest group, comprised mainly of parents—developed in virtually every state in the country (many later morphed into Children and Adults with Attention Deficit/Hyperactivity Disorder, or CHADD, chapters). Legislation was even introduced and almost passed in California mandating that food in school cafeterias be prepared in such a way as to be free of additives, dyes, and colorings.[179]

Finally, sociologist Peter Conrad asserted in a now classic and still widely read article, "The Discovery of Hyperkinesis," that the diagnosis was simply a new example of an old societal tendency to "medicalize" problematic or different but otherwise normal behaviors. As one of the most effective means of social control, Conrad argued, diagnosing hyperactive children with a mental disorder and medicating them with stimulants was akin to silencing political nonconformists and religious heretics.[180] A major factor in the disorder's growing popularity with teachers and clinicians, he maintained, was the profit-driven marketing efforts of the pharmaceutical industry (particularly Ciba-Geigy, the maker of Ritalin).[181] Conrad also singled out the Association for Children with Learning Disabilities for playing an influential lobbying role in expanding this "medicalization of deviant behavior" to include "hyperkinetic" children.[182] Conrad's alternative suggestion—that the children's school or home environment might be the root cause of their deviant behavior—found a receptive audience among the antiauthoritarian spirit of the time and has remained popular to this day.[183]

These publications and the congressional hearings and conferences that preceded them triggered a vigorous political debate over pediatric psychopharmacology. By 1976, several states had established committees to investigate the use of stimulants in children.[184] Five states instituted guidelines for the use of stimulant medications (Delaware, Iowa, Minnesota, New Hampshire, New York); four others issued revised administrative regulations for their use (Connecticut, Hawaii, Indiana, Oregon); and three states passed legislation that either *banned* research on pediatric psychopharmacology altogether (Massachusetts) or prohibited the administration of any drug to a child for experimental purposes unless by written consent of both the child's parent(s) and the family physician (New Jersey, New Hampshire).[185] At the same time, the number of U.S. children estimated to be receiving stimulant medications rose to roughly 600,000 in 1978 (a three- to fourfold increase from when the decade began).[186] Thus, even though the public debate over hyperactive children and stimulants increased over the course of the 1970s, so too did the number of children diagnosed with the disorder and using the drugs.

Finally, a discovery in 1978 further complicated the relationship between the diagnosis and the drugs, and added to the controversy over both. For decades, a hyperactive child's positive response to stimulants was often considered strong supporting evidence for the child having the mental disorder. Clinicians and researchers would often work backward from a poststimulant improvement in a child's behavior to a confirmation of the diagnosis. However, Judith Rapoport—a researcher at the NIMH's Biological Psychiatry Branch whose work was one of the first to receive government funding back in the early 1960s—found that stimulants had effects on normal children that were very similar to those on excessively hyperactive children or children with other related behavior problems.[187] After giving Dexedrine and dextroamphetamine to hyperactive and normal children, she found that both groups experienced similar improvements in attention and on math tests.[188]

Rapoport's work called into question the validity of using drug response as a diagnostic tool. Moreover, if most children's behavior and performance benefited from taking stimulants, how hyperactive did a child have to be to qualify as having a genuine mental impairment? Rapoport and her colleagues' findings demonstrated the need for clinicians to develop more accurate and reliable diagnostic criteria for distinguishing children who truly had the disorder from the majority, who did not. As the next chapter explains, larger efforts along these lines were already under way.[189]

## Conclusion

As the preceding review demonstrates, the historical evolution of the diagnosis that we now refer to as ADHD and the use of stimulants by children were profoundly affected by major episodes of disease and illness, medical research and discovery, political controversies, and shifting cultural perspectives on childhood and education. While the children in question have remained more or less the same over the last century—in terms of their behavioral description—the labels affixed to them changed frequently. From social Darwinism to eugenics, "Influenza 1918," the rise of special education programs, Freud, and America's first "war on drugs" in the 1970s, especially hyperactive and inattentive children have been (and remain) a population of enormous clinical, parental, and educational concern. There are many reasons for the controversy that developed over ADHD and stimulants, but perhaps the key and irresolvable factor, Keith Conners has argued, is that at the core of the disorder is a "black box": the child's brain.[190] Only today are researchers beginning to be able to peer into it with new diagnostic imaging technology and incorporate genetic analyses. For virtually all of the twentieth century, however, whatever was fundamentally amiss in a child's brain (if anything) had to be "taken on faith."[191]

# CHAPTER FOUR

# The Transformation of Mental Disorders in the 1980s

*The DSM-III, Managed Care, and "Cosmetic Psychopharmacology"*

The development and publication of DSM-III represents a fateful point in the history of the American psychiatric profession . . . The decision of the American Psychiatric Association first to develop DSM-III and then to promulgate its use represents a significant reaffirmation on the part of American psychiatry of its medical identity and its commitment to scientific medicine.

—GERALD KLERMAN, *AMERICAN JOURNAL OF PSYCHIATRY*, APRIL 1984

As Prozac's success stories mount, so does the sense that depression and other mental disorders are just that—treatable illnesses, not failings of character. The stigma is receding, and the search for still better treatments is accelerating. Sooner or later, notes Dr. Peter Kramer, there may even be a drug that can "change people in ways they want to be changed—not just away from illness but toward some desirable psychological state."

—*NEWSWEEK*, MARCH 26, 1990

A major transformation occurred within psychiatry and the larger field of mental health in the 1980s, resulting in dramatic changes in how mental disorders were defined and diagnosed. In a relatively short period of time, mental disorders went from broad, causally described entities that were continuous with normality to more symptom-based, categorical medical entities.[1] The publication of the American Psychiatric Association's third edition of its *Diagnostic and Statistical Manual of Mental Disorders* (DSM-III) in 1980 was responsible for much of this change.[2] Disorders such as major depression, social phobia, and

ADHD—and the extent to which their treatments have changed over the past three decades—cannot be well understood without first comprehending what led to, and then resulted from, the DSM-III.[3] For example, attention deficit disorder (ADD; the *H*, for hyperactivity, was added later, in the DSM-III's revised version, in 1987) made its first appearance, as the clinical diagnosis for inordinately impulsive, hyperactive, and/or inattentive children, in the DSM-III.

While most clinicians do not use the current version of the DSM (IV) as thoroughly as the manual outlines when they make ADHD diagnoses,[4] they do use 1 set of the manual's 5 total criteria for the disorder virtually every time: the list of 18 total ADHD symptoms. This truncated use of the current DSM is important because the DSM-II (1968) did not have any of the current criteria—including the arrangement of symptoms—that the DSM-III and DSM-IV have. Also, the DSM is important in general, even though clinicians often use it selectively and arbitrarily,[5] because its numbered diagnoses trigger an array of different policy responses and are a precursor to prescribing psychotropic drugs.[6]

The DSM-III solidified and then accelerated changes in the field of mental health that had begun in the 1960s. Biological psychiatry, with its emphasis on the brain and neurochemistry, displaced environmental psychiatry—which focused on the mind, childhood, unconscious motivations, psychotherapy, and parenting—as the dominant paradigm.[7] The DSM-III was an important factor in bringing about what has been referred to as the "remedicalization" of American psychiatry.[8] In the process, the trend toward greater use of psychotropic medications increased sharply in the latter half of the 1980s.[9]

The DSM-III was not solely responsible, though, for the rapid growth of psychopharmacology. A number of clinical trends originating in the 1960s converged with major new developments in the field of mental health in the mid- to late 1980s, which eventually gave rise to managed behavioral health care and a growing reliance on psychotropic drugs.[10] Over the course of the 1980s, the prevalence of children diagnosed with ADHD and those using stimulants increased modestly. Around 400,000 children were diagnosed with the disorder in 1980; 10 years later, in 1990, the number expanded to roughly 900,000.[11] The key difference, however, and the one that illustrates much of the change that occurred in the field of mental health in the 1980s, is that only about a quarter (28%) of the children diagnosed with ADHD in 1980 were prescribed stimulants, whereas the vast majority (86%) of them were by 1990 (Table 4.2, p. 94).

This chapter focuses on how and why the field of mental health underwent significant change from the 1970s to the early 1990s. It endeavors to explain the pressures and incentives that led to the DSM-III, and the manual's consequences for clinical diagnosis and treatment of mental disorders in the United States.[12] The chapter also traces the major research trends and clinical developments related to ADHD and stimulants that converged in the latter half of the 1980s, which set the stage for a massive increase in ADHD diagnoses and stimulant use in the 1990s.

## The Creation of the DSM-III: Political and Economic Aspects of Mental Diagnoses

In 1980, the DSM-III fundamentally changed the formal definitions of mental disorders. It imported a model from medicine in which diagnosis, based on symptoms, is the keystone of clinical practice and research.[13] The new manual emphasized categories of mental illness rather than fuzzy dimensions, and overt symptoms rather than underlying etiological (or causal) mechanisms.[14] The DSM-III's symptom-based categorization of mental disorders reflected the growing standardization of psychiatric diagnoses that began in the 1970s.[15] This standardization was the product of several factors, including professional politics within the mental health community, increased government involvement in mental health research and policy making, mounting pressure on psychiatrists from health insurers to demonstrate the cost-effectiveness of their practices, and pharmaceutical companies' need to market their products to treat specific diseases.[16]

The basic transformation in the DSM-III was its development and use of a model that equated measurable symptoms with the presence of diseases. This symptom-focused orientation allowed clinicians to develop a standardized system of measurement and resulted in more specific diagnoses and a longer manual (see Table 4.1).[17] It utilized additional criteria from the disease model to define mental disorders, such as a patient's age of onset, as well as the disorder's natural history and developmental course, responses to treatment, role of impairment, and environmental context. This diagnostic classification system did not rely "on identifiable genetic or biological markers," noted Kimberly Hoagwood, but on observations that research has shown "can be biased by clinical assumptions or by historical or social determinants."[18]

The new system, however, did benefit numerous interests. The DSM-III allowed research-oriented psychiatrists, a small but highly in-

*Table 4.1* DSM I, II, III, III-R, IV, 1952–1994

| Version | Year | Total number of mental diagnoses | Total number of pages |
|---------|------|----------------------------------|------------------------|
| I | 1952 | 106 | 130 |
| II | 1968 | 182 | 134 |
| III | 1980 | 265 | 494 |
| III-R | 1987 | 292 | 567 |
| IV | 1994 | 297 | 886 |

*Source:* American Psychiatric Association, *Diagnostic and Statistical Manual of Mental Disorders*, 1st, 2nd, 3rd, 3rd rev., 4th eds. (Washington, DC: American Psychiatric Association, 1952, 1968, 1980, 1987, 1994).

fluential group in the profession, to measure mental disorders in more reliable and reproducible ways.[19] It also helped silence the critics of the previous system, who argued that mental illnesses could not be defined in any objective, scientific way. And because the manual defined disorders mostly through symptoms without regard to causes, it was more theory neutral than its predecessors and thus could be used by clinicians of different theoretical persuasions (Freudian, cognitive behavioral, neurobiological).

Many pressures and controversies came together to force psychiatrists to consider changing the definitions of mental disorders: psychiatry's marginal status within the medical profession, the increasing reluctance of insurance companies and the government to reimburse long-term talk therapy, the need to treat formerly institutionalized seriously mentally ill persons in the community, the growing influence of medication treatments, and the mounting professional threat from nonphysicians (such as clinical psychologists, counselors, and social workers).[20] What is of particular interest and relevance to the primary arguments of this book is the extent to which politics and economics permeated the DSM-III's drafting, passage, and widespread acceptance in the 1980s.

The first step in the process of developing the DSM-III came in 1974, when Robert Spitzer, a leading psychiatrist at Columbia University and consultant to the development of DSM-II, was appointed by the American Psychiatric Association (APA) to coordinate the DSM-II's revision.[21] Initially, the only purpose in revising the DSM-II was to make its nomenclature consistent with the International Classification of Disease, which was scheduled to be modified by the World Health Organization.[22] Those who appointed Spitzer, however, including Melvin Sabshin (medical director of the APA at the time), and Spitzer himself, had entirely different intentions.[23] In 1973, the prestigious journal *Science* published a seminal article, "On Being Sane in Insane Places," by David Rosenhan, which graphically illustrated the lack of validity and reliability associated with that era's dominant approach to psychiatric classifications and diagnoses.[24] The article incensed Spitzer.[25] A 1975 review in the prestigious *New England Journal of Medicine* described psychiatry as "the battered child of medicine . . . born in witchcraft and demoniacal possession, feared by the public, often scorned by the family of medical specialists, and dependent for much of its existence upon handouts from public agencies."[26] Spitzer and several of his colleagues were eager to change this image, and significantly revising the DSM was viewed as critical for doing so.[27]

In determining what would and would not be considered a mental disorder, the membership of Spitzer's task force was hugely consequential. He selected a group of psychiatrists and psychologists who were committed primarily to research, not to clinical practice.[28] Clinicians with other, nonmedical backgrounds were included later in the process, but only after the DSM-III's medically oriented and symptom-focused ground rules had been set.[29] The psychologists who were included in the work on the DSM-III were equally eager to see the field of mental health become less subjective and impressionistic.

Instead of Sigmund Freud, Spitzer and most of his colleagues favored the approach promulgated by Emil Kraepelin, a German psychiatrist of the late nineteenth century whose teachings had been controversial at the time, briefly popular, and then for decades subsequently marginalized in the United States, aside from a few psychiatry departments (that is, Washington University, the University of Iowa, and Columbia University).[30] Rather than focusing on any underlying psychological causes for mental disorders, Kraepelin stressed classifying them according to their unique symptoms, course of development, and eventual outcome. In his view, "Depression, schizophrenia, and so forth were different just as mumps and pneumonia were different."[31] Science inherently requires classification schemes. Using infectious diseases as an example, for scientists to be able to identify and treat tuberculosis or malaria, they first need to be able to distinguish the two from each other and then from other diseases. Epidemiology represents the formal study of classifying diseases according to empirical criteria. For psychiatry to be a medical science, it had to devise a similar epidemiological scheme for classifying mental disorders (known as a "nosology"). Kraepelin's approach to psychiatric classification, explains Allan Young, was based on three arguments: (1) that mental disorders are best understood as analogues with physical diseases, (2) that the classification of mental disorders demands careful observation of visible symptoms instead of inferences based on unproven causal theories, and (3) that empirical research will eventually demonstrate the organic and biochemical origins of mental disorders.[32]

With Kraepelin's theories as his guiding framework, Spitzer became committed to the controversial belief that "mental disorders are a subset of medical disorders."[33] This view was repugnant to psychologists, social workers, and counselors, who saw it as a "power play" by psychiatry to try to preempt the mental health field and lay exclusive claim to diagnosing and treating mental disorders. When put to an official task force vote, the phrase was defeated and substituted with "in the DSM-III each of the mental disorders is conceptualized as a clinically significant behavioral or psychological syndrome."[34]

Nevertheless, the phrase "mental disorders are a subset of medical disorders" represented the intention of Spitzer and several of his colleagues to define mental disorders with testable diagnostic criteria. In their desire to reduce reliance on the vagaries of diagnosticians' subjective understandings, their approach replicated the positivistic drive in the behavioral sciences toward operational definitions of concepts.[35] The result, Spitzer and his colleagues hoped, would be diagnoses that could be reliably verified by a standard classification scheme that focused on describing the symptoms of disorders with the least amount of inference necessary. Increasing the DSM's reliability meant, for instance, that if 10 psychiatrists saw the same depressed patient separately, all 10 should conclude—based on the patient's observable symptoms—that the patient had a depressive disorder. At the time, the DSM-II's reliability was "horrifying low" because not all users of it were equally familiar with the disorders and because definitions of many of the disorders included untestable opinions about their underlying causes.[36] With the DSM-II's lack of formal criteria for determining diagnostic boundaries, clinicians were forced to rely on global descriptions and subjective assumptions about a disorder's origin.

Spitzer and his colleagues made their disdain of the diagnostic status quo—as well as their intent to classify disorders on the basis of their symptoms—clear from the beginning.[37] For Spitzer, the etiologically driven DSM-II brought too many unproven conditions within the realm of psychiatric diagnosis. He expected that the new symptom-based system would narrow, rather than expand, the criteria for defining mental disorders.

## "Homosexuality" as a Harbinger of the Political Conflict Ahead

A precursor to the politics involved in the DSM-III's drafting that strongly motivated Spitzer and his colleagues to redefine psychiatry's area of prime responsibility was the embarrassing public debate over homosexuality's status in DSM-II as a mental "disorder."[38] Was homosexuality fundamentally similar to other diseases such as depression or psychosis? Psychiatrists had enormous difficulty defending this pathological definition of homosexuality. Annual protests by gay activists at the APA's convention from 1970 to 1973 questioned psychiatry's criteria for defining disorders.[39] The controversy suggested that psychiatric diagnoses were strongly influenced not solely by scientific criteria but by public opinion, social constructions of deviance, and political pressure.

As a harbinger of the role he would play in the DSM-III's creation, Spitzer's participation in the homosexuality debate demonstrated his adroit political skills in mediating conflict.[40] Spitzer himself wanted a middle-ground position of defining homosexuality as an "irregular sexual behavior"—not a disorder, but not normal either. After discerning that the APA's task force preferred to completely delete homosexuality from the DSM as a disorder, he acquiesced to gay activists' demands and dropped his preference for a middle-ground position. The APA membership voted in a referendum to confirm the decision to delete homosexuality in 1974 as a disorder and to replace it with a much milder description as a "sexual orientation disturbance."[41] The seventh printing of DSM-II in July 1974 included the following "Special Note" on page vi:

> Since the last printing of this Manual, the trustees of the American Psychiatric Association, in December 1973, voted to eliminate Homosexuality *per se* as a mental disorder and to substitute therefore a new category titled Sexual Orientation Disturbance. The change appears on page 44 of this, the seventh printing. In May, 1974 the trustees' decision was upheld by a substantial majority in a referendum of the voting members of the Association.

The political expediency underlying an otherwise scientific debate over diagnosis was expressed in a stroke, Edward Shorter observed, when "what had been considered for a century or more a grave psychiatric disorder ceased to exist."[42]

The debate over homosexuality demonstrated to Spitzer and his colleagues how difficult it would be to entirely remove social and political considerations from any process of defining mental disorders. Nevertheless, it reinforced their desire to move away from the reigning approach to psychiatric classification, "because the debates about homosexuality could have been about most other diagnoses, had there been strong differences of opinions and hungry media," noted Stuart Kirk and Herb Kutchins. "The debates had nothing to do with the ability of psychiatrists to identify homosexuals, but everything to do with a conceptual and theoretical problem, namely, whether homosexuality constituted a disorder. In order to address that question, psychiatrists would have to define disorder convincingly."[43] The use of narrow, symptom-based definitions could make diagnostic criteria appear more objective and, therefore, avoid political conflicts that exposed the field to widespread ridicule.

## Passage of the DSM-III

By the end of 1975, Spitzer's task force had produced its first draft of the new manual, which included more diagnoses and much more lengthy and comprehensive descriptions of each diagnosis than its predecessors had. At first, the preliminary drafts of the DSM-III triggered relatively modest interest among rank-and-file clinicians. There were a few expressions of opposition by those who favored the field's current psychodynamic orientation.[44] But psychoanalysts, the group with the most to lose with the revised manual, did not immediately register any formal response.[45] The notion that the DSM-III would become *the* textbook for all mental health clinicians—as opposed to the "little manual" (less than 140 pages) its two predecessors had been since 1952—was slow in developing.[46]

Between 1977 and 1979, Spitzer and his colleagues ran field trials of the DSM-III sponsored by the National Institute of Mental Health (NIMH). As a government institution, the NIMH played an important supportive role in creating the DSM-III through financing its research and then legitimating the results by granting them the government's seal of approval.[47] Approximately 500 psychiatrists from across the country used preliminary drafts of the DSM-III in diagnosing more than 12,000 patients. Around 300 psychiatrists were paired and their evaluations compared for consistency.[48] The results were mildly encouraging and agreed upon as a success.[49]

The publication of the DSM-III was declared a "victory" by its advocates, as the change it wrought was quick, thorough, and irreversible. Within 6 months of its publication, more orders were received for the DSM-III than for all the previous DSM editions combined, including their 30-plus reprintings. The DSM-III greatly expanded professional and financial incentives for clinical researchers and pharmaceutical companies.[50] It gave them specific diagnoses to target their research and development efforts at for prospective treatments. Under DSM-I and II, large-scale clinical research was very difficult, because the manuals' lack of reliable diagnostic categories precluded replication by multiple researchers. Researchers responded enthusiastically to the DSM-III in part because they could collaborate with colleagues at other locales using the same diagnostic language. They were also able to submit grant proposals to the government that satisfied standardized scientific criteria. Government funding of mental health research increased considerably after the introduction of the new manual.[51] During the 1980s, a period when President Reagan and Congress slashed funding for community mental health services and Social Security disability benefits for the mentally disabled, the NIMH's research budget grew 84% to $484 million annually.[52]

Finally, even though few of those involved in Spitzer's task force were associated with work on psychopharmacology, the biological default in what they proposed came about as one of the assumptions of neo-Kraepelinians: that the core symptoms of mental disorders stemmed from some form of brain malfunctioning best treated with psychotropic drugs.[53] Consequently, psychotherapy became the primary domain of clinical psychologists, counselors, and social workers, who appeared to practice it as effectively as psychiatrists but who charged less. And psychotropic drug treatment remained the private "turf" of medically trained physicians. By the latter half of the 1980s, the same critics who had lambasted the DSM-III as parochial, reductionist, overly simplistic, and adynamic were publicly lamenting that any attempt to reintroduce pre-DSM-III guiding principles was futile: "Apparently, we have gone so far down the biomedical pathway that psychotherapy, which used to be the only psychiatric intervention, is now rarely even considered."[54] Over the course of the 1980s, psychotropic medications became the first-line, and increasingly only, treatment for the majority of mental disorders.

## The DSM-III and Mental Disorders in Children and Adolescents

A particularly important area of change with the DSM-III was the heightened attention attributed to children. The greatest expansion of diagnoses had to do with childhood disorders, an area relatively ignored in DSM-I (1952) and DSM-II (1968). No distinction was made between childhood and adult disorders in DSM-I; childhood was simply characterized by "transient situational disturbances" described as adjustment disorders.[55] The number of pages devoted to childhood and adolescent categories increased from two in the DSM-II to 65 in the DSM-III.[56] Similar to all disorders in the DSM-III, childhood disorders were listed with and accompanied by significantly more elaborate description and diagnostic criteria than the one paragraph provided by DSM-II. ADHD is a striking example (see Figure 4.1). Instead of the one-paragraph general overview of "Hyperkinetic reaction of childhood," the DSM-III's description of attention deficit disorder ran to three pages with far more extensive and measurable criteria for clinicians to use. In contrast to the DSM-I and DSM-II, the information on each childhood diagnosis in the DSM-III provided a framework for researchers within which empirical data could be systematically introduced: the diagnosis's essential features and, where reasonably reliable data were available, age of onset, course, impairment, complications, predisposing factors, sex ratio, familial pattern, and differential diagnosis.

The increased attention paid to childhood mental disorders in the DSM-III reflected the growing political and clinical interest in children's health that occurred in the 1960s and 1970s.[57] Much of this increased interest was due to the postwar baby boom, in which upwards of 77 million children were born between 1946 and 1964.[58] Pediatrician Benjamin Spock's publication of *Baby and Child Care* in 1946, with its sales of more than 50 million and its subsequent editions, influenced and reflected growing public and parental concern over children's health and development.[59]

In 1967, a new health services benefit for all Medicaid children under age 21 was established: Early and Periodic Screening, Diagnosis and Treatment (EPSDT).[60] Among other primary health care services, the EPSDT benefit required periodic, comprehensive health exams and a developmental assessment of all children enrolled in Medicaid.[61] The new program grew slowly at first, but it eventually resulted in millions of children receiving diagnostic and evaluative services for the first

*Figure 4.1*    Description of ADHD diagnosis in DSM-II and DSM-III

| | |
|---|---|
| DSM-II<br>(1968) | **BEHAVIOR DISORDERS OF CHILDHOOD AND ADOLESCENCE (308)**<br><br>**308.0\* Hyperkinetic reaction of childhood (or adolescence)**<br><br>This disorder is characterized by overactivity, restlessness, distractibility, and short attention span, especially in young children; the behavior usually diminishes in adolescence. If this behavior is caused by organic brain damage, it should be diagnosed under the appropriate non-psychotic *organic brain syndrome* (q.v.). |

| | |
|---|---|
| DSM-III<br>(1980) | **ATTENTION DEFICIT DISORDER**<br><br>The essential features are signs of developmentally inappropriate inattention and impulsivity. In the past a variety of names have been attached to this disorder, including: Hyperkinetic Reaction of Childhood, Hyperkinetic Syndrome, Hyperactive Child Syndrome, Minimal Brain Damage, Minimal Brain Dysfunction, Minimal Cerebral Dysfunction, and Minor Cerebral Dysfunction. In this manual Attention Deficit is the name given to this disorder, since attentional difficulties are prominent and virtually always present among children with these diagnoses. In addition, though excess motor activity frequently diminishes in adolescence, in children who have the disorder, difficulties in attention often persist.<br>    There are two subtypes of the active disorder, Attention Deficit Disorder with Hyperactivity, and Attention Deficit Disorder without Hyperactivity, although it is not known whether they are two forms of a single disorder or represent two distinct disorders. Finally, there is a residual subtype for individuals once diagnosed as having Attention Deficit Disorder with Hyperactivity in which hyperactivity is no longer present, but other signs of the disorder persist. |

**314.01 Attention Deficit Disorder with Hyperactivity**

The essential features are signs of developmentally inappropriate inattention, impulsivity, and hyperactivity. In the classroom, attentional difficulties and impulsivity are evidenced by the child's not staying with tasks and having difficulty organizing and completing work. The children often give the impression that they are not listening or that they have not heard what they have been told. Their work is sloppy and is performed in an impulsive fashion. On individually administered tests, careless, impulsive errors are often present. Performance may be characterized by oversights, such as omissions or insertions, or misinterpretations of easy items even when the child is well-motivated, not just in situations that hold little intrinsic interest. Group situations are particularly difficult for the child, and attentional difficulties are exaggerated when the child is in the classroom, where sustained attention is expected.

    At home, attentional problems are shown by a failure to follow through on parental requests and instructions and by the inability to stick to activities, including play, for periods of time appropriate for the child's age.

Hyperactivity in young children is manifested by gross motor activity, such as excessive running or climbing. The child is often described as being on the go, "running like a motor," and having difficulty sitting still. Older children and adolescents may be extremely restless and fidgety. Often it is the quality of the motor behavior that distinguishes this disorder form ordinary overactivity in that hyperactivity tends to be haphazard, poorly organized, and not goal-directed.

In situations in which high levels of motor activity are expected and appropriate, such as on the playground, the hyperactivity seen in children with this disorder may not be obvious.

Typically, the symptoms of this disorder in any given child vary with situation and time. A child's behavior may be well-organized and appropriate on a one-to-one basis but become dysregulated in a group situation or in the classroom; or home adjustment may be satisfactory and difficulties may emerge only in school. It is the rare child who displays signs of the disorder in all settings or even in the same setting at all times.

**Associated features.** Associated features vary as a function of age and include obstinacy, stubbornness, negativism, bossiness, bullying, increased mood lability, low frustration tolerance, temper outbursts, low self-esteem, and lack of response to discipline.

Specific Developmental Disorders are common, and should be noted on Axis II.

Nonlocalized "soft" neurological signs, motor-perceptual dysfunctions (e.g., poor eye-hand coordination), and EEG abnormalities may be present. However, in only about 5% of the cases is Attention Deficit Disorder associated with a diagnosable neurological disorder, which should be coded on Axis III.

**Age at onset.** Onset is typically by the age of three, although frequently the disorder does not come to professional attention until the child enters school.

**Course.** There are three characteristic courses. In the first, all of the symptoms persist into adolescence or adult life. In the second, the disorder is self-limited and all of the symptoms disappear completely at puberty. In the third, the hyperactivity disappears, but the attentional difficulties and impulsivity persist into adolescence or adult life (Residual Type). The relative frequency of these courses is unknown.

**Impairment.** Academic difficulties are common; and although impairment may be limited to academic functioning, social functioning may be impaired as well. Infrequently children with this disorder require residential treatment.

**Complications.** School failure, Conduct Disorder, and Antisocial Personality Disorder are the major complications.

**Predisposing factors.** Mild or Moderate Mental Retardation, epilepsy, some forms of cerebral palsy, and other neurological disorders may be predisposing factors.

**Prevalence.** The disorder is common. In the United States, it may occur in as many as 3% of prepubertal children.

*(continued)*

*Figure 4.1* *(continued)*

**Sex ratio.** The disorder is ten times more common in boys than in girls.

**Familial pattern.** The disorder is apparently more common in family members than in the general population.

**Differential diagnosis. Age-appropriate overactivity,** as is seen in some particularly active children, does not have the haphazard and poorly organized quality characteristic of the behavior of children with Attention Deficit Disorder. Children in **inadequate, disorganized, or chaotic environments** may appear to have difficulty in sustaining attention and in goal-directed behavior. In such cases it may be impossible to determine whether the disorganized behavior is simply a function of the chaotic environment or whether it is due to the child's psychopathology (in which case the diagnosis of Attention Deficit Disorder may be warranted).

In **Severe** and **Profound Mental Retardation** there may be clinical features that are characteristic of Attention Deficit Disorder. However, the additional diagnosis of Attention Deficit Disorder would make clinical sense only if the Mental Retardation were Mild or Moderate in severity.

Many cases of **Conduct Disorder** have signs of impulsivity, inattention, and hyperactivity. The additional diagnosis of Attention Deficit Disorder is frequently warranted.

In **Schizophrenia** and **Affective Disorders with manic features** there may be clinical features that are characteristic of Attention Deficit Disorder. However, these diagnoses preempt the diagnosis of Attention Deficit Disorder.

**Diagnostic criteria for Attention Deficit Disorder with Hyperactivity**
The child displays, for his or her mental and chronological age, signs of developmentally inappropriate inattention, impulsivity, and hyperactivity. The signs must be reported by adults in the child's environment, such as parents and teachers. Because the symptoms are typically variable, they may not be observed directly by the clinician. When the reports of teachers and parents conflict, primary consideration should be given to the teacher reports because of greater familiarity with age-appropriate norms. Symptoms typically worsen in situations that require self-application, as in the classroom. Signs of the disorder may be absent when the child is in a new or a one-to-one situation.

The number of symptoms specified is for children between the ages of eight and ten, the peak age range for referral. In younger children, more severe forms of the symptoms and a greater number of symptoms are usually present. The opposite is true of older children.

A. **Inattention.** At least three of the following:
  (1) often fails to finish things he or she starts
  (2) often doesn't seem to listen
  (3) easily distracted
  (4) has difficulty concentrating on schoolwork or other tasks requiring sustained attention
  (5) has difficulty sticking to a play activity

B. **Impulsivity.** At least three of the following:
   (1) often acts before thinking
   (2) shifts excessively from one activity to another
   (3) has difficulty organizing work (this not being due to cognitive impairment)
   (4) needs a lot of supervision
   (5) frequently calls out in class
   (6) has difficulty awaiting turn in games or group situations

C. **Hyperactivity.** At least two of the following:
   (1) runs about or climbs on things excessively
   (2) has difficulty sitting still or fidgets excessively
   (3) has difficulty staying seated
   (4) moves about excessively during sleep
   (5) is always "on the go" or acts as if "driven by a motor"

### 314.00 Attention Deficit Disorder without Hyperactivity

All of the features are the same as those of Attention Deficit Disorder with Hyperactivity except for the absence of hyperactivity (criterion C); the associated features and impairment are generally milder. Prevalence and familial pattern are unknown.

### 314.80 Attention Deficit Disorder, Residual Type

**Diagnostic Criteria for Attention Deficit Disorder, Residual Type**

A. The individual once met the criteria for Attention Deficit Disorder with Hyperactivity. This information may come from the individual or from others, such as family members.

B. Signs of hyperactivity are no longer present, but other signs of the illness have persisted to the present without periods of remission, as evidenced by signs of both attentional deficits and impulsivity (e.g., difficulty organizing work and completing tasks, difficulty concentrating, being easily distracted, making sudden decisions without thought of the consequences.)

C. The symptoms of inattention and impulsivity result in some impairment in social or occupational functioning.

D. Not due to Schizophrenia, Affective Disorder, Severe or Profound Mental Retardation, or Schizotypal or Borderline Personality Disorders.

---

*Source:* American Psychiatric Association, *Diagnostic and Statistical Manual of Mental Disorders,* 2nd and 3rd eds. (Washington, DC: American Psychiatric Association, 1968, 1980), 50 and 41–45, respectively.

time, which contributed to the growing awareness of significant unmet physical and mental health needs among poor children.[62] For example, a major, 800-page report in 1969 from the Joint Commission on the Mental Health of Children, entitled *Crisis in Children's Mental Health: Challenge for the 1970's*, resulted in White House conferences on the subject in 1970 and 1971.[63]

The DSM-III's enhanced focus on childhood mental disorders reflected the progress that came not only from federal policy initiatives, but also from the clinical and scientific growth in pediatric research that had occurred since the 1960s.[64] In 1975, Congress passed the landmark Education of all Handicapped Children Act (now called the Individuals with Disabilities Education Act), which mandated a right to a free and appropriate education for all children with disabilities.[65] A number of new journals on child issues began in the 1970s (*Journal of Abnormal Child Psychology*, *Journal of Clinical Child Psychology*), as did new child psychiatric and clinical psychology training programs.[66]

## The Rapid Growth in Inpatient Mental Health Services for Children and Adolescents

An unintentional consequence of the growing attention paid to children's mental health needs was a rapid growth in hospitalizations for those with youth-related and substance-abuse disorders.[67] The phenomenon occurred during an era of significant changes in family structure in the United States.[68] The workforce participation rate of married women with children under the age of 6 increased from 18% in 1960 to 30% in 1970 to 64% by 1995.[69] When both mothers and fathers work outside the home, there is often increased parental stress and decreased tolerance for behaviors in children that are considered disruptive.[70] In addition, joint custody, blended families (stepfamilies), and parents in cohabiting relationships all became much more common beginning in the 1970s,[71] and over time contributed to a dramatic increase in child custody litigation.[72] Research suggests that it takes about 2 years for a child to adjust psychologically to parental divorce and upwards of 5 years to having a stepparent in the household.[73] A number of these children were diagnosed with ADHD and/or another mental disorder (often conduct disorder).[74]

The phenomenon of increased adolescent hospitalizations in the 1980s also stemmed in part from financial reimbursement issues and clinicians' struggles with how best to deal with clinical uncertainty:

mild, borderline, or subthreshold conditions in pediatric and adolescent patients who did not fit neatly into specific mental diagnoses.[75] With third-party payers favoring inpatient treatment over community-based alternatives—in the form of better insurance coverage and more generous reimbursement rates—general community hospitals substantially expanded their psychiatric-medical units and number of nonpsychiatric ("scatter") beds reserved for patients with mental diagnoses.[76] Similarly, the number of private, for-profit psychiatric hospitals increased by almost 50% in just 3 years (1983–1986), after growing 43% between 1982 and 1983 (from 105 to 151 investor-owned hospitals).[77] As a result, in the mid-1980s the number of beds in private psychiatric hospitals rose by more than 40%.[78] In 1985 alone, the total number of public and private hospital beds reserved for psychiatric patients in the United States increased by 37%.[79] And by 1988, 64% of all inpatient psychiatric facilities were privately owned, the most rapid growth being in corporate hospital chains.[80]

The majority of the new mental services in general and private psychiatric hospitals were marketed directly to youths and their parents.[81] Ad-psych (adolescent psychiatry) units—with their low overhead costs (little to no need for expensive medical equipment) and long average lengths of stay—were so profitable that many hospitals closed units that provided other types of services in order to establish more profitable ad-psych units.[82] From 1980 to 1986, the number of children admitted to private psychiatric units increased fourfold and the total days of care provided more than tripled.[83] The mean length of stay of children and adolescents was approximately 50% longer than that for adults, which made minors an especially expensive (or lucrative) patient population.[84] Rates for a bed in an intensive psychiatric care unit at the time could run as high as $1,500 per day.[85]

The substantial growth in the number of children and adolescents hospitalized with psychiatric diagnoses raised a growing number of concerns and complaints.[86] Many of the beds in private psychiatric hospitals were filled, wrote the then president of the APA, Mary Jane England, "through sophisticated marketing campaigns targeting adolescents and substance abusers, resulting in many unjustified and even harmful hospitalizations as well as sharply increased costs."[87] With commercial insurance coverage and the summer months out of school—which allowed for longer hospitalizations—children and adolescents became prime targets of psychiatric exploitation with unnecessary hospitalizations.[88] Researchers found that upwards of 40% of youngsters were being admitted inappropriately,[89] "served inadequately, and had their stay in the hospital controlled by the coverage limits of their insurance policy rather than by actual need."[90] Several corporations used parental fear and guilt as advertising models to induce demand for their institutions. Advertisements for private psychiatric hospitals often encouraged parents to admit their children for conditions that did not meet "medical necessity" standards of inpatient care, such as engaging in premarital sex, using marijuana, or failing to perform adequately in school.[91] A high percentage of minors were diagnosed with adjustment disorders, substance use that rarely rose to the level of abuse let alone dependence (frequently one–two episodes of experimenting with marijuana or alcohol), ADHD (not warranting inpatient care), and less severe mood disorders such as dysthymic disorder (chronic mild-to-moderate depression).[92]

One of the most problematic aspects of the growing number of children hospitalized with mental disorders was the financial conflicts of interest that arose and that contributed to the growth in admissions.[93] Private psychiatric hospitals implicitly (and sometimes explicitly) viewed physicians as business partners,[94] who were encouraged to use their admitting privileges to increase revenue for the hospitals and the investors who owned them.[95] Children with garden-variety behavior problems, substance-abuse issues, psychosomatic illnesses, and mild eating disorders became prime candidates for lengthy and unnecessary psychiatric hospitalizations.[96] Many observers noted the extraordinary "coincidence" by which minors often experienced a remarkable and full recovery from their mental disorder at just the time when their health insurance benefits for hospitalization ran out.[97]

For-profit private psychiatric hospitals were not the only institutions tempted by the generous reimbursement rates for inpatient psychiatric care. Public community hospitals faced their own set of economic incentives and pressures. In particular, Medicare—the nation's single largest purchaser of hospital care—fundamentally transformed its method for reimbursing hospitals to a prospective (set-rate) system in late 1983. This major change limited hospitals' ability to charge for whatever services they provided.[98] Under the program's new reimbursement model, hospitals would receive a flat-rate sum for patients' individual diagnoses regardless of the costs the hospital actually accrued in delivering care to Medicare patients. The program's new payment system, however, exempted psychiatric units. These units could (and did) continue to bill for services as long as they provided them.[99] Thus, hospitals had an incentive to keep psychiatric patients hospitalized longer in order to receive greater reimbursement,[100] and to supplement other inpatient revenues that became limited by Medicare's new hospital payment system.[101]

## The Managed-Care Response, Changes in the Pharmaceutical Industry, and Prozac

Eventually, third-party payers became increasingly unwilling to fund long-term psychiatric hospitalizations,[102] so they began to turn to managed behavioral health-care organizations in the late 1980s in an effort to contain costs.[103] Insurers and employers would assign (or "carve out") their mental health coverage by contracting with these new organizations that, in turn, contracted with cheaper and limited numbers of psychiatric nurses, social workers, and psychologists to oversee and authorize the use of mental health and substance-abuse services (particularly inpatient hospitalizations).[104] According to Saul Feldman, a former executive of the federal Community Mental Health Center program, who later went on to run one of the largest managed behavioral health companies (U.S. Behavioral Health), "The greatest contributors to the development of managed mental health, a development they now bemoan, have been the service providers themselves, [fee-for-service] practitioners and facilities. By not paying sufficient attention to or not caring about costs and lengths of treatment, they killed or at least seriously wounded the goose that laid the golden egg."[105]

After limiting coverage of inpatient hospital days (by substituting more outpatient services), managed behavioral health companies found it easy to negotiate discounted daily rates from hospitals for inpatient care due to the oversupply of psychiatric beds in public and private hospitals.[106] Occupancy rates at private psychiatric hospitals dropped from more than 70% in the mid-1980s to less than 50% (loss-making territory) by the late 1980s,[107] while psychiatric patients' average length of stay decreased markedly to 10.6 days—down from 30 days in 1986.[108] Children with an ADD diagnosis experienced the largest decline in inpatient bed days and costs per treated child beginning in the late 1980s.[109] More and more of these children (as this chapter explains) were switched to stimulants. Many private psychiatric hospitals closed during this period, while others teetered on the verge of bankruptcy.[110]

Managed behavioral health companies' biggest cost-control strategy included making rapid psychopharmacological intervention (and limited short-term psychotherapy if necessary) the dominant treatment model in the field of mental health.[111] With psychotherapy costing anywhere from $50 to $150 per visit—depending on which mental health professional provided the service—and a week's worth of Prozac costing roughly $14 to $21, the shift to emphasizing psychotropic drugs was, pardon the pun, a no-brainer, especially when primary-care physicians could write prescriptions for them.[112] As health maintenance organizations, in general, and managed behavioral health companies, in particular, began to increase their share of the health insurance market in the late 1980s, the use of prescription drugs (including psychotropic medications) expanded dramatically.[113] By 1990, for example, most psychiatrists were reimbursed for treatment only if it involved prescribing psychotropic medications.[114]

The pharmaceutical industry itself was experiencing massive changes in the latter half of the 1980s. In 1984, Congress passed the Drug Price Competition and Patent Term Restoration Act (also known as the Hatch-Waxman Act for its cosponsors, Senator Orrin Hatch [R-UT] and Representative Henry Waxman [D-CA]).[115] The Hatch-Waxman Act revolutionized the use of pharmaceuticals in the United States by essentially creating the market for generic drugs. The fledgling industry's much cheaper versions of brand-name drugs dramatically lowered the cost of pharmaceuticals. Prior to the Hatch-Waxman Act, the military was one of the very few organizations allowed to buy and use generic drugs.[116] Following the Thalidomide scandal in the 1950s, in which thousands of children in Europe were born with horrendous birth defects after their mothers used the drug in an attempt to relieve morning sickness and as a sleep aid, in 1962 Congress passed amendments to the federal Food, Drug, and Cosmetic Act making it a requirement that all new drugs—both brand-name *and* generic—be proven safe and effective.[117] The clinical trials needed to demonstrate safety and efficacy were ordinarily too expensive for the few generic drug companies in existence at the time; only brand-name companies could afford them.

As a result, by the early 1980s there were 150 drugs whose exclusive patents had expired but for which there were no generic versions.[118] At the same time, the period required for clinical testing of new drugs had been increasing from approximately 30 months in 1960 to 120 months by 1980.[119] Consequently, as generic drug companies and a handful of elected leaders in Congress and the Reagan administration were seeking ways to introduce more competition into the drug industry, major pharmaceutical companies were seeking ways to extend patents over (and, therefore, increase revenue from) their products that were requiring more and more time to receive approval from the FDA.[120]

The Hatch-Waxman Act that emerged from these cross-cutting political pressures provided one of the best political horse trades ever: generic drug companies received a significantly less expensive and abbreviated drug application process for generic versions of drugs with expired patents, while brand-name companies got the right to apply for a patent extension of up to 5 years for drugs whose approval was delayed by the FDA.[121] The act also provided one important additional incentive for both generic and brand-name drug companies: Hatch-Waxman allowed generic companies to file an application to make a patent-protected generic version of a brand-name drug and to sell it exclusively for 180 days before other generic competitors could join the market with their own generic versions. And brand-name companies could receive an extra 6 months of patent protection for a new drug if they conducted clinical trials to study its use by children.[122]

After Hatch-Waxman went into effect, scores of new and significantly cheaper generic drugs entered the market. The pharmaceutical industry consolidated extensively, with eight major mergers in the latter half of the 1980s.[123] Before the act, only 35% of brand-name drugs with expired patents had generic competition; by the early 1990s, virtually all of them did.[124] As a result, even as the use of pharmaceuticals increased substantially beginning in the late 1980s,[125] their share of total medical expenditures in the United States decreased from 16% in the 1960s to 7% by the beginning of the 1990s.[126] Prescription drugs were being used much more, just as they were becoming much cheaper. Health maintenance organizations and managed behavioral health companies embraced the use of generic and brand-name drugs with enthusiasm.[127] Initially, pharmaceutical firms refused to deal with managed-care organizations because they imposed restrictions on sales representatives and insisted on discounted drug prices. But with managed care rapidly gaining market share, all major U.S. pharmaceutical companies had designated units within their marketing departments by the late 1980s that dealt with managed-care clients.[128]

Pharmaceutical companies also changed their traditional "one-price policy," by which they refused to discount their products. With so little generic or other competition, they seldom had to discount the price of their drugs prior to Hatch-Waxman. By 1990, all U.S. drug companies provided discounts, with substantial ones to large managed-care plans and for product lines with major competition.[129] The companies did so because of an effective tool increasingly being used by managed-care plans for obtaining pharmaceuticals at reduced prices: drug product formularies.[130] Until the late 1980s, pharmaceutical companies had marketed their products directly to physicians, who were free to prescribe virtually whatever drugs they wanted.

Under the new formularies, which were simply lists of drugs for which managed-care plans had negotiated discounts from drug companies, physicians would ordinarily prescribe from a preapproved selection of drugs.[131] Patients bore full financial responsibility for any nonformulary prescribed drugs. Formularies themselves were facilitated by a new corporate organization—drug wholesalers—that emerged in the latter half of the 1980s as middlemen between pharmaceutical manufacturers and retail pharmacies.[132] Drug wholesalers aggregated the purchasing power of individual retail pharmacies and, in the process, were able to extract larger discounts from drug companies.[133]

One new drug in particular, Prozac, had a major impact on how clinicians and much of the general public viewed mental disorders, as well as how they perceived it best to treat them.[134] Officially approved by the FDA on December 29, 1987, after more than a decade of research, the new drug for treating depression quickly became a financial blockbuster for its manufacturer, Eli Lilly. It also became something of a cultural icon, with references to the drug in *New Yorker* cartoons and sitcoms, as well as articles about it in publications ranging from the *Archives of General Psychiatry* to *Good Housekeeping*.[135] By the early 1990s, Prozac had become 1 of the top 5 best-selling drugs in the world, with annual sales of $1.2 billion and between 900,000 and 1 million prescriptions per month.[136] These figures far exceeded Lilly's initial expectations—back when it was a $600 million company that focused primarily on producing antibiotics—that the drug would top out at no more than $70 million in annual sales.[137]

There were two aspects of Prozac's unprecedented success that influenced the use of other psychopharmacological agents, including stimulants.[138] First, Prozac was not addictive. The extremely popular sedatives (or minor tranquilizers) from the 1950s to the 1970s, Librium and Valium, treated the diagnostic forerunner to the modern version of major depression: anxiety. Eventually, however, the dangers of these drugs' addictive properties became well-known and physicians severely curtailed their prescribing of them, particularly among women.[139] Second, unlike previous antidepressant and mood-elevating drugs (but similar to Ritalin), Prozac had fewer side effects (apart from sexual dysfunction). The original drugs used to treat depression—the tricyclics, including imipramine (sold under the brand name Tofranil), and the monoamine oxidase inhibitors, including iproniazid—were equally effective for many depressed patients, but they also increased the risk of blurred vision, dizziness, cardiac arrest, blood pressure problems, substantial weight gain, psychotic reactions, and even death from overdose.[140]

Prozac's popularity gave rise to the claim—and ultimately the term—that the use of certain psychotropic drugs could, in the form of "cosmetic psychopharmacology," *enhance* a person's character and personality as much as they could alleviate the symptoms of a mental disorder.[141] Or, as Peter Kramer famously stated, they could make a person feel "better than well."[142] As a quintessentially American drug, Prozac did not increase pleasure or bring happiness. Rather, it promoted "adroit competitiveness."[143] The introduction of paroxetine (Paxil) in late 1992 to treat social anxiety disorder—a marked, persistent, and excessive fear of various social situations—provided more fuel to the debate over "cosmetic psychopharmacology."[144]

## CHADD, Ritalin, and the Evolving Diagnosis of ADHD

Prozac's introduction coincided with another major public controversy over ADHD and stimulants.[145] By 1987, the number of children diagnosed with the disorder (around 750,000) and using stimulants (roughly 400,000) had increased somewhat from 1980 (around 400,000 and 185,000, respectively).[146] But 20 highly publicized lawsuits and a negative media blitz spearheaded by the major national television talk show hosts of the time—Oprah Winfrey, Geraldo Rivera, Phil Donahue, and Morton Downey, Jr.—contributed to an almost 40% decrease in the number of Ritalin prescriptions from 1988 to 1990.[147] The lawsuits were orchestrated largely by the Church of Scientology, behind a front organization called the Citizens Commission on Human Rights.[148] They targeted local physicians, school districts, and individual school personnel around the country for alleged "inappropriate use of Ritalin."[149]

In this sense, they were similar to the debates and lawsuits in the early 1970s, when doctors and school officials were charged with "coercion, amid suspicion that teachers and principals were dumping unruly, bored students on local clinicians who routinely prescribed amphetamine maintenance as a way out."[150] One of the lawsuits in the late 1980s was a class-action suit for $125 million against the American Psychiatric Association for aiding and abetting the "inappropriate" use of Ritalin.[151] The controversy and lawsuits led to a special "commentary" in the *Journal of the American Medical Association* in October 1988, which reveals the timeless quality of the debate over children's use of stimulants to treat ADHD:

> One possibility, of particular concern not only to physicians and educators but to parents of affected children and to legislators interested in public policy, is that methylphenidate is now being prescribed for children who may not require it. The increased use of methylphenidate raises the possibility that rather than reflecting the real strides that have been made in our conceptualization of neurobehavioral disorders, current treatment practices ignore such advances and represent a reversion to an antiquated, simplistic approach that views all school behavioral problems as one. In such a view, the diagnostic process is replaced by the reflex use of a particular treatment, in this case stimulants, prescribed for almost any child presenting with a behavioral or learning problem.[152]

The lawsuits, all of which were eventually dismissed for lack of merit, and the negative media blitz obscured less sensational but more important developments regarding the diagnosis of ADHD and stimulants. First, the APA's newly revised manual that came out in 1987, the DSM-III-R, altered the disorder's symptomatic criteria. The previous DSM-III (1980) arranged the 14 symptoms of ADD into three groups, to match what were considered to be the basic aspects of the disorder: *inattention* (5 symptoms), *impulsivity* (5 symptoms), and *hyperactivity* (4 symptoms). At least 3 symptoms of inattention, 3 of impulsivity, and 2 of hyperactivity were required for a patient to receive a diagnosis of ADD with hyperactivity.[153] If a case presented 3 or more symptoms from both the inattention and the impulsivity groups, but only 1 symptom or none from hyperactivity, the case received the diagnosis of ADD without hyperactivity. Criticism by clinicians and researchers that this method for diagnosing ADD was too complex led to the DSM-III-R (1987), which contains a single list of 14 inattentive, impulsive, and hyperactive symptoms, any 8 of which were sufficient to receive a diagnosis of attention deficit/hyperactivity disorder (ADHD).[154] By simply changing the way in which the same symptomatic criteria were counted, the DSM-III-R's diagnosis of ADHD became 15% more prevalent among children than the DSM-III's diagnosis of ADD.[155]

Second, Children and Adults with Attention Deficit/Hyperactivity Disorder (CHADD), a new mental health advocacy organization, was founded in 1987 by a small group of parents of children with the disorder and two clinical psychologists in Plantation, Florida (near Miami). Partly financed by the company that manufactured Ritalin, Ciba-Geigy (a fact that has caused CHADD considerable embarrassment at times and accusations of a major conflict of interest),[156] the organization quickly grew in membership and influence, with annual meetings drawing upwards of 1,500 people from hundreds of local chapters that formed across the country. In fact, many CHADD chapters were formerly Feingold parent support groups—as discussed in Chapter 3—which arose in the 1970s, but which eventually morphed into CHADD groups when evidence against Feingold's diet claims (for the cause of hyperactivity in children) emerged in the 1980s.[157] As Chapter 5 explains in detail, CHADD was critical in successfully lobbying Congress and the Department of Education in 1990 and 1991 for ADHD to be officially included as a protected disability under a major federal law—the Individuals with Disabilities Education Act (IDEA)—that made individuals diagnosed with the disorder eligible for special educational services.[158]

Finally, access to a much larger group of clinicians (pediatricians) who could make a diagnosis of ADHD and prescribe stimulants expanded substantially over the latter half of the 1980s. With the growth of managed care, which discouraged expensive referrals to specialist physicians (such as child psychiatrists), pediatricians increasingly diagnosed ADHD and prescribed stimulants themselves.[159] As a result, psychosocial problems were becoming the centerpiece of pediatric primary care by the end of the 1980s, the most common chronic condition that pediatricians treated, surpassing asthma and heart disease.[160] But managed-care incentives also encouraged pediatricians and family doctors to see greater numbers of patients and spend less time with each of them.[161] Consequently, an increasing proportion of children diagnosed with ADHD began being treated exclusively with stimulants (Table 4.2), while the provision of psychotherapy and follow-up visits to children diagnosed with the disorder decreased significantly beginning in the late 1980s.[162] Already inexpensive, especially compared to hospitalization and long-term psychotherapy (neither of which proved particularly effective in treating children with ADHD),[163] methylphenidate and related stimulants became even cheaper after Ritalin's patent ran out in the mid-1980s.[164]

*Table 4.2* Characteristics of patient population diagnosed with ADHD, 1980–1990 (in percent)

|  | 1980 | 1983 | 1985 | 1987 | 1990 |
|---|---|---|---|---|---|
| *Patient sex* |  |  |  |  |  |
| Male | 69 | 71 | 76 | 72 | 83 |
| Female | 31 | 29 | 24 | 28 | 17 |
| *Geographic region* |  |  |  |  |  |
| East | 35 | 24 | 26 | 17 | 21 |
| Midwest | 13 | 22 | 21 | 27 | 27 |
| South | 24 | 32 | 31 | 28 | 39 |
| West | 28 | 22 | 22 | 28 | 13 |
| *Physician specialty* |  |  |  |  |  |
| Pediatrician | 21 | 22 | 27 | 38 | 40 |
| Psychiatrist | 65 | 68 | 59 | 49 | 40 |
| Neurologist | 3 | 3 | 2 | 4 | 6 |
| Family practitioner | 5 | 5 | 6 | 7 | 4 |
| Others combined | 6 | 2 | 6 | 2 | 10 |
| *Treatment prescribed* |  |  |  |  |  |
| Stimulant drugs | 28 | 32 | 45 | 57 | 86 |
| No stimulant drugs | 72 | 68 | 55 | 43 | 14 |

*Source:* IMS Health, "National Disease and Therapeutic Index," 1980, 1983, 1985, 1987, 1990.

## Conclusion

Unlike in the early 1980s, children with a diagnosis of ADHD by the end of the decade were becoming less likely to be seen *without* a stimulant prescription being made (Table 4.2). With the growth of pediatric research and cost-conscious managed care, the decreased cost of pharmaceutical drugs, and the well-established effectiveness and relative safety of stimulants, drug treatment for ADHD was becoming the rule rather than the exception.[165] And as it did so, social acceptability of Ritalin and related stimulant use by children increased.[166] The growing perception of ADHD as a neurologically based behavioral disorder best treated by medicine (stimulants) received an additional boost by the *New England Journal of Medicine*'s lead article for its November 1990 edition, authored by researchers at the NIMH, who, as the *New York Times* reported, "for the first time have found that a specific brain abnormality could explain why some children and adults are hyperactive and cannot pay attention or be still."[167] The study, which examined individuals' brains with positron emission tomography scanning, found that "adults who have been hyperactive since childhood had markedly low brain activity in areas that are used to control attention and movement."[168] The authors of the article were more cautious about the implications of their findings,[169] and subsequent studies on adolescents failed to replicate the strength of the original findings.[170] But as Chapter 5 explains in greater detail, the convergence of economic, advocacy, clinical, and scientific research trends by the end of the 1980s left the massive increase in ADHD diagnoses and stimulant use a "tipping point" waiting to happen. It needed only a spark.

# CHAPTER FIVE

# ADHD and the Politics of Children's Disability Policy

As I walked with some children in a parade, one six-year-old boy intrigued me. He was precocious, energetic and a delightful companion. When I dropped him off at his home, I mentioned these traits to his mother. She startled me when she replied, "That's not what his teacher says. She told me he has ADHD and needs to be put on Ritalin" . . . He was so bright, and his level of energy seemed normal for a little boy. What if he just needed a more challenging curriculum or a different learning environment?

—PATTI JOHNSON, "TOO MUCH RITALIN," THE INDEPEN-
DENCE INSTITUTE, DENVER, COLORADO, OCTOBER 20, 1999

You ask any parent who has an ADHD child how tough they've tried to parent their kids, and they work their fingers to the bone and still can't fix 'em. They need medical help. They need other kinds of help, and that's what SSI is for.

—DR. BENNET LEVENTHAL, DIRECTOR OF CHILD AND
ADOLESCENT PSYCHIATRY, UNIVERSITY OF CHICAGO,
"DISABLING BENEFITS," *NEWS HOUR WITH JIM LEHRER,*
NOVEMBER 18, 1997

As the 1990s began, the American public was still generally unaware of ADHD. That would change by the end of the decade. In the intervening years, government programs for individuals with disabilities became more accepting of children with behavioral and learning disorders like ADHD. Soon critics began faulting the government for encouraging children to disobey teachers, fight with peers, and fail in school in order to secure the benefits and accommodations afforded children who were found mentally disabled. For these critics, ADHD was emblematic of the "perverse" incentives created by programs that granted privileges to individuals with disabilities but did not tightly police the boundaries between those with disabilities and those without.

This chapter looks at developments in two programs in particular: special education and Supplemental Security Income (SSI). Reforms to both programs have their roots in the patients' rights movement and the disability rights movement of the late 1960s and early 1970s. These movements championed the closing of mental health asylums and integration of individuals with disabilities into the community, the ending of discrimination against individuals with disabilities, the modification of architectural barriers to provide equal access to public facilities, and to a lesser extent, the creation of alternative sources of income support and social services that would enable individuals with severe disabilities to live their lives outside institutions and hospitals. Mental health and disability activists championed expansions to a number of social welfare programs (for example, Medicaid, Medicare, Social Security Disability Insurance, and SSI) and the enactment of civil rights protections for people with disabilities (for example, Section 504 of the Rehabilitation Act of 1973 and the Americans with Disabilities Act of 1990, or ADA).

These transformations in disability policy had a profound effect on children's programs. During the early 1990s, a diverse coalition of children's advocates, disability activists, mental health professionals, and antipoverty groups spearheaded the expansion of SSI and special education to children with learning and behavioral problems. Although children with ADHD were not the focal point of these reform efforts, they benefited nonetheless. The identification and diagnosis of children with learning and behavioral problems, however, can be fraught with error, and the children exhibit behaviors that most people find difficult to sympathize with or understand. As a result, as special education and SSI became more accepting of children with learning and behavioral disorders, the media alleged that parents and school officials were seeking to have children labeled with ADHD or other mental disorders because of the advantages that such a diagnosis would bring: money for schools; welfare payments for families; and accommodations, individualized attention, and services for students. Although these allegations were difficult to substantiate, they set the stage for program retrenchment, particularly in SSI, as well as a broader backlash against ADHD in the mid- and late 1990s, which is explored further in Chapter 6. The reforms to children's disability policy intersected with the changes to health-care financing described in Chapter 4 and an expansion of Medicaid in the late 1980s and early 1990s. Together, these changes increased the number of children, low-income and middle-class alike, who were identified with

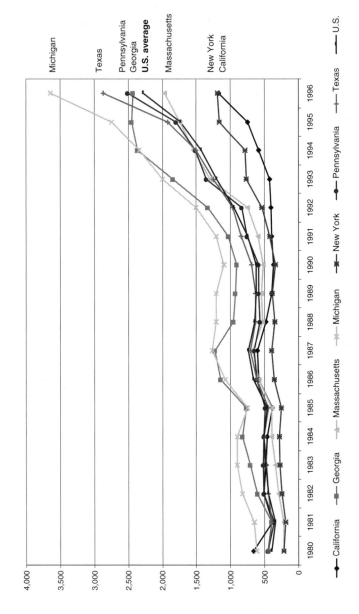

*Figure 5.1* Stimulant (methylphenidate and amphetamine) distribution rate in grams per 100,000 individuals from selected states and U.S. average, 1980–1996

*Table 5.1* Diagnosis and treatment of ADHD and U.S. production of methylphenidate (Ritalin), 1990–1993

| Variable | 1990 | 1991 | 1992 | 1993 |
|---|---|---|---|---|
| Number of patients diagnosed with ADHD | 902,000 | 1,161,000 | 1,701,000 | 2,019,000 |
| Number of outpatient visits for ADHD | 1,687,000 | 2,256,000 | 3,168,000 | 4,195,000 |
| Amount of methylphenidate produced (kilograms) | 1,784 | 3,162 | 3,884 | 5,110 |

*Source:* J. Swanson, M. Lerner, and L. Williams, "More Frequent Diagnosis of Attention-Deficit Hyperactivity Disorder," *New England Journal of Medicine* 333 (October 5, 1995): 944.

ADHD and prescribed stimulants. As a result, throughout the 1990s, the nation's spending on stimulants and prescription drugs in general grew dramatically (see Figure 5.1 and Table 5.1)

## Who Advocated for Disability Reform?

The groups advocating for the expansion of children's disability programs in the early 1990s represented a broad array of interests. SSI attracted antipoverty advocates, particularly Legal Services attorneys and lawyers for the Bazelon Center for Mental Health Law (called the Mental Health Law Project before 1990), a public interest law firm that specialized in mental health and poverty litigation. Although SSI is the cash benefit program for the aged poor and poor people with disabilities administered by the Social Security Administration (SSA), prior to the 1980s antipoverty groups had paid little attention to the SSA since its largest program, Social Security, served a largely middle-class clientele. But in the early 1980s, these groups came to recognize the importance of the SSA's disability programs for the poor people they represented. In 1981, President Ronald Reagan tried to slash spending for Social Security Disability Insurance, resulting in hundreds of thousands of disabled workers losing their sole means of financial support as well as their access to Medicare coverage (which is tied to eligibility for Social Security). Because it is a smaller version of Social Security, SSI was caught up in the budget-cutting endeavor. Since Social Security Disability Insurance and SSI use the same disability criteria, when the SSA tightened its administration of disability insurance, it also threw off the disability rolls thousands of impoverished SSI recipients. The Reagan administration's purge of the disability rolls ended in 1984, when Congress enacted the Social Security Disability Benefits Reform Act, which relaxed the standard of disability the SSA used to evaluate adults. But Legal Services and the Bazelon Center remained active in Social Security disability issues, turning their attention next to expanding SSI's program for children with disabilities, which used the same stringent standard of disability that had governed the adult disability program prior to 1984.

Because special education is a program for all children with disabilities, not just the poor (as is the case with SSI), debates over the Individuals with Disabilities Education Act (IDEA; formerly the Education for All Handicapped Children Act) mobilized a broad range of groups. Entering the fray were groups that represented children with specific impairments, such as autism, deafness, developmental disabilities, and learning disabilities, as well as groups that claimed to speak for a wide range of impairments (the Council for Exceptional Children, or CEC, for example). Special education politics also included education professionals, such as school administrators, teachers, school nurses, psychologists, and school counselors.

The disability community, therefore, is diverse, with varied concerns and needs, a fact that, in the past, had impeded cooperation among groups. That changed with the rise of the disability rights movement in the early 1970s. The movement altered the terrain of disability politics in three important ways that, in turn, profoundly influenced the course of SSI and special education in the 1990s.

First, thinkers and activists associated with the movement articulated a trenchant critique of society that questioned the prevailing government approach to disability. Prior to the 1970s, the federal government and the states had pursued programs that sought either to rehabilitate individuals with impairments so that they could return to their jobs and rejoin society (for example, physical therapy, occupational therapy, and vocational rehabilitation) or, in the case of individuals too impaired to find gainful employment, to provide alternative means of care and support, through welfare programs, residential schools, hospitals, and asylums. Disability rights activists regarded the rehabilitation and caring approach with disdain, however. The only reason society provided assistance, they argued, was because it viewed individuals with disabilities as inherently incapable of productive activity.[1] Moreover, accepting social assistance was not without cost. Individuals with disabilities who were institutionalized were stripped of their decisionmaking authority, placed under the control of physicians, and denied the opportunity to vote, marry, have a family, and hold a job—all privileges that able-bodied individuals took for granted. Individuals with disabilities, in short, were expected to adapt to the world of the able-bodied or else remove themselves from it, a policy that, according to historian Paul K. Longmore, "created a large stigmatized and segregated category of persons" who lived as wards of the state.[2]

In the past, disability groups had lobbied the government for increased funding for research into diseases and injury, welfare and vocational rehabilitation programs, and the construction of hospitals and asylums. Disability rights activists, however, were not interested in asking for more money; they wanted government to end discrimination against individuals with disabilities.[3] Discrimination entailed not only blatantly prejudicial acts against individuals with disabilities but also any social convention that was premised on the view that individuals with disabilities were weak, helpless, or otherwise functionally incapacitated. The problem, in their eyes, was that society was structured in such a way that people who did not function in a "normal" manner were rendered "incapable," even though these individuals were not inherently unproductive. Frank Bowe, former executive director of the American Coalition of Citizens with Disabilities, best described this subtle form of discrimination in the following manner: "Buildings went up before their 'inaccessibility' was 'discovered'—and then it was too late. During America's periods of greatest growth, when subways were constructed, television lines laid, school programs designed, and jobs manufactured, disabled people were hidden away in attics, 'special' programs, and institutions, unseen and their voices unheard."[4] The able-bodied structured society's physical spaces and cultural practices (for example, schooling, employment, and family life) in ways that excluded individuals with disabilities from full participation, and because individuals with disabilities had been "hidden away" in the first place, no one protested. "Day by day, year by year," Bowe wrote, "America became ever more oppressive to its hidden minority."[5] To activists, the fact that individuals with disabilities could not function outside of hospitals and asylums or without accommodations was indicative, not of their inherent inferiority, but of society's desire to exclude people with functional differences.

Advocates for the rights of mental patients applied the logic of disability rights to individuals with mental disabilities. In his famous 1972 book, *Prisoners of Psychiatry*, Bruce Ennis argued that the concept of mental illness was nothing more than society's way of controlling individuals deemed "useless, unproductive, 'odd,' or 'different.' "[6] Judi Chamberlain, a former mental patient turned activist, supported the sentiment. People with mental illness, she argued, were "an oppressed group, oppressed by laws and public attitudes, relegated to legalized second class citizenship" by practices such as involuntary commitment and forced treatment.[7]

If, as disability rights activists argued, people with disabilities were held back more by the prejudicial attitudes of an able-bodied society than by their own functional capacities, then the solution was not more funding for programs that perpetuated the discriminatory belief that individuals with disabilities were inferior and needed special help. Such an approach would only reinforce the social exclusion of individuals with disabilities.[8] What activists demanded instead was a government mandate that all public facilities and social institutions be made compatible with the needs and capabilities of people with disabilities. As political scientist Harlan Hahn pointed out, if society were "compatible with a broad range of human capabilities" or "designed to meet the needs of each of its members," disability would no longer have meaning; it would no longer be a disadvantage.[9] But until that day came, activists believed that architectural modifications, adaptive devices, and special services such as personal attendants, tutors, or extra time on assignments were reasonable and just accommodations that permitted people with "different modes of functioning" equal access to spaces that had been designed without attention to their abilities and for the purpose of enforcing their exclusion.[10] The demand that government policy be reoriented to further equal access for individuals with disabilities led to the enactment of the IDEA and ADA and spilled over into the politics of programs like SSI, which had been premised on the older view that people with disabilities needed income support because they were incapable of performing paid work.

The second major transformation brought about by the disability rights movement was the attenuation of the stigma associated with disability. Prior to the movement, people viewed disability as a tragedy, a condition to be feared and pitied; people were ashamed of their own disabilities or of their family members who had disabilities. Many parents were blamed for their children's condition or were pressured to institutionalize or otherwise socially isolate their offspring with disabilities.[11] Leaders of the disability rights movement, however, argued that disability was an identity, like race or sex, and as such, it was an essential part of a person's being that should be celebrated rather than a tragic defect to be ashamed of, healed, or concealed. It did not mark the inadequacy of a person, but merely his or her functional diversity.[12]

The emphasis that the disability rights movement placed on disability as an identity had special relevance for many adults with ADHD and for many parents of children with ADHD. Just as the larger community with disabilities promoted slogans such as "Disabled and Proud," "Deaf Pride," and "Disability Cool," so too did the logic of disability rights lessen the stigma associated with mental disorders such as ADHD. In fact, some individuals with ADHD came to reinterpret their lives and their sense of self in light of their condition.[13] For instance, Karenne Bloomgarden, a 43-year-old gym teacher diagnosed with ADHD as an adult, recounted her academic struggles in college for *Time* magazine in 1994. Describing what it was like to be diagnosed finally, she said, "It's been such a weight off my shoulders . . . I had 38 years of thinking I was a bad person. Now I'm rewriting the tapes of who I thought I was to who I really am."[14] Similarly, Edward Hallowell and John Ratey, whose 1994 book, *Driven to Distraction*, brought ADHD to a popular audience, proudly proclaimed that they were two adults suffering from the very disorder of which they wrote, and they underscored the constructive attributes of their disordered brains. Impulsiveness was redefined as spontaneity and decisiveness; hyperactivity became energy and enthusiasm; distractibility, alertness.[15] Hallowell and Ratey were not alone. One psychologist characterized children with ADHD, whom others might view as recalcitrant and selfish because they would not follow rules or wait their turn, as "wild, funny, and effervescent" rather than "bad." Adults with the disorder he described as "incredibly successful," with a tendency to excel at creative endeavors and to grow restless at monotonous desk jobs.[16] Another author called ADHD a "gift" that bestowed on those with the disorder a knack for inventiveness and creativity.[17] Some chapters of Children and Adults with Attention Deficit/Hyperactivity Disorder (CHADD) even went so far as to draw up lists of famous historical figures who ostensibly had had ADHD, a list that included Benjamin Franklin, Winston Churchill, Socrates, Isaac Newton, Amadeus Mozart, Leonardo da Vinci, Albert Einstein, and Bill Clinton (notwithstanding the mountain of evidence showing that ADHD was not a disorder to be taken lightly and that it put sufferers at risk for academic failure and professional disappointments).[18] The label of ADHD was no longer a stigma to be avoided but an affirming identity to be embraced. This was an ideolog-ical shift of profound consequences. Not only did it lay the foundation for the coalescing of groups like CHADD in the 1980s, but it also could have removed the reticence of parents who in the past would have avoided labeling their children with any disabling condition, especially a mental disability.

Finally, the disability rights movement allowed people with disabili-ties, regardless of their impairment, to ally in common cause, a devel-opment that aided people with controversial and suspect disorders such as ADHD. In the past, each disease, impairment, or disorder had its own champion, and groups tended to compete for government funding for medical research and programs. In addition, well-organized and sympathetic groups—such as the wheelchair-bound veterans with dis-abilities, or parents of children with developmental disabilities—avoided association with less popular groups, such as adults with mental illness.[19] The logic of disability rights, however, helped to bring down the barriers between people with disabilities, as they came to see themselves all as victims of societal discrimination, regardless of their impairments.[20] Moreover, with the demand for accommodations framed in terms of civil rights, disability groups no longer regarded one another as competitors for funding. Because a right is a moral claim, not easily subjected to a cost-benefit calculus, once the political de-mands of individuals with disabilities were reframed in terms of rights, explained Robert Katzmann, "questions of cost became irrelevant: each group could champion the demands of others without financial sacrifice."[21]

People with ADHD—indeed, people with mental disorders, in general—greatly benefited from the cross-impairment alliance spawned by the disability rights movement. People with mental disorders were never as vocal or well organized as other disability groups.[22] But they could piggyback on the gains that the movement's more powerful groups helped secure. Policy makers, for instance, did not enact the re-forms made to SSI specifically with the purpose of helping children with ADHD, but children with ADHD became the beneficiaries of these changes. Similarly, civil rights laws that granted individuals with dis-abilities the right to accommodations and services—the IDEA, Section 504, and the ADA—were not enacted with individuals with ADHD in mind, but because ADHD is regarded as a medical condition, children and adults with the disorder can request modifications to school and job requirements under these laws (though there is no guarantee that these requests will be granted). Nevertheless, the fact that CHADD was unable to convince members of Congress to make children with ADHD explicitly eligible for special education services attests to the doubts about ADHD that persist and the political weakness of ADHD proponents when the broader community of individuals with disabilities does not support them.

## How Did the IDEA Become More Open to Children with ADHD?

The development of special education illustrates the triumph of the disability rights logic. Prior to the 1970s, school systems discouraged parents of children with severe disabilities from sending their offspring to neighborhood schools. Parents kept their children at home and educated them privately, if at all.[23] In large cities, children who were less severely impaired could attend school, but they were isolated from able-bodied schoolchildren in separate classrooms called "ungraded school," "crippled classes," or "special education." Within these separate classrooms, children with physically handicaps were divided from children deemed "backward," "mentally defective," or "feeble-minded."[24] According to historian Judith Sealander, the teachers who managed ungraded classrooms for children who were mentally impaired had little interest in educating their pupils. Such classes were "a place of exile for disruptive students. 'Repeated failures' and 'naughty boys,'" she noted, "dominated classrooms which were primarily punishment halls."[25]

By the early 1970s, this long-established system of segregated classrooms was under attack. Drawing from the Supreme Court's assertion in *Brown v. Board of Education* that a "separate but equal" education was "inherently unequal," parent advocacy groups challenged the ungraded classroom in court. In 1971, in *Pennsylvania Association for Retarded Children (PARC) v. Pennsylvania*, a district court held that the state of Pennsylvania could no longer write off children with disabilities as "uneducatable"; such children, even those with severe disabilities, were entitled to an education in the public schools. Schools, therefore, could no longer turn away children with disabilities; they had to educate them, and if schools placed children in ungraded classrooms, they had to ensure that the education provided was meaningful. These classrooms could not serve as mere "holding pens" for bothersome students.[26]

Because in principle it established that children with disabilities had the right to equal access to the education that able-bodied children enjoyed, *PARC* laid important legal and political groundwork for the budding disability rights movement.[27] The next year, in another landmark case, *Mills v. Board of Education*, a Washington, D.C., district court struck down the city's practice of assigning children, most of whom were racial minorities, to ungraded classrooms. Finding the practice discriminatory, the court noted that little real learning occurred in such classrooms, a clear violation of *Brown's* dictum against "separate but equal" education.[28] By the early 1970s, more than 20 states found their system of educating children with disabilities under legal challenge.[29] Desperate, the states turned to the federal government, hoping Congress would provide the financial assistance necessary to cover the burgeoning costs of meaningfully educating students with disabilities.

In 1975, Congress enacted the Education for All Handicapped Children Act, a law that one of its chief proponents, Senator Edward Kennedy (D-MA), argued would "rewrite one of the saddest chapters in American education."[30] Renamed the Individuals with Disabilities Education Act in 1990, the law requires schools to provide children with disabilities a "free and appropriate public education" according to an "individualized education plan" drawn up by a team of school officials, teachers, counselors, psychologists, and social workers and in consultation with parents. The law also grants parents extensive due process guarantees, including the right to sue the school district in federal court if they disagree with its placement of their child. To placate states, the Education for All Handicapped Children Act gave states some funds for the supplemental services schools would need to offer in order to accommodate the needs of children with disabilities. However, for many school districts, the federal money has not been enough to cover the costs of educating children with disabilities in a manner that is meaningful, "appropriate," and sufficiently satisfactory to parents.[31]

Nevertheless, as extensive as the IDEA's legal guarantees for students with disabilities and their parents were, advocates for children with ADHD long believed that such children were ill served by the program. Efforts to reform special education so that schools would become more accepting of children with ADHD began in the late 1980s and continued into the following decade. In 1987, the U.S Interagency Committee on Learning Disabilities convened the National Conference on Learning Disabilities. The conference recommended changes to the definition of learning disabilities that would have treated ADHD as a distinct condition recognized by federal law.[32] Advocates sought to incorporate this new understanding of ADHD into special education. The crux of the controversy was not whether children with ADHD could be disabled by their condition. No one disputed that. Rather, opposing sides disagreed over whether the children were receiving the assistance to which they were entitled under the IDEA.

The dispute was related to the IDEA's listing of impairments. The law specifically mentions several impairments that fall under its protection: autism, hearing impairments (including deafness), visual impairment (including blindness), concomitant deafness and blindness, mental retardation, orthopedic impairment, multiple disabilities, serious emotional disturbance, specific learning disabilities, speech or language impairment, developmental delay, and other health impairments.[33] These classifications are *not* diagnostic labels; they are impairment classifications based largely on functional capacity. Though a child must have a medical diagnosis to qualify for the IDEA, the diagnosis of a disorder is not enough to qualify a child for special education services. Services are provided only if the child meets the functional standard required by the IDEA. According to the law, a child's medical condition must result in an impairment that limits functioning so severely that "special education and related services" are needed. In other words, the impairment must be severe enough that the student cannot function in a regular classroom without supplemental services or modifications, which will vary from student to student depending on his or her particular needs.[34] A child, therefore, must both have a qualifying medical diagnosis and meet the functional standard of severity in order to be a candidate for special education.

In 1990, Congress debated whether to add separate impairment listings for autism, traumatic brain injury, and ADHD. Adding the new impairment categories was not meant to change the substance of education policy. Children with these disorders already qualified for special education services under the category of "other health impairment," a catchall listing designed for children with limited strength, vitality, or alertness because of a chronic or acute health problem that adversely affected academic performance.[35] Children with ADHD could also qualify as having a "specific learning disability" or "serious emotional disturbance," depending on whether the children exhibited emotional, behavioral, or learning problems, or some combination of the three.

Advocates, however, were dissatisfied with the prevailing approach of evaluating the disorders under the existing classifications. They pointed out that educators poorly understood ADHD, autism, and traumatic brain injury, and that the existing diagnostic categories did not make it adequately clear to school officials that students with these conditions were protected under the IDEA. As a result, these students were either not identified or, once identified, not provided the services and accommodations appropriate to their medical conditions.[36] More-over, the catchall categories for ADHD served only to confuse teachers, counselors, and school officials further. As the House report on a re-form bill explained, "ADD is not the result of serious emotional distur-bance, learning disability, gross brain damage, psychosis, autism, per-vasive developmental disorder, or mental retardation." As such, ADHD deserved its own listing. "Because of the unique nature of their dis-order, children with ADD will frequently require educational interven-tions that are very different from those commonly used with children with . . . other disabling conditions."[37] Listing the disorders as separate and distinct impairments, the House argued, would ensure that stu-dents with ADHD received medical and educational interventions de-signed to meet the specific challenges posed by their disorder.[38]

Even though children with ADHD were technically already eligible for services, CHADD officials realized that having a distinct category for ADHD would change special education in practice, making it easier than was currently the case to get children with ADHD special educa-tion services. In hearings before the House Subcommittee on Select Ed-ucation (of the Committee on Education and Labor), a mother affili-ated with the organization told lawmakers, "As currently written, children with attention deficit hyperactivity disorder . . . are currently excluded from needed special education services."[39] Citing a study con-ducted by the Professional Group for Attention and Related Disorders, an ADHD advocacy group comprised of educators and health special-ists, she explained that 90% of children with ADHD did not meet the criteria for learning disabilities, and unless they showed another handi-capping condition, they were not admitted into special education pro-grams or allowed accommodations in regular classroom settings. De-scribing the prejudice that students with ADHD encountered, she explained that "these children are perceived as lazy and . . . not trying hard enough" and, as a result, "are often penalized for exhibiting the symptoms of their disorder."[40] Creating a separate impairment cate-gory for ADHD would increase the visibility of the disorder and reduce the possibility that educators would ignore children with its symptoms. It would also mean that children diagnosed with ADHD who suffered from academic troubles would no longer need to satisfy the qualifying criteria of additional impairment categories. Meeting the benchmarks in the ADHD impairment category would suffice.[41]

Although disability groups frequently work together, the question of adding ADHD to the IDEA bitterly divided them—a prelude to the intense controversy the disorder would engender later in the decade. While CHADD pressed for a separate listing, a number of well-respected disability and education groups opposed the move. These included the National Association of State Directors of Special Education, the National Education Association, the National Association of School Psychologists, the Council for Exceptional Children, and the NAACP Legal Defense and Education Fund. Motivating their opposition was a concern that school administrators would never be able to contain the number of students with ADHD receiving special education services. Explaining its position, the CEC argued that ADHD was a disorder with amorphous symptoms, the medical validity of which had not been thoroughly researched. There would be no way that school officials would be able to distinguish children with functional deficits stemming from a real medical disorder from those whose academic troubles were the result of the child's attitude or environment. Given the potential size of the ADHD population, the CEC contended that making children with ADHD explicitly eligible for the IDEA would divert resources away from children with more severe impairments.[42] In addition, the NAACP Legal Defense and Education Fund worried that explicit recognition of ADHD would further encourage the overidentification of African American boys as learning or behaviorally disabled. Preferring to adopt a "better safe than sorry" approach, opponents argued that students with ADHD could already receive services under current arrangements provided that their symptoms were severe enough.[43]

As IDEA reform worked its way through Congress, there was little disagreement that ADHD children should be eligible for special education services; the question was how best to evaluate their impairment. The Senate and House included language, either in the bill or in accompanying reports, stating that ADHD was a qualifying condition. But in the face of strong opposition from national disability and educational groups, the conference committee dropped references to ADHD as a specifically covered disability. In amendments to the IDEA enacted in 1991, lawmakers added autism and traumatic brain injury to the list of qualifying impairments but left out ADHD. CHADD, however, did arouse enough concern that lawmakers called for the U.S. Department of Education to look further into whether schools were meeting the needs of children with ADHD. Congress required the department's Office of Special Education Programs (OSEP) to solicit comments on ADHD from the public, study further the nature of ADHD and the need for services for students with the disorder, report the findings to Congress, and establish information centers that would share the research findings with parents and educators.[44]

As it prepared to carry out Congress's mandate, the Department of Education found advocates and educators intensely organized around ADHD issues. In response to the request for public comments on the disorder, more than 2,000 responses poured into the department, an unusually large number, which reflected the contentious feelings ADHD elicited. Many letters came from parents who believed that schools were not adequately meeting their children's needs and who urged the department to do more. Comments from educators and medical professionals, however, were mixed. Many noted that the existing criteria were sufficient to ensure that the special education needs of children with ADHD were accommodated, but they also believed that the law's ambiguity meant that some eligible students were falling through the cracks.[45] At the same time, CHADD organized a lobbying campaign that generated 4,000 letters sent to lawmakers, the education committees in Congress, and the Department of Education. In response, several members of Congress pressed the department to find some way of making sure that children with ADHD were not improperly denied services.[46]

The Department of Education was caught in an irreconcilable dilemma. On the one hand, should it treat ADHD liberally, thus ensuring that schools did not unjustly deny educational assistance to children with real medical impairments? This approach risked giving services to children who were struggling in school but whose troubles did not rise to the level of a medical impairment (however that was defined). Or should the department adopt a stringent approach, setting strict standards to make sure that assistance was targeted at only those children who "truly" had severe functional limitations because of ADHD? This approach would turn down an unknown number of children who were genuinely in need of assistance but who, for whatever reason, could not provide proper clinical proof of a medical disorder. In September 1991, the Department of Education issued a report that tried to balance the conflicting demands of parents and CHADD with the concerns voiced by cautious health and education professionals. The OSEP concluded that school districts were properly meeting the needs of children with ADHD despite the fact that the IDEA did not have a stand-alone listing for the disorder. But it also noted that educators would find more information useful. Thus, the OSEP, together with the department's Division of Rehabilitation and the Office of Civil Rights, issued a joint memorandum to states and local school districts clarifying the rules regarding the eligibility of students with ADHD for special education.[47] Under the revised guidelines, the offices underscored that students with ADHD could qualify for IDEA services if they met the criteria for a "serious emotional disturbance," "learning disability," or "other health impairment." But, OSEP reiterated, even those students who did not meet IDEA standards might still be entitled to accommodations in an integrated setting through the broader definition of disability used by Section 504 of the 1973 Rehabilitation Act. Unlike the IDEA, Section 504 did not require a specific clinical diagnosis of a qualifying disorder, nor did it list specific functional standards a child had to meet; instead, it protected any student who could demonstrate "a physical or mental impairment which substantially limits one or more major life activities."[48]

The prevalence of ADHD among children receiving special education services quickly grew. During the 2000–2001 school year, more than 5.7 million students ages 6 years old to 21 years old were covered under the IDEA, an increase of more than 28% since the 1991–1992 school year.[49] Although the department's clarifications were not meant to automatically qualify children with ADHD for educational assistance or disability accommodations, the number of children with behavioral or learning programs who were enrolled in special education programs increased rapidly after 1991, a development some critics and program specialists attributed to the policy changes made in relation to ADHD. The proportion of special education students 6 years old to 21 years old who were classified as learning disabled, for example, grew from 2.2 million to nearly 2.9 million, a 28% increase between the 1991–1992 and 2000–2001 school years.[50] Similarly, over the same time period, the number of students eligible for reasons of an "emotional disturbance" rose by 18%, from 400,000 to well over 473,000.[51] The most dramatic growth, however, occurred in the listing for "other health impairment." Of the three IDEA classifications used for ADHD, this listing showed the largest increase between the 1991–1992 and 2000–2001 school years, growing from approximately 58,700 students to more than 290,000, an astounding fourfold increase.[52] This expansion occurred despite the fact that, in 1990, Congress removed children with autism and traumatic brain injury from the "other health impairment" classification (where they had previously been grouped) when it created stand-alone impairment listings for them. Although the category of "other health impairment" also encompasses children with heart conditions, asthma, diabetes, and rheumatic fever, state officials reported to Department of Education officials in 2002 that these conditions made up only a small proportion of children in the category and that much of the expansion in the listing was attributable to increased identification of children with ADHD.[53] Reviewing data on adolescents served by the IDEA, researchers at the Department of Education likewise concluded that the growing share of special education students who were listed under an "other health impairment" largely reflected "the increase in the number of students diagnosed with attention deficit/hyperactivity disorder as a primary disability."[54] As a result of these trends, currently, specific learning disabilities represent half of all students in special education, followed by speech or language impairments (19%), mental retardation (11%), emotional disturbance (8%), and other health impairments (5%). These are the 5 largest categories of the IDEA, together representing 93% of all school-age children granted special education accommodations and services.[55]

Thus, even though neither Congress nor the Department of Education believed it was making substantial changes to special education policy when the OSEP clarified the status of ADHD in its 1991 policy memorandum, the clarification changed educational practices in ways that, in turn, led to an increase in the number of children labeled with ADHD.[56] First, the rule clarification alerted many teachers and school administrators to the fact that ADHD was indeed a qualifying disorder for special education.[57] Also, the publicity surrounding the rule change itself could have increased awareness of the disorder among teachers and education officials, leading them to pay closer attention to children who may be eligible.[58] Moreover, the Department of Education's announcement encouraged states to do a more thorough job of identifying students with subtle impairments like ADHD and to locate children with disabilities at an earlier age in order to provide preventative and adaptive services.[59]

## How Did SSI Become More Open to Children with ADHD?

At the same time that policy makers became more willing to offer special education services to students with learning and behavioral deficits, antipoverty advocates and health professionals sought to expand SSI to children who were being excluded from benefits because of the SSA's strict disability standards. These reform efforts were part of a long-running campaign that antipoverty advocates had pursued since the Reagan administration tried to cut spending for Social Security disability payments. Between 1981 and 1984, at the urging of the White House, the Social Security Administration conducted a large-scale review of the Social Security disability rolls for the purpose of removing anyone deemed "no longer disabled," either because the person had recovered and could now work or because the disability assessment had been flawed and the person had been erroneously granted benefits in the first place. One of the children cut from Supplemental Security Income was a young boy named Brian Zebley, who suffered from numerous physical and mental ailments and had been placed on SSI as a toddler. His family sued, and in 1990, his Legal Services attorneys argued his case before the Supreme Court.[60] In February 1991, in the case of *Sullivan v. Zebley*, the justices struck down the SSA's process for evaluating childhood disability, ruling that it did not offer the individualized assessment mandated by the Social Security Act. *Zebley* laid the groundwork for a rapid increase in the number of children receiving SSI payments, and by 1994, SSI spent more on benefits to low-income families than either Aid to Families with Dependent Children (AFDC) or the Earned Income Tax Credit, two much more widely known antipoverty programs.[61]

That SSI would become a major source of support for low-income families is somewhat surprising, for there is no evidence that Congress intended for SSI to become a safety net for children with disabilities and their families. When Congress enacted SSI in 1972, lawmakers decided to permit children to receive cash assistance if they had an impairment that was of "comparable severity" to one that would disable an adult—that is, an impairment so debilitating that if an adult had it, he or she would no longer be able to work. Why lawmakers made children eligible for SSI was never entirely clear. The 1971 House report on the legislation argued that children with disabilities should qualify for aid because "their needs are often greater than those of nondisabled children."[62] The Senate, however, disagreed. It countered that only the "health care expenses" of children with disabilities were greater than those of able-bodied children, and these expenses were largely covered under Medicaid. "Disabled children's need for food, clothing, and shelter," the Senate concluded, "are usually no greater than the needs of nondisabled children" and thus should be covered by AFDC—the public assistance program for poor families—not SSI, which it wanted to reserve for aged adults and adults with disabilities.[63] Members of Congress never resolved this dispute. Instead, the conference committee ironing out differences between the House and Senate versions of a large omnibus bill, of which SSI was one small part, glossed over the children's program. It simply accepted the House language, which made children with disabilities eligible for SSI, but it did not explain why such payments were necessary.[64]

From the beginning, the Social Security Administration found the SSI children's program administratively problematic for two reasons. First, childhood disabilities are notoriously difficult to assess with accuracy. Though children are less likely to be disabled than are adults, the range of medical disorders that plague children is vast. Some disorders occur only rarely in the general population, and their causes, prognosis, and treatment are not well understood. However, the most common disorders found in children—cognitive, emotional, and mental impairments—tend to rely on diagnostic criteria that are more subjective than those used for physical ailments.[65] And it is not uncommon for children to have multiple impairments, thus complicating efforts to diagnose disorders, measure disability, and determine treatment. As the Surgeon General explained in a 2000 report, "children with pervasive developmental disorders often suffer from" attention deficit/hyperactivity disorder, and children with conduct disorders are frequently afflicted with depression and learning disabilities as well.[66]

In addition, the ongoing process of development "presents an ever-changing backdrop that complicates" diagnosis and disability evaluation. Some behaviors, such as temper tantrums, "may be quite normal at one age but suggest mental illness at another age."[67] At the same time, the child's social environment also exerts a profound influence on impairment "such that some afflicted children improve . . . as a result of healthy influences" while "at-risk" children "develop full-blown forms of disorder."[68] Because sharp distinctions between "normal" and "abnormal" childhood behavior are difficult to make, clinicians tend to consider childhood mental disorders not as pathological illnesses but as marked deviations from statistical norms of "cognitive, social, and emotional development."[69] The special challenges posed by children's disorders greatly complicated the SSA's efforts to draw a bright-line distinction between children who were and were not disabled. This does not mean that childhood mental disorders are not real, but it does mean that accurately diagnosing a real medical disorder and thus evaluating disability—never easy, even in the case of adults—was especially problematic in the case of children. ADHD, a disorder that exists along a continuum of severity and that includes extreme variants of normal childhood behavior, is illustrative of this ongoing problem with evaluating disability in children.

A second difficulty with the SSI children's program was the fact that SSI had been based on disability assistance programs for adults and was only later expanded to children, in 1972. Because of this, SSI assessed disability against employment, a standard that clearly did not apply to the new child beneficiaries. The Social Security Administration judged the severity of an adult's impairment according to whether it prevented him or her from finding and keeping employment. If it did, then the impairment was deemed severe enough to qualify the adult for benefits. But because children are not expected to work, the SSA had a difficult time determining what constituted an impairment of "comparable severity." In 1977, the SSA devised a makeshift process for evaluating disability in children. It required children to show the specific clinical signs and symptoms of one of hundreds of illnesses, injuries, and disorders compiled in the agency's Listings of Medical Impairments. Adults were also required to show a medical impairment that matched the listings in order to receive SSI payments. But if they did not, they could still qualify if after an individualized assessment an agency examiner determined that the functional restrictions imposed by the impairment precluded work. Since they did not work, children were not afforded this second opportunity to qualify. SSA officials, of course, recognized that the approach was not necessarily "comparable" to the adult process, but according to one official, they concluded that "it's better than nothing."[70]

Throughout the late 1970s and early 1980s, the SSA's restrictive interpretation of disability kept the SSI children's program small. But in 1990, a broad coalition of medical professionals, antipoverty activists, and disability and children's advocates banded together to compel the SSA to loosen its interpretation of childhood disability. The coalition supporting the liberalization of SSI was a veritable honor roll of medical and disability groups that included the American Medical Association, the American Academy of Pediatrics, the American Psychiatric Association, Mental Health America (formerly the National Association of Mental Health), the Bazelon Center, Easter Seals, the Arc, and the March of Dimes. Although Congress had not created the SSI children's program for the specific purpose of integrating children with disabilities into community settings, reformers recognized that SSI had become an important source of support for families with children with disabilities, allowing parents to purchase needed medical supplies, make structural modifications to their homes, or cut back on work hours to provide around-the-clock-care for their children—key considerations for parents who wanted to keep children at home rather than institutionalize them.[71] Children disabled by ADHD require neither structural modifications nor constant medical care, and reformers were not focused on ADHD in particular. But because their efforts loosened the SSA's evaluation of childhood disability overall, children with ADHD benefited from the policy changes instituted in the wake of *Zebley*.

Brian Zebley's attorneys argued that the SSA did not pay enough attention to the functional impact of children's impairments. By looking only at the severity of a child's clinical signs and symptoms, the SSA disadvantaged any child whose medical condition prevented adequate functioning but whose symptoms were not obviously disabling: children with multiple impairments that were not fully cataloged in the Listings of Medical Impairments, children with rare disorders that were not discussed in the listings, and infants and toddlers, who were too young to take part in many of the clinical tests discussed in the listings.[72] In fact, Brian Zebley, the named plaintiff in the coalition's class-action lawsuit, was the perfect example of the kind of child who was disadvantaged by the SSA's approach. Admitted into SSI in the early 1970s when adjudicators were not as strict, Zebley was later dropped when examiners discovered that none of his separate medical problems rose to the level of severity described in any of the SSA's listings. The SSA, meanwhile, did not have any means for assessing the overall functional impact of Zebley's many different impairments: congenital brain damage, mental retardation, visual problems, developmental delays, and partial paralysis. Though none of them was severe enough on its own to disable Zebley, it is hard to imagine that a child with so many impairments at the same time was not severely functionally limited.[73]

In addition, mental health advocates argued that the SSA's methods for examining childhood disability disadvantaged children with learning and behavioral problems unless those impairments were utterly incapacitating. To illustrate the point, the Bazelon Center filed an amicus brief that gave examples of children with the symptoms of ADHD. The brief pointed out that "a hyperactive child who could not attend school" would be judged "not disabled" under the SSA's restrictive disability standard because such a child could still "engage in appropriate self-care skills." Also excluded would be "a child with emotional and behavioral disorders who cannot adapt to special education classes but who has self-care skills."[74] Because the standard for adults was not nearly as restrictive, the Bazelon Center and other advocates concluded, there was no way the children's program was "comparable" to the adult program, as Congress had required when it created SSI in 1972.[75]

By a vote of 7–2, the Supreme Court agreed. In his opinion for the majority, Justice Harry Blackmun stated that the SSA could not look at clinical signs alone. In addition to medical symptoms, it was required to look at how each specific child functioned in his or her environment. Although gainful employment—the standard used in SSI's disability program for adults—could not be used as the yardstick to measure disability in children, the court suggested that the SSA examine instead a child's ability to feed and dress himself or herself, learn, and play—all activities that the court deemed the "work" of children. The operative standard would be whether the child performed these activities in an "age-appropriate" manner.[76]

In light of the *Zebley* decision, the SSA made several important changes to its childhood disability rules that affected children with ADHD. To start, the agency added an Individualized Functional Assessment (IFA), a test that was designed to assess the extent to which a child's medical condition hampered his or her ability to reach developmental milestones, perform like children of the same age, and acquire the skills necessary to become a productive and self-sufficient adult. Thus, measuring a particular child against his or her age peers, SSA's disability examiners rated whether the child performed in an "age-appropriate" manner in 7 functional areas: response to stimuli; cognition; communication; motor functioning; social functioning; personal and behavioral functioning; and concentration, persistence, and pace. A child was disabled if examiners determined that he or she had limitations in 2 or 3 of the 7 functional areas.[77]

In addition, shortly before the Supreme Court handed down its decision in *Zebley*, the SSA issued rules that required examiners to pay greater attention to a child's functioning when evaluating the severity of a child's medical symptoms under the Listings of Medical Impairments. The agency also released updated rules for assessing a number of complicated childhood impairments, including Down syndrome, phenylketonuria, fetal alcohol syndrome, psychoactive substance abuse disorders, and of course ADHD, which appeared in the SSA's medical listings for the first time. The updates were meant to bring the children's medical listings in line with the changes in diagnostic language that had taken place with the publication of DSM-III, and they went into effect at the same time that the SSA launched the IFA.[78] The combined impact of these reforms, especially the IFA, was to open SSI to children with behavioral and learning disorders, including ADHD.

Nevertheless, the IFA became the key point of access for children with learning and behavioral disorders for three reasons. First, as an evaluation of individual functioning, the IFA helped those children with disorders that were not cataloged specifically in the listings or that lacked tangible physical markers, in particular children with mental disorders, multiple impairments, or rare diseases, who all tended to fare poorly under the listings. Infants and toddlers also benefited from the addition of the IFA. Previously, if examiners suspected that an infant had hearing problems, they had to wait until the child was old enough to respond to auditory tests. But now under the IFA, the examiner needed only to see if the infant reacted to stimuli in the same way as did children of a similar age. The IFA also expanded SSI to children with mental disorders, especially those whose impairments were difficult to classify under one particular listing (a common problem given the subjectivity of diagnostic criteria and the high rate of comorbidity in children with mental disorders). Under the IFA, children alleging conditions such as ADHD no longer had to show the specific clinical signs and symptoms included under a particular medical listing; they could instead qualify under the IFA simply by demonstrating functional deficits, irrespective of the diagnosis with which those deficits were associated.[79]

Second, the IFA set a lower standard for qualification than the listings in the case of mental disorders. This was due to the fact that, when designing the IFA, the SSA's Office of Disability made a fateful choice. It decided to lift the functional domains for the IFA from its medical listings for childhood mental disorders. The reason for doing so was simple. Officials at the agency had no idea how to adapt the work-oriented adult standard for disability to a children's program, but they were forced to come up with a way in a very short period of time. (Only a year elapsed between the time the Supreme Court handed down its *Zebley* decision and the SSA drew up and tested the IFA, trained its examiners how to use it, and fully implemented the new rules.) "All we knew to do," one SSA official explained, "was provide some way that a child ... who has a less severe impairment than it takes to meet the Listings could be found disabled" under an individualized evaluation of functioning, as was the case when adults who do not meet the criteria in the medical listings were examined to see if they were capable of working.[80] Without guidance from the Supreme Court and under enormous time constraints, the SSA's Office of Disability patterned the IFA after the functional measures included in its medical listings for childhood mental disorders, reasoning that those measures could apply just as easily to physically impaired children.[81]

The IFA, therefore, contained the same functional domains used in the listings for mental disorders, but it lowered the standard for qualifying. The listings generally required that an impairment cause "marked" restriction in functioning, whereas, in some circumstances, the IFA allowed children with only "moderate" functional limitations to qualify for payments. Thus, in some cases, a child who could not meet the functional standard in the listings would be evaluated a second time under the same functional domains in the IFA but with a lower threshold to qualify.[82] It was little surprise then that a 1995 study found that 42% of the children with mental disorders who entered SSI after *Zebley* had qualified through the IFA, while only 7% of the children with physical impairments did.[83]

Finally, the IFA was a broader inquiry into functioning than the adult test, which pegged its standard to work capacity. Rather than limiting itself to one domain, the IFA measured functioning across virtually every activity in which children could participate: studying, playing, socializing, communication, dressing and feeding oneself, and carrying out pursuits in school as well as at home. The children's assessment, therefore, was a global evaluation of functioning (unlike the adults'), and because more domains of functioning were addressed, there were more chances for children to qualify.[84]

Because of these policy changes, enrollment in SSI grew significantly and quickly. In 1989, fewer than 300,000 children qualified for SSI payments. By June 1994, when participation in the children's program hit an all-time high, just over 1 million children were receiving disability benefits nationwide.[85] Of the children who entered SSI through the new rules, 84% had a mental disorder listed as their primary limitation.[86] Both the addition of an ADHD listing and the IFA appeared to have an especially marked effect on the number of children with ADHD who were able to qualify for assistance. An analysis of SSI and Medicaid in four states found that enrollment of children with ADHD in SSI increased by almost threefold in the few short years between 1989 and 1992.[87] Nevertheless, it is important to keep these program trends in perspective. Even after the number of children receiving benefits based on a diagnosis of ADHD grew significantly, these children represented no more than 6% of new enrollees, a rather small segment of the children newly eligible for SSI.[88] Similarly, in 1993, children with ADHD, learning disabilities, and mental impairments other than mental retardation represented no more than 22% of total SSI enrollment.[89]

## SSI: From Underserved Children to Undeserving "Disabled"

The rapid increase in the number of children with learning and behavioral problems eligible for SSI benefits and IDEA services instigated a backlash against generous treatment of individuals with disabilities. In February 1994, Benjamin Weiser and Bob Woodward, famous for having broken the Watergate scandal, ran a story in the *Washington Post* entitled "Costs Soar for Children's Disability Program: How 26 Words Cost the Taxpayers Billions in New Entitlement Payments."[90] The story detailed several examples of fraud and abuse in the SSI children's program: children who intentionally flunked exams, fought with teachers and classmates, and misbehaved in school, all in an effort to qualify for SSI payments under a mental disability. Soon newspapers across the country ran sensational stories of children who put gum in their hair to act crazy and parents denying medication to their sick children, all of which caused an uproar in Congress.[91]

Although Republicans intent on cutting social welfare spending were among the most vocal of SSI's critics, the effort to rein in the program's growth was bipartisan. Indeed, at the same time that the *Post* ran the Woodward story, President Clinton was contemplating far-reaching reforms to AFDC, the cash benefit program for poor families. He asked his advisers to glean money from other antipoverty programs in order to pay for the expanded job-training and child-care initiatives that he envisioned as part of his welfare reform plan. One of the first programs they focused on was SSI.[92] Given the rapid growth in the children's program and media allegations of rampant fraud and abuse, SSI's political status as a program for the "deserving" disabled had been badly damaged. Surveying the run-up in children's benefits after the *Zebley* decision, one SSA field director summed up the public's and Congress's view of the situation when she stated, "It would make one think that almost any adolescent or pre-adolescent child going through the typical socialization experiences and 'growing pains' may qualify for SSI."[93]

Clinton failed to convince fellow Democrats in Congress to enact welfare reform during their terms, and when Republicans took control of the House and Senate following the 1994 midterm elections, efforts to cut SSI and welfare took on new life. Congressional critics of SSI were outraged by what they saw as the program's incentives for children to misbehave and fail in school. The new Speaker of the House, Newt Gingrich, derisively called SSI payments "crazy checks" and "dumb checks." "The U.S. government is encouraging child abuse by encouraging children to perform below their levels in order to qualify for a check," he complained. "Now this is just sick."[94]

To critics, because of its relatively generous payments to low-income families and its lax standards for evaluating mental disorders, SSI provided children with an incentive to feign their disabilities and their parents with an incentive to encourage this deceit. This was the story line behind the *Boston Globe*'s 1994 portrayal of single mother Lisa T. Lisa T.'s eight-year-old son struggled in school, frequently threw temper tantrums, and fought with his classmates. Academically weak, he was placed in a class for children with special needs. Although she freely admitted that she did not consider her son disabled—"I just think he needs help in terms of his attitude," she explained—Lisa T. was able to enroll him in SSI. Asked to justify her actions, the young woman shrugged her shoulders and stated simply, "We need the money." The SSI checks amounted to $480 a month, far more than what most of the families in their South Boston neighborhood received from AFDC.[95]

Anecdotal stories like Lisa T.'s were supported by a handful of studies that showed that obtaining SSI benefits was indeed financially rewarding for cash-strapped families. One analysis estimated that a family of three living in Maryland could increase its annual income by more than $3,500 if one of the children transferred from AFDC to SSI.[96] Another study traced SSI's dramatic growth in the 1990s to the fact that, in most states, eligibility for SSI allowed children to enroll automatically in Medicaid (the government's health insurance program for the poor), not an insignificant benefit given the difficulty low-income parents often face securing health-care coverage from their employers.[97] Nonetheless, even if studies confirmed that families were better off on SSI than on AFDC, there was little evidence that a significant number of families consciously made this financial calculation when applying for SSI. Instead, many were diverted to SSI by state governments. During the late 1980s and early 1990s, many states both tightened eligibility for general assistance and AFDC (for which they paid all or roughly half the costs) and provided legal assistance to families trying to switch their children to SSI (for which the federal government paid virtually the entire tab). Some states even required families to apply first for SSI before being eligible for general assistance and AFDC.[98]

Nevertheless, to critics, a generous approach to children with learning and behavioral impairments sent the wrong message about personal responsibility. The General Accounting Office (GAO) explained in its report to Congress, "Children who cannot function at an age-appropriate level may be able to develop so that they can work by the time they reach adulthood." This was especially the case since many of the children with mental disabilities who had just entered SSI did not have impairments that were completely incapacitating.[99] But, the GAO argued, self-sufficiency was not likely to occur unless the SSA shifted its focus from sending out checks to "work[ing] with recipients more actively to help them increase their self-sufficiency"—a task that agency officials viewed as well beyond their mission and expertise.[100] Conservatives balked at the idea that SSI should pay cash benefits indefinitely to children who were not completely unable to function. Noting that Congress was currently contemplating ending the entitlement to cash assistance for poor families and compelling impoverished single mothers to work, Carolyn Weaver, a fellow at the conservative think tank the American Enterprise Institute, explained, "SSI does not present problems at the forefront of the welfare reform debate—teen pregnancy, out-of-wedlock births, and the cycle of dependency." But the program was inherently flawed, just the same, Weaver argued. "SSI discourages work and in providing cash support with basically 'no strings attached,' tends to perpetuate the very conditions that preclude work and promote dependency."[101]

In the summer of 1996, shortly before the presidential elections, congressional Republicans passed a welfare reform bill that Clinton promptly signed. Despite the fact that the debate over cutting assistance to needy families had been exceedingly contentious, one of the few points of agreement between Republicans and Democrats was the need to restrict the growth of SSI. Congress tightened the SSI eligibility rules for children, specifically targeting children with learning and behavioral difficulties by eliminating both the individualized functional test and the ability of children to qualify for benefits based on "maladaptive" behavior. It also deleted the statement that children qualified for benefits if their impairment was of "comparable severity" to one that would disable an adult. In its place, lawmakers required children to show "marked and severe" impairments before they could qualify for SSI. Not surprisingly, then, after the SSA implemented the cutbacks, it found that those children most likely to lose benefits were children with learning disabilities, ADHD, and conduct disorders.[102] Yet the dispute over ADHD was not settled. Concerns about children with learning and behavior troubles receiving special education services soon arose as well.

## The IDEA: Incentives to Label Children with ADHD

The Americans with Disabilities Act was barely a decade old when conservatives began disparaging the "perverse" incentives and unfair advantages disability rights law gave to individuals who were not really disabled.[103] Conservatives were especially critical of the IDEA for creating incentives for teachers to label students with conditions like ADHD. According to Patti Johnson, Denver's representative on the Colorado State Board of Education, "financial incentives exist for schools to label children with learning disorders." An outspoken critic of both public schools and special education, Johnson disapproved of the fact that the IDEA provided local school districts with federal funds to cover a portion of the costs of educating children with disabilities, including children with disorders like ADHD, for which there were no objective clinical tests with which to separate legitimately impaired students from questionable cases. So long as schools received money for special education students, Johnson explained to members of Congress during a hearing in 2000, "so-called learning disorders" will "become a way for financially strapped schools to make ends meet." Pointing to the example of the California special education program, she argued that "tens of thousands of . . . students were placed there not because they have a serious mental or emotional handicap, but because they were never taught to read properly."[104] Bob Schafer, a Republican congressman from Colorado, agreed. "When the federal government provides billions of dollars in incentives," he explained, "it is expected that the local administrators and teachers will follow the money . . . Without a doubt, we are subsidizing the aggressive pursuit of disabilities, and it's resulted in overdiagnosis of these [learning and behavioral] conditions."[105] Prominent social conservative Phyllis Schlafly jumped on the bandwagon as well, arguing to the readers of her newsletter, "Since this labeling brings more money into the schools, it's not surprising that schools often pressure parents to get an ADHD diagnosis and put their child on Ritalin."[106]

Other critics blamed, not the federal government's funding of the IDEA per se, but how the states distributed special education money among school districts. According to Jay Greene and Greg Forster of the Manhattan Institute, a conservative think tank, states used 1 of 2 methods for funding special education.[107] In a state that used lump-sum funding, a school district's special education funds were based on the total student population in the district.[108] "Bounty" funding states, in contrast, allocated funding according to the size of a district's special education program, either the number of students or the number of teachers in the program.[109] Greene and Forster argued that the bounty funding system offered a financial incentive for school districts to seek larger programs and, thus, more money.[110] In response, they proposed overhauling the IDEA to limit incentives to expand special education.[111] Among the changes they recommended were caps on the amount of money the federal government provided for IDEA services, formulas that distributed money to states or districts based on the overall student population (rather than on the number of students in need of services), and scholarships for disabled students to attend private schools so that they would not bring money into the public school system.[112] David Schnittger, a supporter of capping a state's IDEA funding, argued, "The practical effect of not having this cap is that states would have a financial incentive to overidentify children for special education. This is unacceptable. Children should be identified for educational services based on their individual needs, not based on financial considerations."[113]

The conservative critique of disability policy extended beyond the IDEA to the very principle of granting accommodations to students alleging a mental disorder or any other impairment that could not be objectively verified. Students who did not meet the criteria for disability specified in the IDEA might still be eligible for accommodations to standard academic requirements under the Americans with Disabilities Act and Section 504. Unlike the IDEA, Section 504 and the ADA do not list the specific impairments that qualify for protection but instead use a looser, functional definition of disability. Both laws define a disability as a physical or mental impairment that substantially limits one or more major life activities, such as learning.[114] They require colleges, universities, and elementary and secondary schools (public and private) to accommodate the functional limitations of students through modifications to the academic standards and procedures that otherwise nondisabled students have to abide by.[115]

To critics of disability rights law, these accommodations constituted unfair competitive advantages, granting qualifying students the right to do less homework than their peers, view instructors' notes for class, and take extended time to complete exams. What was worse, many of the disorders students were claiming were subjective.[116] In a 1997 article in the conservative magazine *The New Republic*, skeptic Ruth Shalit lambasted disability rights law for having encouraged the proliferation of a "number of boutique disorders," and she singled out as prime examples of this trend ADHD as well as many new, lesser known learning disorders, including dyscalculia (an inability to do math); dysgraphia (an inability to write); dyssemia (an inability to properly socialize); and dysrationalia (an inability to reason).[117] Calling learning disabilities "an opportunistic tautology," Shalit argued, "The fact that one displays a marked lack of aptitude for a particular intellectual discipline or profession establishes one's legal right to ensure at least a degree of success in that discipline or profession" through the accommodations mandated by the ADA (a charge that fails to take into account the fact that lack of enforcement and judicial narrowing of key provisions have scaled back the real protections available under the ADA).[118] Likewise, Schlafly listed "extra time to complete the SATs, MCATs and LSATs" as among the key "advantages of an ADHD classification" for high school and college students, and she pointed derisively to the example of "an Ivy League school [where] a student can merely present a doctor's letter and some pills to obtain extra time for routine assignments."[119] Moreover, doubts about the validity of many of the learning disorders students claimed were not limited to conservative writers and activists. After Educational Testing Services decided to stop flagging the SAT tests of students who had requested extended time, Princeton University's dean of admissions Fred Hargadon maintained, "I have little doubt there will now be more students without legitimate reasons seeking some sort of documentation from physicians or psychologists that, for example, their simple inability to add and subtract is really a disability for which an appropriate medical term can be found."[120]

## Did SSI and Disability Rights Create Incentives to Claim the ADHD Label?

The common theme that runs through criticism of SSI, the IDEA, and the ADA is the belief that the vagueness and subjectivity of psychiatric diagnoses provide an opening for schools to label students or students to label themselves with a mental disorder in order to obtain extra funding, income support, or disability accommodations—benefits not available to children who are not disabled. For some critics, the mere correlation between the timing of reforms to disability policy and ADHD's increase was enough to prove causation. For instance, as Patti Johnson wrote for the conservative think tank the Independence Institute, "In 1991, the federal Department of Education said schools could get hundreds of dollars in special education grant money each year for every child diagnosed with ADHD. Since then ADHD diagnosis shot up an average of 21% a year. These data suggest a link between money and Ritalin use."[121]

Reality is more complicated, however. While there is no question that the increase in rates of ADHD diagnosis and stimulant use occurred at the same time that the ADA was implemented and at the same time that the IDEA and SSI expanded to cover more behaviorally and cognitively impaired children, it is also the case that these reforms could reflect the fact that government policy was finally catching up to the unmet needs of millions of children significantly limited by legitimate medical disorders. Under this scenario, SSI, the IDEA, and the ADA do not represent "perverse" incentives for otherwise healthy children to claim a disability label. Instead, children with real and significant needs are at last receiving the services and accommodations they deserve, and their families are getting the income support they need to facilitate their children's functioning in an integrated setting—precisely the intention of disability rights advocates. Program expansion and concerns about program integrity, therefore, have little to do with fraud, abuse, or "perverse" incentives. Instead, they result from the inherent subjectivity of programs based on a functional understanding of disability.

### Little Evidence of "Perverse Incentives," Fraud, and Abuse

Advocates for individuals with disabilities protested that reports of fraud and abuse in the SSI children's program were overblown and misleading.[122] Jonathan Stein, one of the attorneys who litigated the *Zebley* case, called criticisms of the SSI program "a cheap shot."[123] He and other advocates could point to the fact that despite numerous investigations, congressional researchers were unable to verify accusations of deceit. After exhaustively examining allegations that parents were encouraging children to act disabled, the General Accounting Office noted, "Unless parents admit it, coaching is almost impossible to substantiate." It also acknowledged that "the extent of coaching cannot be measured with much confidence," and in cases where coaching or malingering might be present, only a handful had resulted in an award.[124] Thus, there was little systematic evidence that SSI altered the incentives of poor parents so that they were now willing to have their children feign mental and behavioral disorders.

The dearth of evidence for widespread fraud and abuse in the SSI children's program, however, did not negate the fact that even anecdotal reports of dishonesty had great political significance. Alarmed by the burgeoning costs of SSI, lawmakers felt compelled to act on the media allegations. Between 1994 and 1996, President Clinton and Republican congressional leaders pushed for restrictions to several antipoverty programs. With many programs for the poor on the chopping block, lawmakers were forced to make difficult choices between needy and sympathetic groups of the poor. In this political climate, singling out SSI for budget cuts was easy, for as political scientist R. Kent Weaver explained, "Concerns about the deservingness of entitlement recipients are closely tied to policy makers' concern for avoiding waste, fraud, and abuse and gaining good value for expenditures."[125] What mattered for the reform debate was not whether allegations of fraud, abuse, and perverse incentives were true. The fact that they existed at all undermined the perceived "deservingness" of beneficiaries with mental disabilities, directing attention away from their needs and toward the problematic aspects of the parents' and the children's behavior. Urging Congress to address the matter, the GAO contended that even the perception of impropriety was unacceptable. "Regardless of the actual extent of such abuse," it stated, "reports [of abuse] can significantly erode public confidence in the program's integrity."[126]

Yet it is unlikely that SSI led to the expansion of ADHD diagnosis through "perverse" incentives. SSI is a small program; it pays benefits to fewer than 1 million of the approximately 73 million children who live in the United States. Given its size and the lack of any systematic evidence of widespread fraud, it is difficult to imagine that SSI itself could have had a dramatic impact on national diagnostic trends for ADHD. Instead, it is more likely that the children identified with learning and behavioral disabilities in SSI did indeed have significant functional deficits that legitimately qualified them for benefits, though whether they met the clinical definition of ADHD is another matter. The reforms made in the early 1990s merely allowed them to finally receive disability payments for their conditions.

Likewise, the argument that schools have a "perverse" incentive to label students with ADHD so that they can obtain federal funding falls flat given the modest subsidies that the federal government provides for special education. In fact, the financial assistance the federal government offers schools to educate children with disabilities is far short of the amount promised in 1975. Today the federal government covers only 7.5% of total special education costs at the local level, even though it is authorized to pay for up to 40% of the national average for per-pupil expenditures.[127] Defenders of special education also point out that the current allowance of roughly $827 per child with disabilities is paltry when compared to the enormous sums—roughly $12,000 annually—it takes to educate the average special education student.[128] Other studies have estimated that the costs of educating a child with ADHD range from $2,511 in an integrated setting to more than $7,400 in a segregated setting.[129] "How can that small amount of IDEA funds be an incentive for us to overidentify kids as needing special services?" asked Bruce Hunter, a director for the American Association of School Administrators.[130] Moreover, as a Department of Education official pointed out to lawmakers, the number of students on stimulants did not necessarily increase the amount of IDEA money a state received. Indeed, Congress had addressed this issue in 1997, when it altered the formula for determining a state's IDEA grant. To reduce incentives for overidentification, lawmakers decided to base special education funding on a state's total population and poverty rate, rather than on how many disabled students its school districts served.[131]

### The Problem with DSM and Impairment Classification

The expansions of SSI, the IDEA, and the number of children diagnosed with ADHD are in all likelihood tied to a common cause: the emergence of a functional approach to disabilities and disorders. Prior to the late 1980s, the SSA examined the severity of a claimant's clinical signs and symptoms when determining whether the claimant met the agency's standard of disability. For example, in the case of a mental disorder, the SSA required that the claimant show the active signs of the disorder—hallucinations, hyperactivity, paranoia, and so forth—at the moment of examination. In addition, the symptoms had to be so debilitating that the claimant was utterly incapable of caring for him- or herself or socializing with others.[132] One physician affiliated with the SSA protested that the rules were so restrictive that it was "practically impossible . . . for any individual whose thought processes are not completely disorganized, is not blatantly psychotic, or is not having a psychiatric emergency requiring immediate hospitalization" to qualify.[133]

Advocates for the poor and for individuals with disabilities agreed, and between 1982 and 1984, they lobbied Congress to force the SSA to revise its rules for evaluating mental impairments. The publication of DSM-III provided a staging ground for their efforts. In a letter to the SSA presented to Congress in 1982, 2 years after the release of DSM-III, James Folsom of the American Psychiatric Association explained that the SSA's disability standards were outdated and flew in the face of "good clinical practice," which indicated that most of the individuals the SSA deemed "not disabled" in fact suffered from severely incapacitating mental illnesses. So long as the SSA's descriptions of mental disorders did not match DSM-III, Folsom maintained, the agency had made "evaluation of such disability unnecessarily difficult" for both its own examiners and the thousands of psychiatrists around the nation whose medical notes examiners used as the basis of their decision making.[134] The argument was a compelling one. Noting that "serious questions" had been "raised by the old listings," Congress in 1984 ordered the SSA to revise its criteria for evaluating mental disorders and bring its rules in line with professional diagnostic standards. What emerged from those meetings was a set of rules that lowered the threshold for qualifying (claimants now had to show "marked" limitations in functioning rather than utter incapacity) and that focused attention on an individual's ability to function in his or her environment (for example, whether an employer would actually hire a mentally deranged individual rather than tolerate one as a customer), a move that resembled DSM-III's symptom-based approach to diagnosing disorders.[135]

This is an approach that might work well for severe mental illnesses, such as schizophrenia, but disorders, like ADHD, that were not completely debilitating were revamped along functional lines as well. In doing so, however, policy officials made it extraordinarily difficult for examiners to tell the difference between children who were impaired because of a medical condition and children who faced social disadvantages but were not medically incapacitated. The difficulty is clearly seen in the SSA's struggle to implement a rigorous, reliable, and valid test of individual functioning for children applying for SSI during the early 1990s. While many of the children whom the SSA accepted into SSI after 1991 *were* substantially incapacitated, the agency had a difficult time making that case because the IFA was in disarray. Studies by congressional investigators found that, despite extensive training, the SSA's examiners had trouble placing children's impairments into the correct functional categories and, in fact, tended to see more functional deficits than investigators thought appropriate.[136] For example, if a child lied, behaved aggressively toward peers, and fought in school, examiners had to decide whether the child suffered from impaired social functioning, impaired personal and behavioral functioning, or both. By classifying the child as having both social deficits and personal and behavioral deficits, rather than just one or the other, the examiner could be overstating the extent of the child's impairment.[137] Yet drawing these boundaries was almost impossible for disability examiners. While the functional domains were conceptually distinct, in the real world, they were hopelessly entangled.

Moreover, SSA examiners could not adequately distinguish the degree of a child's impairment in borderline cases or properly differentiate between impairments caused by a medical condition and impairments caused by social conditions (such as a poor home environment). Examiners were supposed to allow awards only for impairments that caused a "marked" limitation in one functional domain and a "moderate" limitation in another domain or "moderate" limitations in three domains. The agency found, though, that examiners could determine if an impairment was "extreme" or "mild," but they struggled to discern the difference between "marked" and "moderate" impairments.[138] Furthermore, the SSA discovered that its examiners were basing awards on limitations that officials at the Office of Disability regarded as rooted in the child's living circumstances rather than his or her medical condition. While SSI would compensate children for the latter, it would not do so for the former.[139] Yet asking examiners to parse the difference between medical handicaps and social disadvantage was a theoretical exercise that did not make sense in the real world, where the two were interconnected.

In addition, the SSA was unclear about how to apply the rules it had devised for the IFA. One the one hand, clear and specific rules gave examiners guidance that ensured that children evaluated by different examiners were treated the same. Yet even the SSA was uncomfortable with mechanistic rules that failed to consider the child as a whole and how that child's medical condition interacted with the demands of his or her surroundings. The Office of Disability had told examiners that SSI awards were justifiable in the case of three moderate impairments as long as they were "three good, solid moderates." But the office was reluctant to make this a bright-line rule; it cautioned examiners that this was a "general guideline, not a firm rule." Instead, it encouraged examiners to take a "step back" and consider whether "other possible combinations of ratings, such as two strong moderates" might meet SSI's overall standard of disability once the individual child's circumstances were taken into account.[140] But this only reintroduced the subjectivity that the SSA had hoped to remove with clear guidelines.

As the SSA's troubles with the IFA illustrate, mental disorders such as ADHD posed irreconcilable problems for a disability determination system that sought to provide an individualized evaluation of each person's functioning but still hold the line on benefits or services granted. This was the concern that split disability groups like the CEC from CHADD during the debate over adding ADHD to the IDEA's list of qualifying impairments. The dispute over whether administrators could contain the growth in special education focused on administrators' inability to accurately measure and evaluate behavioral or learning impairments. Clinicians could engage in comprehensive evaluations of children and apply diagnostic criteria rigorously if they chose. But there was nothing in the IDEA's rules that required doctors to follow the diagnostic criteria contained in DSM-IV (which superseded DSM-III in 1994), much less apply them in an exacting manner. To the contrary, studies of pediatricians found that they were not strictly abiding by DSM when diagnosing patients, preferring instead to rely on holistic assessments and intuitive judgment, much like SSA's examiners felt compelled to do when evaluating children for SSI.[141] In addition, sociological studies showed that clinicians were more likely to err on the side of "false positives" (decreeing a healthy person sick) rather than "false negatives" (finding a sick person well), making them unreliable agents of restraint.[142]

Similarly, evidence showed that professionals from outside the field of medicine varied when using the diagnostic criteria, if they used them at all. For example, when epidemiologists tried to identify children with ADHD, they tended to fall back on symptom-based measures divorced from other criteria (such as age of onset) that might limit the number of children identified. This led to widely varying estimates of the number of children who could become eligible for special education should Congress make ADHD a stand-alone listing.[143] Indeed, during debate over reforming the IDEA, congressional investigators reported to lawmakers that depending on the criteria used to identify children, as many as 3% to 5% of all school-age children have ADHD. Other estimates ranged as high as 10%.[144] Other efforts to determine the precise number of children with ADHD who were in special education were, by the researchers' own admission, "fraught with potential error."[145] Thus, the variations in estimates made it difficult for lawmakers to anticipate how much changing IDEA to explicitly include students with ADHD would affect special education costs.

Without strict diagnostic barriers in place, the only remaining screen was the functional standard that the child's impairment be severe enough to adversely affect school performance. But this merely raised anew questions about what distinguished medical impairments from common childhood struggles. In the case of a learning or behavioral impairment, such as ADHD, the functional standard is redundant with the diagnosis; a significant part of a child's diagnosis is based on his or her poor functioning in school. Opponents of creating a stand-alone listing for ADHD simply did not believe that doctors or program administrators could prevent struggling, though not medically impaired, children from receiving services. A special education official for the Department of Education voiced this concern when he argued that listing ADHD as a separate impairment "may result in the inclusion of some children who may have learning problems, but who do not have disabilities."[146]

In sum, while DSM-III was the foundation for reform efforts to expand children's disability programs, and while a comprehensive examination of children using a rigorous application of all the DSM criteria might limit the number of children identified with the disorder, in the real world of clinical practice, busy classrooms, and financially strapped families, DSM was only a starting point. Clinicians, like disability examiners, perhaps even teachers and school officials, were likely to take a holistic and intuitive view of a child's problems, one that collapses clinical symptoms with functioning, and medical conditions with environmental and social circumstances.

While the failure to abide by DSM is disconcerting, it is also understandable. For disability examiners, program administrators, teachers, school officials, and parents, the overriding concern may not be what a child's specific diagnosis is but the fact that there is a diagnosis of something. This makes the task of the disability examiner fundamentally different from the task of the clinician, who seeks a specific diagnosis in order to determine treatment. For the disability examiner, however, it does not matter what the diagnosis is so long as there is one; all diagnoses, regardless of what they are for, open the door to services, accommodations, and benefits. Thus, for example, SSA's disability examiners do not attempt to make awards and classify children according to which impairment is most responsible for the child's disability. Instead, they code children according to which impairment is the easiest to develop a medical record for, because in the end, the result is the same: If found eligible, the child will receive disability payments. Those payments are adjusted for his or her family's income but not for the nature and severity of the child's impairment.[147] Likewise, in the area of special education, high rates of comorbidity between ADHD and learning and conduct disorders make it difficult to determine the precise diagnosis of children classified under specific learning disabilities, emotional disturbance, and other health impairment.[148] In addition, in the case of ADHD and learning disabilities, precise diagnosis did not necessarily influence accommodations made at school. Contrary to CHADD's assertions during congressional debate that children with ADHD need tailored services, studies have found that students with ADHD tend to benefit from educational interventions that are not markedly different from those that benefit children with other learning and behavioral problems.[149] As a result, what specific disorder a child has (whether it is ADHD or learning disability or both, for instance) makes little difference when one is determining services and benefits rather than medical treatment.

## Underdiagnosing and Overdiagnosing

Despite the dramatic increase in the number of children with learning and behavioral problems who enrolled in SSI and special education during the 1990s, there should be little reason for alarm if program expansion represented government policy finally recognizing the vast unmet needs of children suffering from a legitimate medical dysfunction. Given how prevalent learning disabilities and behavioral problems are among poor and low-income children, the growth in SSI following *Zebley* is to be expected.[150] As one SSA official later explained, given the restrictiveness of disability rules in the past, and the aggressive outreach campaigns the SSA and children's and mental health advocacy groups launched in the wake of *Zebley*, it should have come as no surprise that there would be a huge influx of children with mental disabilities into SSI. "It was more surprising," the official argued, "that there were times when we had only a quarter of a million kids on the rolls."[151]

Like SSI payments, the accommodations and services provided under IDEA assist a large number of needy schoolchildren. In 2000, there were approximately 50.1 million elementary and secondary school students; the IDEA enrolled 5.7 million, or roughly 10%, of these children.[152] Studies find that students who receive help through the IDEA have a host of social disadvantages that can complicate their medical impairments. Compared to young people in the general population, adolescents receiving special education services are more likely to live in a single-parent household (one-third compared to roughly one-quarter for the general population), come from a household in which the family head lacked a high school education (22% compared to 13%), and live in a household with an annual income of less than $25,000.[153] The expansion of the IDEA in the 1990s, therefore, is the result not simply of schools labeling children to take advantage of federal funds but of services expanding to underserved communities. The outreach that states conducted following the Department of Education's 1991 memorandum is especially important given the lack of awareness of ADHD among some disadvantaged groups. Indeed, studies of ADHD in poor, urban, and minority communities found that parents and educators were more likely to attribute children's shortcomings to individual failings or social factors rather than to children's medical conditions, hardly a case of parents and schools succumbing to "perverse" incentives to label children.[154]

The story, however, may be different for disability accommodations that students receive through the ADA. In this case, such policies may encourage the overidentification of learning disabilities and disorders like ADHD among students who are relatively advantaged to begin with, are knowledgeable about the legal mandates for disability accommodations, and face strong competitive pressures to succeed. Take, for instance, college-bound students taking standardized entrance exams such as the SAT. A study conducted by the Los Angeles Times in 2000 found that the number of students requesting additional time to take the SAT because of a learning disability had increased by more than 50% in recent years.[155] Yet the typical student who asked for an accommodation was a rather privileged individual. He was white and male and came from a family with annual earnings of more than $100,000. He was also likely to come from an elite private or public school in one of the affluent suburbs along the Boston–Washington, D.C., corridor.[156] In contrast, students who one would think would be most in need of disability accommodations were the least likely to get them. Although learning problems are prevalent among poor and low-income children, the Los Angeles Times study found that not one of the 1,439 students from Los Angeles's 10 inner-city high schools received any extended time to take the SAT.[157]

## Medicaid: How Policy Changes Lead to Increased
## Stimulant Use among the Poor

As SSI and the IDEA expanded to serve more children with mental disorders, Medicaid, the nation's health insurance program for the poor, grew to serve more children, a move that provided millions of low-income children with behavioral and learning disorders access to medical treatment for their conditions. Medicaid expansion took place in the late 1980s as part of a broad bipartisan congressional initiative to expand social welfare benefits to the "deserving" poor.[158] Representative Henry Waxman (D-CA) led efforts to extend Medicaid coverage to pregnant women and young children, while in the Senate, Republicans John Chaffee (R-RI) and John Heinz (R-PA) sought to expand SSI and health care to needy children and their families.[159] In addition, after Clinton agreed to cuts to SSI in 1996, he urged congressional Republicans to extend health-care coverage to low-income children, including the children who would otherwise lose Medicaid coverage when they were dropped from AFDC and SSI as a result of welfare reform. In response, Congress "grandfathered" former SSI children into Medicaid as part of the 1997 Balanced Budget Act, a law that also created the State Children's Health Insurance Program, which provided states with $40 million through 2007 to expand public health care coverage to low-income children not otherwise eligible for Medicaid.[160]

As lawmakers enacted these expansions to public health insurance, ADHD and stimulants were far from their minds, and yet these policy reforms had a dramatic effect on the ability of low-income children to access prescription medication. Between 1991 and 2001, Medicaid spending for prescription drugs increased by more than fivefold, from $4.7 billion to $24.1 billion, and a large share of the growth was driven by spending for psychotropic medications, which grew by more than tenfold, from $0.6 billion to $6.7 billion.[161] Spending increases for stimulants were also striking. Over the same time period, after controlling for inflation, Medicaid's expenditures for stimulants per enrollee grew ninefold, while the number of prescriptions for children covered by Medicaid grew sixfold.[162] In recent years, state officials have tried to curb Medicaid spending by switching from fee-for-service to managed-care health insurance coverage, especially for mental health services. In turn, however, managed-care plans that cover mental health services

*Table 5.2* Characteristics of patient population diagnosed with ADHD, 1991–2000 (in percent)

|  | 1991 | 1993 | 1995 | 1997 | 1999 | 2000 |
|---|---|---|---|---|---|---|
| *Patient age* | | | | | | |
| 2 years and under | 1 | 1 | 1 | 1 | 1 | 0 |
| 3–9 years | 49 | 45 | 49 | 41 | 40 | 40 |
| 10–19 years | 48 | 51 | 50 | 58 | 59 | 60 |
| 19+ years | 2 | 3 | 0 | 0 | 0 | 0 |
| *Physician specialty* | | | | | | |
| Pediatrician | 41 | 42 | 49 | 50 | 53 | 55 |
| Psychiatrist | 36 | 31 | 31 | 25 | 23 | 23 |
| Neurologist | 10 | 8 | 6 | 7 | 6 | 5 |
| Family practice | 5 | 10 | 7 | 12 | 10 | 9 |
| Others combined | 8 | 9 | 7 | 6 | 5 | 8 |
| *Treatment prescribed* | | | | | | |
| Stimulant drugs | 88 | 91 | 93 | 92 | 94 | 93 |
| No stimulant drugs | 12 | 9 | 7 | 8 | 6 | 7 |

*Source:* IMS Health, "National Disease and Therapeutic Index," 1991–2000.

made greater use of pharmaceutical interventions rather than psychotherapy, thus further encouraging the turn toward medication.[163]

The trends in Medicaid matched an overall increase in psychotropic drug prescription among the general population. Studies showed that, in 2000, 62% of children under the age of 18 using outpatient mental health services received psychotropic medications.[164] Between 1996 and 2001, the number of Americans taking prescription drugs for mental disorders grew by 5.5 million.[165] Prescription drug spending grew by an average annual rate of 20%, an increase fueled by more individuals using prescriptions, the switch to newer and costlier medications, and general inflation.[166]

Table 5.2 illustrates the results of these far-reaching transformations in children's disability policy, Medicaid, and (as discussed in Chapter 4) health-care financing. In 1991, nearly half the children diagnosed with ADHD had been seen by a specialist (a neurologist or psychiatrist). But by the end of the decade, less than one-third (28%) of children had been diagnosed in this manner. Instead, almost three-quarters of children with ADHD were being diagnosed by pediatricians, family practitioners, or some other physician whose specialty was not mental disorders. While the DSM-III and later editions of the diagnostic manual were developed to make the identification of disorders such as ADHD more reliable, the diagnostic criteria are difficult to apply in the real world, especially when a large share of the physicians using the DSM are general practitioners not specifically trained in the diagnosis and treatment of mental disorders.

## Conclusion

It is too simplistic, therefore, to conclude, as the media and social conservatives did in the mid- and late 1990s, that SSI and the IDEA encouraged parents and teachers to label children with ADHD. While the two programs may play some role in the growth of ADHD, that role is difficult to quantify with any precision. Program administrators do not make thorough diagnostic examinations (though this does not mean that the children are not disabled in some way), nor do the SSA and Department of Education use impairment classifications that correspond to diagnostic labels. They are in the business of identifying impairments, not illnesses. Nevertheless, in an effort to provide benefits and services to needy children, program administrators may have inadvertently contributed to the growth of ADHD by using the disorder as a residual category, a handy place to put children until clinicians, educators, and parents can better determine how to best assist them. These actors are not responding to incentives so much as they are struggling to fit needy children into the classifications and categories that policy provides. Without a medical diagnosis, the child simply cannot access assistance.

Medicalizing academic and social problems is not an ideal approach to the problems that plague many of the children enrolled in SSI and the IDEA, especially for the children labeled with ADHD, who are influenced more by social and environmental factors than by their inherent medical condition. But the compunction to do so is understandable. Indeed, this is an old dilemma. In the 1970s, antipoverty advocates asked SSA officials to loosen the definition of disability and fold into the determination process an assessment of social factors in recognition of the fact that poor people, even if not physically or mentally incapable of work, are often not able to secure a remunerative job because of inadequate job skills, disorganized living and family arrangements, and lack of education. In response, one SSA official asked "whether a disability 'oriented' approach is really the way to deal with the underlying problem" of poverty and social disadvantage. He explained further,

> Is the basic problem . . . an unrealistic assessment of their medical conditions and the effect on their lives, or is it basically the fact that there are a

group of socially disadvantaged or disoriented people who . . . find themselves in a state of dependency which must be dealt with as a matter of policy? If . . . it really is the latter situation which prevails, then isn't trying to bring these people under the umbrella of a "disability" program really attempting to solve a problem with the wrong tool and shouldn't efforts be made to deal with the problem more directly?[167]

To the extent that families still lack social support and disability programs are the only way they can obtain them for their children, parents and program administrators alike will face pressure to apply diagnostic labels liberally.

The reasons behind the growth in the number of children with learning and behavioral disorders in SSI and the IDEA, therefore, are complex. While policy changes that opened benefits and services to children with disabilities probably encouraged parents to have their children diagnosed so that they could apply for benefits, it is also the case that many of these children and their families legitimately needed the help. We might regard Lisa T. as a "welfare cheat" because she signed her son up for SSI even though she did not regard him as disabled. But we might also applaud her as a mother who endeavors to secure assistance for her son, who is clearly troubled, the only way she knows how—through disability programs. Moreover, policy was not the only cause of ADHD's growth. In fact, the increasing number of children enrolled in SSI and the IDEA and the growing numbers of children diagnosed with ADHD and similar learning and behavioral disorders are attributable to the same larger social and political forces, namely, changes to the criteria used to diagnose ADHD that may have contributed to a more expansive definition of the disorder; the declining stigma associated with being a child with a disability; and a growing awareness of such disabilities among parents, educators, clinicians, and children's advocates. Not all of these transformations—in particular, society's more accepting attitude toward disability and increasing understanding of mental disorders—are negative. Yet as Chapter 6 explains, the uproar over behaviorally troubled children in SSI was merely a prelude to the much larger controversy over ADHD and stimulants that arose in the mid- and late 1990s.

# CHAPTER SIX

# The Backlash against ADHD and Stimulants

If your child is running the show at your house, your problem isn't that he or she is sick. It's that you are too lenient . . . [M]any kids misbehave because they can get away with it. These kids are not hyperactive or conduct disordered—they're spoiled. Put them in a situation where they can't get away with being brats, and their brain dysfunction miraculously vanishes.

—SYDNEY WALKER, *THE HYPERACTIVITY HOAX*, 1999

Parents want their kids to excel in school, and they've heard about the illegal use of stimulants such as Ritalin and Adderall for "academic doping." Hoping to obtain the drugs legally, they pressure pediatricians for them. Some even request the drugs after openly admitting they don't believe their child has ADHD . . . And some pill-eager parents aren't just seeking to level the playing field, they're trying to make their kids superstars.

—VICTORIA CLAYTON, "SEEKING STRAIGHT A'S, PARENTS PUSH FOR PILLS," MSNBC, 2006

As a result of our daughter's label, I have struggled with the ambiguity of my own guilt, my desire for some way (any way) to help our child, my cynicism about the "nature" of her problems, my hope for a so-lution to them regardless of their etiology, and my de-spair at finding none that fully satisfies . . . At times, I have complied with the label, at others I have resisted the psychiatric and educational strategies that were os-tensibly designed to help her. Throughout, I have been guided by a desire to protect her while acknowledging that what I do has the potential to do her harm . . . I would be lying if I said it has been easy.

—CLAUDIA MALACRIDA, *COLD COMFORT*, 2003

The controversy over children with behavioral and learning problems receiving SSI benefits or disability accommodations was a prelude to a much wider debate over the diagnosis and medication of children with mental disorders in general. By the mid-1990s, critics voiced three concerns about ADHD and Ritalin. First, more fanatical critics tied to the antipsychiatry movement of the 1970s questioned whether ADHD was a valid medical disorder at all. Their objections were not confined to ADHD but related to their belief that there was no such thing as a mental illness, that the concept was entirely a social construct. Second, these same critics questioned whether any psychotropic drug, stimulants included, had therapeutic value and could be administered safely at any dose. Third, more moderate critics raised questions about the overidentification of children with ADHD and the overuse of stimulant medication. Thus, even though these critics believed that ADHD was a valid mental disorder and that stimulants were a valuable part of treatment, they nevertheless expressed unease about the large numbers of children labeled with ADHD and taking prescription drugs.

Sorting fact from fiction during the public debates over ADHD and stimulant use was complicated by the divisiveness of the topic. Disagreements over ADHD and stimulants were not just about ADHD and stimulants; they also involved people's views on a wide range of vexing social and political issues: drug abuse, government regulation of consumer products, the role of for-profit companies in humanitarian endeavors such as medicine, the ability of the state to override parental authority, and the ability of the nation's schools to meet the needs of children, especially young boys. The fact that so many of the participants in the debate—clinical researchers, pharmaceutical companies, and purveyors of alternative treatments—had material stakes in how the dispute was resolved served to complicate matters for parents struggling to choose the proper course of treatment for their children's social and academic woes.

## Who Were the Opponents and Supporters of Medicating Children?

The critiques ADHD's detractors articulated were not based on new knowledge of the disorder or stimulants; they were instead a reprise of criticisms that had been around since the antipsychiatry movement of the late 1960s and the 1970s, which drew from the works of Thomas Szasz and adherents of "labeling theory," and the political ideology of the patients' rights movement. In his 1961 landmark book, *The Myth of Mental Illness*, Szasz gave voice to today's contemporary criticism that psychiatry "medicalizes" common human foibles and shortcomings. Mental illnesses, he claimed, were not illnesses at all but instead were behaviors rooted in the conflicts endemic to human relationships; they represented individuals' attempts to deal with common problems with living. Society found these conflicts troubling but dealt with them by pathologizing them so as to justify therapeutic intervention.[1] Borrowing from Szasz's critique of psychiatry, sociologists who worked with labeling theory, most notably Thomas Scheff, further undermined the medical underpinnings of mental illness. Scheff argued that mental illnesses were not pathological diseases, but labels society used to control people who deviated from social conventions. These labels, once given, justified intrusions into the individual's autonomy that citizens would otherwise find intolerable, including involuntary commitment, compulsory medication, and indefinite confinement in a mental hospital.[2] Thus, according to proponents of labeling theory, the real harm to an individual was not an internal pathogen or a physiological or anatomical abnormality, but the individuals in authority whom society had empowered to label (that is, diagnose) and treat the "mentally ill."[3]

Labeling theory offered the budding patients' rights movement much to support activists' contentions that psychiatry was a form of political oppression rather than a scientific and humane endeavor. In his 1972 book, *Prisoners of Psychiatry*, Bruce Ennis, a lawyer affiliated with the Mental Health Law Project and the American Civil Liberties Union, laid the intellectual foundations of the patients' rights movement in language that sounded reminiscent of Szasz and Scheff. (In fact, Szasz wrote the book's preface.) Psychiatry, Ennis asserted, was the majority's instrument to "tame our rebellious youth, rid ourselves of doddering parents, or clear the streets of the offensive poor." Psychiatry was not a therapeutic profession but a device for stripping individuals of their rights and sending them to mental hospitals where "sick people get sicker and sane people go mad." Therefore, Ennis argued, the goal of patients' rights reformers should be to empower mental patients with legal rights that prevented physicians from having complete control of their lives.[4]

By the 1990s, labeling theory had faded into scholarly obscurity, but its critique of psychiatric medicine was resurrected with the anti-Ritalin crusade. The most extreme of the critics denied that ADHD was a medical disorder, attributing its symptoms instead to a host of environmental, social, or dietary causes. Richard DeGrandpre's *Ritalin Nation*, for instance, argued that children's hyperactivity and inattentiveness were the result of their living in a competitive, fast-paced, and media-saturated world.[5] Sydney Walker's *The Hyperactive Hoax*, in contrast, blamed parents' lack of discipline for ADHD.[6] Mary Ann Block, an osteopathic healer whose clinic promoted "natural" alternatives to drug therapy, published two books—*No More Ritalin* and *No More ADHD*. She attributed ADHD to children's intolerance for certain foods and a host of vague biological abnormalities, including low blood sugar and undetected thyroid conditions.[7] Similarly, Thomas Armstrong's *The Myth of the ADD Child* and Fred Baughman's *The ADHD Fraud* denied that ADHD was a disorder of biological and neurological origin.[8] Divorced from the mainstream medical community, these authors simply restated the same critiques about hyperactivity, inattentiveness, and Ritalin that had been floating around for decades, and all of them urged parents to think twice before accepting a diagnosis of ADHD and placing a child on medication.

Certainly one of the more prolific of the critics was Peter Breggin, a psychiatrist by training whom *Forbes* magazine in 2001 credited with "almost single-handedly reenergizing the anti-Ritalin contingent."[9] Allied with the antipsychiatry movement, Breggin as early as the late 1960s questioned the biological model of mental illness and psychiatric practices such as involuntary commitment, psychotropic medications, and electroshock therapy.[10] In the 1990s, Breggin questioned the safety of the new SSRI antidepressants with books such as *Toxic Psychiatry* and *Talking Back to Prozac*. After taking on depression, Breggin made a name for himself as an outspoken critic of ADHD and Ritalin with dozens of articles on the subject and two books written for a popular audience, *Talking Back to Ritalin* and *The Ritalin Fact Book: What Your Doctor Won't Tell You*.[11] In his works, Breggin repeated the assertions that surface again and again in the arguments of the skeptics, including the claims that ADHD is not a real medical condition, that the disorder is the creation of overstressed parents and teachers who cannot deal with normal childhood willfulness, that Ritalin predisposes a child to future drug abuse, and that stimulants have dangerous side effects, such as growth retardation and irreversible brain damage. Summing up his views in *Talking Back to Ritalin*, Breggin wrote, "The notion of a biochemical imbalance in the brain of children diagnosed with ADHD is wild speculation . . . Diagnosing a child with ADHD is basically harmful and should never be done. Its main purpose is to justify the use of drugs." It would be, he argued, "unethical and illegal in a society that truly valued its children."[12]

Also active in the anti-Ritalin campaign in the 1990s were the Church of Scientology and its front organization, the Citizens' Commission on Human Rights (CCHR). Scientologists retooled their long-standing critique of psychiatry into a new message to fit the growing use of psychotropic medications in children. For instance, on its new Web site, FightForKids.org, the CCHR claimed that it was devoting itself to educating "loving parents" so that they could "prevail in the face of the enormous 'drug children now' pressures so entrenched in society today."[13]

Though the Church of Scientology has long been active in the antipsychiatry movement, many opponents of Ritalin sought to distance themselves from Scientology because of its reputation as a cult and a fringe organization. Breggin is one example. His views echo those of Scientologists, and he has acknowledged having worked with the Church of Scientology in the early 1970s. Breggin is adamant, however, that today he is no longer affiliated with the group. In fact, he has charged that rumors linking him to Scientology were part of a smear campaign orchestrated by Eli Lilly, the maker of Prozac, to punish him for his work with lawyers representing patients allegedly harmed by the company's drugs.[14] Thus, even the most extreme voices in the ADHD debate by no means form a united front; what they share, though, is a profound distrust of psychiatry and psychotropic medications.

In the 1990s, two new groups rose to the fore in the anti-Ritalin movement: aggrieved parents and social conservatives. The first of the parent groups was Parents against Ritalin, founded in 1995 by Debra Jones of Claremore, Oklahoma. Jones claimed that she started her organization after a friend was pressured by a North Carolina school district to put her son on Ritalin. Parents against Ritalin, however, came under scrutiny and disbanded after it became public that Jones worked as a distributor for Enrich International, a company that marketed the herbal supplement ephedra as a "natural" alternative to Ritalin.[15] Several years later, in 2001, Patricia Weathers and Sheila Matthews, two mothers who had contested their sons' ADHD diagnoses, founded Ablechild, an organization that opposes the labeling and medication of children.[16] Meanwhile, Lawrence and Kelly Smith launched the National Alliance against Mandated Mental Health Screening and Psychiatric Drugging of Children after their 14-year-old son, Matthew, died suddenly in 2000, allegedly from heart damage caused by Ritalin.[17] The organization is dedicated to bringing together mothers and fathers who believe that school officials pressured them into placing their children on stimulants after falsely labeling them with a learning or behavioral disorder. The national alliance functions as part political lobby, part tribute and support group. Its Web site—RitalinDeath.com—features the pictures and personal stories of a dozen boys and girls like Matthew Smith, that is, boys and girls who, parents believe, died from the toxic effects of Ritalin and other medications used to treated ADHD.[18]

Conservatives also mobilized against ADHD and Ritalin. What had started out as a critique of SSI and IDEA had grown by the late 1990s into a full-scale attack on the use of Ritalin, which conservatives viewed as a liberal conspiracy to weaken the traditional family and to "drug" children, especially young boys. Antifeminist activist Phyllis Schlafly in particular was a staunch opponent of stimulant use, and she warned that Ritalin was the wedge that would allow government to override parental rights and intrude into the sanctity of the family.[19] In addition, Patti Johnson, Denver's representative on the Colorado State Board of Education, rose to prominence as a vocal critic of the nation's education system, which, she argued, used Ritalin to cover up the failings of corrupt schools and incompetent teachers.[20] Protecting the rights of parents to control the labels educators gave their children and the medical treatment their children received was one area in which anti-Ritalin parents' groups and social conservatives found common cause.

Critics of ADHD and stimulants, therefore, were a varied lot whose doubts about ADHD and stimulants revolved around the validity of the disorder, the ability of clinicians to properly identify children with the disorder, and the safety and effectiveness of stimulants. The most radical of the critics, like Scientologists and Breggin, denied that any mental disorder is a medical condition. Moderate critics of ADHD and stimulants, however, agreed that ADHD was a real medical condition, the result of some biological abnormality, but they were nevertheless concerned about the degree to which childhood behavior had become medicalized. They were also troubled by the possible overidentification of ADHD, the potential overuse of stimulants, and the ever more aggressive tactics pharmaceutical companies used in marketing their products to doctors and consumers.[21]

Behavioral pediatrician Lawrence Diller was perhaps the most widely known of these moderate skeptics. His best-selling 1994 book, *Running on Ritalin*, was a thoughtful rumination on the Ritalin phenomenon, written from the perspective of a doctor with extensive experience treating behaviorally troubled children. In his book, Diller affirmed his belief in the medical validity of ADHD and the need for stimulant medication in some cases for a short period of time, particularly to help a child in imminent danger of academic failure or expulsion from school. However, Diller was deeply troubled by the prospect that parents and teachers—and even some doctors—could come to see stimulants as the sole therapeutic intervention for ADHD when in fact a child's behavioral problems were also usually tied to deep-seated emotional and family troubles. Though he was comfortable prescribing medication as a stopgap measure until a comprehensive multimodal treatment plan could be implemented, Diller explained that he worried that behavioral therapy and family counseling, vital aspects of any child's long-term treatment plan, too often fell by the wayside once a child was placed on stimulants.[22] Yet articulating this moderate position was difficult. In his medical memoir, Diller noted that because he raised the issue of stimulant overuse, when he spoke at public events he felt it necessary to distance himself from the antipsychiatry movement by prefacing his remarks with the introduction "I am not against Ritalin nor am I a member of the Church of Scientology."[23]

The irony of the anti-Ritalin movement is that it occurred at a time of growing evidence that ADHD was a neurologically based disorder and that left untreated, it had devastating effects on a person's well-being. As Chapter 7 explains in greater detail, a growing body of studies confirmed that without medical intervention, children with ADHD did not simply outgrow the problems associated with their disorder. By adulthood, they were at increased risk of depression, drug abuse, failed relationships, and professional disappointment. Furthermore, clinical research showed that stimulants were generally safe and effective (alone or in combination with behavioral intervention). Moreover, pharmaceutical companies had made great strides in developing ADHD medications that were longer lasting and therefore more convenient to administer than Ritalin. Whereas Ritalin's effects wear off in approximately 4 hours, requiring dosing during the middle of the schoolday, new drugs and new preparations of existing drugs (Adderall XR, Metadate CD, and Concerta) require only one dose, and their effects last throughout the day.

Nevertheless, the message that ADHD was real and that medical treatment was imperative was compromised by the close ties between clinical researchers and the pharmaceutical companies that manufactured the drugs under scrutiny.[24] Studies found, for example, that clinical trials sponsored by drug manufacturers (and most trials were financed in this manner) were more likely to declare medication effective than trials conducted without industry backing.[25] As a former editor for the *British Journal of Medicine* noted, one could not blame anyone who questioned the objectivity of medical research given that between two-thirds and three-quarters of the clinical trials published in the major medical journals were financed by drug manufacturers.[26] Troubled by the situation, Richard Horton, editor of the *Lancet*, chided academic medical journals for having "devolved into information laundering operations for the pharmaceutical industry," and former editor of the *Journal of the American Medical Association* Marcia Angell declared that the entire pharmaceutical industry was nothing more than "a marketing machine" with little interest in science or patients' health.[27]

Even advocates for children with ADHD were tainted. Though CHADD sought to serve as an advocate, support group, and information source for families of children with ADHD, the group's credibility was badly damaged when it became evident in 1995 that Ciba-Geigy (now called Novartis), the manufacturer of Ritalin, paid a large share of CHADD's operating expenses. By 2005, donations from pharmaceutical companies totaled almost one-quarter of CHADD's total revenue, casting doubt on the ability of the group to provide unbiased information on stimulant therapy to parents.[28]

By the mid-1990s, therefore, despite the growth in clinical knowledge about ADHD, the position of antipsychiatry critics had barely changed since the 1970s, when Szasz and Scheff argued that mental illnesses were mere social constructs. While there were understandable reasons to be skeptical about the growing numbers of children diagnosed with ADHD and taking stimulants, thoughtful discussion of these trends was precluded by the polarization of the public debate. The divisiveness of the topic intensified once some social conservatives articulated a critique of ADHD that tied the disorder to a larger ideological "culture war."[29] These conservatives saw ADHD as indicative of a society hostile toward men, traditional discipline, the sanctity of the family, and the autonomy of private citizens from state control. Their opposition to ADHD and stimulant use, in other words, extended beyond the disorder and the drugs alone; conservatives were worried about what the increasing prevalence of medicated children said about American society.

Thus, the bitter controversy over ADHD in the late 1990s and early 2000s took place amid a growing wealth of scientific research into the disorder as well as a great deal of misinformation circulating in newspapers, television shows, and popular magazines, and on the Internet. Parents of children with ADHD had to navigate this confusing morass of conflicting claims and conflicts of interest on their own, with little idea of how to evaluate the veracity of what they read or heard. Given some of the more outrageous claims made by antipsychiatry critics, one can hardly blame parents if they felt lost and frightened for their children. Though extreme and few in number, hardened skeptics of stimulant use wielded great influence, launching campaigns against "forced drugging," testifying at congressional hearings, and garnering media attention for their message. They were a powerful countervailing force to the medical community's message that ADHD was a legitimate disorder that could be effectively treated with medication.

## Questions about the Widespread Use of Stimulants

In the 1990s, questions about the availability and safety of Ritalin and other stimulants arose. In arguments reminiscent of those of the 1970s, contemporary anti-Ritalin critics denounced the drug as "kiddie cocaine" and complained that it was too widely distributed and too easily accessible, thus encouraging abuse and "raising kids to be drug addicts."[30] Chapter 7 explores in greater depth the issue of stimulant misuse, but as this chapter explains, concerns about the wide use of stimulants were not confined to extreme anti-Ritalin detractors. Elected officials and federal regulators soon became involved when it became evident that stimulants were being prescribed to very young children. Lawmakers undertook efforts to encourage pediatric drug testing, but this did little to quell concerns that stimulants were being overused.

### Descheduling Ritalin
The dispute over how easily accessible Ritalin should be focused both on the potential for children's misusing the drug and on physicians' practice of prescribing it for children it was not intended to treat. As had been the case with SSI in 1994, the media played a key role in putting abuse of prescription drugs on the public agenda. Beginning in the mid-1990s, journalists began reporting outrageous stories of children misusing Ritalin, snorting it to get high, selling it, or giving it to friends. The *Washington Post* reported the case in Alexandria, Virginia, in 1995, of three students who were expelled for sharing Ritalin with classmates. Meanwhile, that same year, in Bethesda, Maryland, in 1995, a ninth-grader was expelled for offering a friend's pills to

younger students.[31] The problem was not confined to children. Adults were also implicated in the theft and dealing of stimulants. In 2000, *USA Today* reported the story of a principal from Orum, Utah, who was arrested and jailed for stealing Ritalin from his students and replacing the drugs with sugar pills. Meanwhile, in Athens, Georgia, that same year, school employees were asked to submit to urine tests after someone stole nearly 300 Ritalin pills from a locked cabinet at the school.[32] Reporters scouring the nation's colleges and universities found students confessing to wandering the library the night before an exam looking for someone with a Ritalin or Adderall prescription, soliciting or selling Ritalin pills over the campus e-mail system, or mixing stimulants with alcohol to stay up all night partying after a taxing week. A *New York Times* correspondent concluded that while "students in previous eras relied on over-the-counter stimulants like Vivarin, No-Doz, or plain old coffee," among today's students, Ritalin had become the drug of choice.[33]

CHADD cofounder Harvey Parker dismissed the episodes as "isolated incidents" rather than evidence of an "epidemic." Such abuse, he contended, was "an unfortunate statement on society, more than on Ritalin itself."[34] Indeed, as Chapter 7 points out, systematic studies found that stimulant misuse was not widespread. But that was beside the point. Perception is what mattered. Just as media allegations of fraud undermined the integrity of the SSI program and opened the door to tightening of the program, so too did the media's relentless focus on stimulant abuse among young adults create the perception that Ritalin was too freely available. Growing concern about the potential for abuse put a stop to CHADD's efforts to loosen government controls on Ritalin.

A shortage of methylphenidate in the fall of 1993 provided an impetus for ADHD advocates to push for relaxing regulations on Ritalin. That year the Department of Justice inadvertently failed to approve Ciba-Geigy's request to produce additional supplies of methylphenidate. Some pharmacies reported running out of Ritalin and its generic counterpart, and some parents claimed to have trouble filling their children's prescriptions. Dr. Wade Horn, a CHADD spokesperson, expressed frustration at the situation: "We have to find a better way of dealing with Ritalin that prevents these shortages. Why make kids go through this?"[35] In 1995, CHADD petitioned the Drug Enforcement Administration (DEA) to reclassify methylphenidate from a Schedule II to a Schedule III drug. Schedule II is the DEA classification for highly addictive drugs that can remain legal, albeit with tight restrictions on use. The move to Schedule

III classification would have lifted government limits on the annual production of Ritalin and made it easier for doctors to prescribe the drug by eliminating the need for patients to schedule office visits to obtain a refill. Several respected professional organizations in pediatric and psychiatric medicine, including the American Academy of Pediatrics, the American Academy of Neurology, the American Academy of Child and Adolescent Psychiatry, and the American Psychological Association, supported CHADD's petition.[36]

Before the DEA could respond, however, a series of events undermined CHADD's credibility and, as a result, cast doubt on the wisdom of descheduling Ritalin. In October 1995, the Merrow Report, a show aired on PBS stations, ran a story entitled "Attention Deficit Disorder: A Dubious Diagnosis?" Not only was the story highly critical of the burgeoning number of ADHD cases, but it also revealed that Ciba-Geigy, the manufacturer of Ritalin, had contributed almost $800,000 to CHADD between 1991 and 1994. Although the contributions Ciba-Geigy made were not illegal, they did raise the specter of a conflict of interest, a conflict CHADD failed to disclose to either its members or federal drug regulators. Ciba-Geigy did not help matters for CHADD when a company executive characterized the organization to the Merrow Report as the company's "conduit for providing . . . information directly to the patient population."[37] The United Nation's International Narcotics Control Board weighed in, expressing concern that the financial relationship between Ciba-Geigy and CHADD violated the provisions of a 1971 international drug treaty.[38] Meanwhile, the Drug Enforcement Agency noted that it was alarmed by both "the depth of [CHADD's] financial relationship with the manufacturer" of Ritalin and the "abundance of scientific literature which indicates that methylphenidate shares the same abuse potential as other Schedule II stimulants."[39] In 1996, amid a public relations debacle, CHADD withdrew its petition, while Ciba-Geigy issued a letter to doctors reminding them of the potential for Ritalin abuse and asking them to monitor patients' medication use carefully.[40]

*Medicating Toddlers and Preschoolers*
A few years later, a political firestorm erupted over the medicating of toddlers and preschoolers. In February 2000, the *Journal of the American Medical Association* released a study directed by Julie Magno Zito of the University of Maryland, which reported that the number of children ages 2 to 4 taking psychiatric medication had increased markedly

during the 1990s. According to the study, stimulant use in this age group had tripled between 1991 and 1995, while the use of antidepressants had doubled. Overall, the study concluded that as many as 150,000 children, or 1.5% of all preschoolers, were taking stimulants, tranquilizers, antidepressants, or other antipsychotic drugs.[41] This was a small segment of the preschool population. Yet public and elected officials were largely unaware of the practice of prescribing powerful psychotropic medications to such young children prior to the publication of Zito's study. Although many clinicians who worked closely with children knew of the growing use of medication to treat psychiatric problems in the very young, it was a development that took many politicians and policy makers by surprise. (To put these trends in perspective, however, as Table 5.1 illustrates, the children who were taking stimulants in the 1990s were increasingly adolescents, not the young children that stirred up the controversy over the Zito study.)

Zito's study drew attention to several troubling developments that had taken place in pediatric mental health care. First, it became clear that many clinicians were engaging in off-label use of psychotropic drugs. This was because many of the medications children were taking had been designed for and tested on adults. Pharmaceutical companies did not have to conduct pediatric clinical trials for a drug even if children would end up using it. Instead, once a drug was approved, a physician could use it for any patient he deemed fit. Though a pharmaceutical company could conduct pediatric clinical trials for drugs, in the past, the relatively small number of pediatric patients and the limited marketability of pediatric medications led manufacturers to invest little in research into children's drug regimens.[42] As a result, very few of the drugs Zito and her colleagues studied had been approved for use in children under the age of 7, never mind children as young as age 2 or 3. Ritalin, in fact, carried a warning label that specifically cautioned against its use in children under 6 years of age since, according to the label, "safety and efficacy in this age group have not been established."[43]

Furthermore, Zito's study showed that pediatric use of pharmaceutical agents was not confined to Ritalin. The researchers found that young children were taking a host of other drugs, including Prozac, Wellbutrin, or Paxil for depression, anxiety, or aggression, and Zoloft or Luvox to treat obsessive-compulsive disorders. These medications had been developed for an adult market, and until 1997, when Prozac was approved for pediatric use, none had been approved specifically for use in children. At least Ritalin had originally been used for children before migrating to the adult population.[44] Moreover, a follow-up study found that not only were children taking psychotropic drugs at younger ages, but they were taking them for longer periods of time and often in combination with other drugs, either additional psychotropic agents or medications for physical ailments.[45]

Very little was and is known, however, about the use of psychiatric drugs among very young children. For many medications, researchers did not know the proper dosage, the long-term effects of particular medications, or the side effects of taking various drugs in combination. That young children would be given powerful medications about which so little was known troubled critics.[46] Commenting on the results of the Zito study, Dr. Joseph Coyle of Harvard Medical School highlighted the thorny ethical issues raised by administering drugs to very young children. The early years are "a time of extraordinary, unprecedented changes in the brain," Coyle argued. "We have very little information about the long-term impact of treatment with these drugs early in development."[47] More alarmist critics pointed to animal studies suggesting that medications given before puberty could permanently influence brain development.[48] Antipsychiatry critic Peter Breggin claimed, "Stimulants do not 'normalize' the brain; they render it abnormal . . . As a parent, I would be very careful about putting my child on any drug that affects the brain and mind. It's a gamble and we can never be sure of the results."[49] This was an extreme claim, but in the absence of a better understanding of pediatric drug use, it played into the fears of elected officials and the public.

Yet the clinical trials that medical researchers would have liked to conduct to discern the long-term effects of medicating young children were themselves controversial. For instance, in 1998, Dr. Lawrence Greenhill, a child psychiatrist at the Psychiatric Institute in New York City and the author of a landmark study on ADHD in school-age children, proposed research into the effects of Ritalin use among preschoolers. The National Institute of Mental Health (NIMH) agreed to fund the research, but its decision was met with condemnation following the release of Zito's study in the *Journal of the American Medical Association*.[50] Critics who challenged the validity of ADHD feared that Greenhill's clinical trial could end up increasing stimulant use by legitimizing both the disorder and the medication. In fact, Breggin denounced Greenhill's trial as "a tragedy for America's children."[51] Steven Hyman, director of the NIMH, nevertheless defended his agency's decision, arguing that with so many toddlers and preschoolers already taking Ritalin, "we are damnable if we don't do them . . . then every child becomes an uncontrolled experiment of one."[52]

### Efforts to Improve Knowledge of the Effects of Stimulants on Young Children

In response to the ensuing uproar over the results of the Zito study, in March 2000 First Lady Hillary Clinton announced several initiatives to enhance the nation's understanding of psychotropic drug use among children.[53] Clinton's plan included the release of a fact sheet to warn parents and teachers about the risks of Ritalin, Prozac, and other popular psychotropic medications.[54] The NIMH promised to spend $5 million to research the effects of these drugs on children under the age of 7. One of the studies NIMH pledged to fund was Greenhill's research into the long-term effects of stimulant use by preschoolers.[55] (As discussed in Chapter 2, a group of researchers from 6 universities and medical centers, including Greenhill, published the initial findings from the Preschool ADHD Treatment Study [PATS] in November 2006.) Additionally, the Food and Drug Administration (FDA) declared that it would improve the labeling of drugs for young children, and the White House announced the National Conference on the Treatment of Children with Behavioral and Mental Disorders to take place in the fall of 2000—in the eyes of cynics, just in time to coincide with Hillary Clinton's bid for the U.S. Senate seat in New York state.[56]

Clinton's was a moderate approach to the controversies roiling over the medication of children. None of these measures necessarily curbed preschoolers' use of psychotropic medication, but they were meant to encourage parents and professionals who worked with children to be more circumspect about using such powerful drugs on young patients. The measures were also designed to support more research into the effects these drugs had on children.[57] Introducing her initiatives, the First Lady sought to distance herself from the antipsychiatry critics and take a middle-of-the-road position on the issue. She expressed discomfort with the stark increase in the medication of children, particularly in the case of mental disorders, but she also affirmed the need for such drugs in some cases. "We are not here to bash the use of these medications," she noted. But "some of these young people have problems that are symptoms that are nothing more than childhood or adolescence."[58]

The First Lady's efforts were only the first in a long line of initiatives the government pursued to facilitate pediatric pharmaceutical research. In 1993, the FDA issued rules that pushed drug companies to determine and provide basic pediatric dosing information for their products. The agency also established a network of research centers, typically based in university teaching hospitals, that would conduct drug studies among children.[59] In 1997, Congress took these efforts a step further by enacting the Food and Drug Administration Modernization Act, which tightened regulations pertaining to pediatric medications.[60] The law's goal was to encourage drug companies to conduct pediatric tests on both medications that were about to enter the market and drugs that the FDA determined were already being used extensively on children. Under the new law, manufacturers had to provide a pediatric label for any drug that reached a threshold of 50,000 pediatric prescriptions written per year. The FDA Modernization Act also allowed the FDA to require manufacturers whose medications it deemed important to children's health to provide labeling information. The agency quickly developed a list of 450 priority drugs that it wanted more information on; 25 drugs on the FDA's priority list were for psychiatric conditions.[61] Finally, the FDA issued rules calling for manufacturers to submit studies of a drug's effect on children as part of their applications for new drug approvals.[62]

To make these new rules palatable for pharmaceutical manufacturers, the 1997 FDA Modernization Act offered incentives for manufacturers to cooperate with federal drug officials. The most important of these incentives were rules that allowed the FDA to reward companies with an additional 6-month period of patent protection on their pediatric medications if they conducted clinical trials of drugs that would be used on children.[63] These patent extensions could be quite lucrative. The patent extension for Prozac, for example, generated an additional $2 billion in sales for Eli Lilly.[64] Furthermore, even though drug companies were not necessarily required to seek formal approval for many of their products that were already being used by children, they expected approval to boost drug sales substantially. This led many drug companies to seek formal approval for their products even in the absence of government requirements. Eli Lilly, for example, asked the FDA to approve Prozac for patients as young as 7 years of age, and Bristol-Myers Squibb and SmithKline Beecham (now GlaxoSmithKline) began running clinical trials to lay the groundwork for the approval of their antidepressants for use in children.[65] Within a few years of the passage of the FDA Modernization Act, drug companies conducted approximately 300 pediatric clinical studies compared to just three studies prior to the passage of the law.[66] Federal regulators credited the law's incentives for patent extensions with having spurred the additional research, and in 2002, Congress passed the Best Pharmaceuticals for Children Act, reauthorizing the 6-month patent extension for pediatric medications.[67]

## Questions about Regulating Pharmaceutical Companies

For Ritalin's critics, Congress's belated efforts to ensure that pharmaceutical companies were conducting adequate research into the long-term appropriateness and safety of pediatric drugs were far from adequate. Indeed, scandals about prescription drugs pulled from the market once adverse side effects became known cast doubt on the ability of government to regulate effectively the booming pharmaceutical industry. Even as Congress created incentives for drug companies to conduct more research into medications given to children, these companies launched aggressive marketing campaigns promoting Ritalin and a number of new stimulants. In response, anti-Ritalin forces took more drastic measures to rein in the growth of stimulant use, bringing a number of lawsuits that challenged both the validity of ADHD as a true medical disorder and the safety of stimulants.

### Drug Advertising

By the late 1990s and early 2000s, stimulants were big business for the nation's pharmaceutical companies. The story of Shire illustrates how ADHD could transform a drug company's fortunes. In 1994, Shire acquired Rexar Pharmaceuticals and rechristened its diet drug Obetrol, Adderall. The company then asked the FDA to approve Adderall for the treatment of ADHD, which it did in 1996. Overnight, Adderall catapulted Shire from a small-time drug company into a major pharmaceutical giant.[68] Whereas Ritalin had once dominated the marketplace, by 2006 there were more than a half dozen choices available to consumers, including longer-acting stimulants (Adderall XR, Metadate CD, and Concerta) and a nonstimulant medication sold under the brand name Strattera. Drug makers also developed a stimulant that could be delivered through a skin patch rather than a pill. Both the patch and the longer-acting stimulants promised to remove the stigma of frequent dosing that Ritalin necessitated.[69] As a result, Ritalin's market share stagnated after the introduction of long-acting stimulants. Adderall became one of the most popular of the new drugs, eventually securing 25% of the stimulant market. The number of Adderall prescriptions alone grew by an astounding 1,107% between the drug's introduction in 1997 and 2001. By 2006, almost 50 million prescriptions for Adderall and its extended-release version had been written for children and adults.[70]

At the same time that treatment choices for ADHD multiplied, pharmaceutical companies stepped up their marketing campaigns.[71] In 1997, the FDA relaxed rules governing pharmaceutical advertising on television.[72] A few years later, in 2001, several drug companies broke with a 30-year-old voluntary agreement and began marketing ADHD medications directly to consumers, a development that troubled federal drug regulators.[73] In August 2001, Celltech, the manufacturer of Metadate CD, ran a series of print ads in several women's magazines that showed a smiling mother and son under the caption "One dose covers his ADHD for the whole school day." The following month, the makers of Adderall and Concerta ran ads in women's magazines with toll-free numbers that consumers could dial to get more information on ADHD and stimulants. The manufacturer of Concerta supplemented its print campaign with 60-second spots on cable television channels, while Celltech sent to doctors' offices brochures and magnets that featured a superhero with a reference to its drug emblazoned on his chest, a marketing gimmick that critics argued was aimed at children in the waiting room instead of the doctors themselves.[74] Similarly, in 1999, Shire entered into a partnership with CHADD to create a 1-800 hotline staffed by doctors, nurses, and teachers who answered callers' questions about ADHD and stimulant use. Critics viewed the hotline as a thinly veiled attempt to promote Adderall use to the concerned parents who called.[75]

Some critics worried that pharmaceutical manufacturers were targeting their marketing campaigns at the nation's schoolteachers and school nurses.[76] For example, both Shire and Novartis created Web sites for educators, separate from their industry Web sites, which gave information on ADHD and the stimulant treatments available and included advice on how teachers should handle questions about ADHD from parents. In 1997, Novartis teamed up with the National Association of School Nurses to distribute information kits about ADHD and stimulants to 11,000 school nurses, while other companies sponsored and conducted educational programs for teachers. A few drug manufacturers distributed online science education materials with corporate sponsorship, a tactic that medical writer Christine Phillips found especially insidious. Even if these materials did not mention specific brand-name drugs, she argued, "they reinforce the place of the pharmaceutical industry as a benevolent and authoritative presence in the school, much as the provision of branded educational materials to doctors reinforces the position of the pharmaceutical industry within the clinic."[77] On the one hand, these efforts might be viewed as attempts to increase understanding and awareness of ADHD, but as Phillips pointed out, one did not see similar corporate educational efforts on behalf of autism or dyslexia, conditions that "do not have accepted pharmaceutical therapies."[78]

FDA and DEA officials were concerned about the aggressiveness of the pharmaceutical companies' marketing tactics, but they felt hamstrung. Although the FDA monitors drug advertising and requires companies to state the risks of their medications, there was little that government officials felt they could do to stop the direct marketing to consumers. "We don't feel we can legally take action," said one FDA drug official. "We're not the good taste police."[79]

## The Regulation of Drug Safety and the Resurrection of the Ritalin Lawsuits

Should Ritalin be made more easily available? What, if anything, could the government do about the off-label use of prescription psychotropic medications on young children? How should government regulators handle aggressive pharmaceutical marketing tactics? These questions were simply a few of the many that the FDA confronted in the late 1990s and early 2000s—and Ritalin was just one drug. At the same time that FDA, DEA, and NIMH officials struggled with what to do about potential Ritalin overuse, a larger political controversy brewed over the regulation of prescription drugs in general. Policy makers and elected officials were alarmed by media and scientific reports of adverse side effects linked to several popular prescription drugs: heart damage caused by the diet drug combination Fen-Phen, muscle damaged tied to the cholesterol-lowering drug Baycol, and a few years later heightened risk of heart attacks associated with the painkiller Vioxx. For the FDA, the withdrawal of a number of approved prescription drugs from the market after evidence of serious adverse side effects came to light was a public relations disaster, one that badly tarnished the agency's reputation. With some drug safety reviewers and agency heads serving as consultants to pharmaceutical companies and receiving company money for their clinical research, the FDA's detractors argued that agency officials had become so close to the pharmaceutical industry that the FDA could no longer effectively carry out its watchdog role.[80]

Though stimulants had been shown to be safe and effective for the vast majority of children taking them, public concerns about drug safety in general formed the backdrop of critics' attacks on Ritalin. With FDA officials unable or unwilling to rein in pharmaceutical companies, anti-Ritalin forces took matters into their own hands, attempting to accomplish through litigation what they could not accomplish through congressional and administrative lobbying or moral persuasion—the eradication of stimulants from the market. Between 2000 and 2001, entrepreneurial plaintiffs' lawyers filed five class-action lawsuits in Texas, California, New Jersey, Florida, and Puerto Rico against CHADD, the American Psychiatric Association, and Novartis Pharmaceuticals. The lawsuits attempted to break up what critics regarded as a cozy and financially lucrative relationship among advocates, doctors, and business executives. The plaintiffs charged that Novartis had colluded with CHADD and the American Psychiatric Association "to create, develop, promote, and confirm the diagnoses [of ADHD] . . . in a highly successful effort to increase the market for its product Ritalin."[81]

The plaintiffs' attorneys involved in the lawsuits were closely connected to the antipsychiatry movement. For instance, Andy Waters, the attorney who brought the Texas lawsuit, had made a name for himself suing asbestos manufacturers and distributors in the 1980s. He claimed he was motivated to take on Novartis after he read Breggin's book *Talking Back to Ritalin*.[82] Likewise, at the helm of the California and New Jersey lawsuits were John Coale and famed plaintiffs' attorney Richard Scruggs, both of whom had made a fortune in the landmark tobacco settlement between cigarette manufacturers and state attorneys general in 1998.[83] Coale, like Waters, had ties to the anti-Ritalin crusade. In the late 1980s, he had represented LaVarne Parker, a mother who had sued the Atlanta school district, the American Psychiatric Association, and several doctors for $150 million after the Ritalin pills that school officials insisted she give her 10-year-old son allegedly made him hallucinate and contemplate suicide.[84] Breggin served as an expert consultant for the plaintiffs, and Scruggs wrote a laudatory preface in the new edition of *Talking Back to Ritalin*, in which he claimed that reading the book led him to realize that, as had been the case with the tobacco companies, "our vulnerable children were again being targeted for corporate profit."[85]

Although both the Parker lawsuit and the Scientologists' lawsuits of the 1980s were dismissed for lack of merit, Coale, Waters, and Scruggs represented a new breed of plaintiffs' attorneys, more sophisticated and experienced, having honed their skills with the asbestos and tobacco litigation. This time, rather than focusing on the adverse side effects that Ritalin had allegedly caused in a handful of people, like Parker's son, attorneys instead concentrated on attacking the legitimacy of the ADHD diagnosis in the case of most children.[86] Most children on Ritalin, they maintained, were given their diagnosis because of the defendants' continual efforts to promote ADHD and sell Ritalin. "I'm not saying it [ADHD] doesn't exist," Scruggs claimed, but he adamantly maintained that the number of children who were truly sick was much smaller than the number currently taking stimulants.[87] In fact, Scruggs asserted that Big Pharma was even more culpable of wrongdoing than Big Tobacco insofar as the "marketing of stimulants is even more insidious—and ultimately more shrewd and effective" than that of cigarettes. "Stimulants," he observed, "are disguised as 'medicines.' Their imposition on children is called 'treatment.' A 'disorder' has been manipulated to justify their use."[88] The parallel that Scruggs drew between Ritalin and cigarettes was no accident; it was a window into the plaintiffs' legal strategy. As Scruggs later explained, "The turning point in the tobacco litigation was when we showed the tobacco companies were targeting children. And I believe that is going to be the turning point here" with Novartis.[89]

But it was not to be. By 2002, all five of the lawsuits had been either dismissed for lack of merit or withdrawn by the plaintiffs once they realized their cases would not get far.[90] Before long, however, questions about drug safety and the specter of another round of lawsuits loomed on the horizon. Once again, the plaintiffs' bar returned to the issue of adverse side effects, the legal argument that had dominated lawsuits in the late 1980s. Though studies showed that for most children side effects were generally minor, the media and the FDA came to focus on a handful of isolated cases in which children suffered severe reactions allegedly linked to Ritalin. In February 2006, a panel of FDA physicians narrowly voted to recommend a "black box" label for Ritalin, Adderall, and all other drugs used to treat ADHD after reports of sudden death in 19 children and 4 adults who were being treated for the disorder, as well as 54 cases of other cardiac problems, including heart attacks and strokes.[91] The label constituted the strongest possible safety warning the agency can give a drug. In the end, the FDA decided not to issue a black box label because the number of adverse cases was small compared to the millions of adults and children who took stimulants each year and because investigators concluded that the risk of heart problems was not elevated among stimulant users. Moreover, medical professionals, including the members of the American Psychiatric Association and the American Academy of Child and Adolescent Psychiatry, expressed concern that the label could deter patients who needed medication from using it, thus increasing the risk of social and academic failure and later substance abuse (a risk that was much more certain than that of cardiac problems).[92] The FDA's decision did not stop enterprising personal-injury attorneys from wading into the fray, scouring for plaintiffs in order to instigate the third wave of Ritalin class-action lawsuits.[93] To date, however, none of these lawsuits has come to fruition.

## Questions about the Educational Demands Placed on Children

ADHD is a disorder closely tied to a child's performance in the classroom. According to standard diagnostic criteria, a child must exhibit symptoms of hyperactivity, inattentiveness, or impulsiveness in at least two settings, typically at home and at school, in order to qualify. Moreover, the symptoms of ADHD may not become fully evident until a child is placed in a learning environment in which demands on his or her ability to concentrate, pay attention, and keep pace with peers increase.[94] Not surprisingly, teachers may be the first to notice, perhaps even confirm parents' suspicions of, something amiss, making teachers vital partners in efforts to identify and manage children with ADHD.[95] Yet for many of ADHD's detractors, especially conservatives, this is the crux of the problem: Teachers were too eager to label children with ADHD in order to hide their own failings as educators, and schools were compelling parents to place their children on stimulants, whether they liked it or not. While critics focused much of their ire on ADHD, their true animus was against larger social trends, including the decline of the traditional family, the rise of progressive educational pedagogy, and the influence of the liberal feminist movement. ADHD, in other words, was a convenient vehicle for conservatives to attack all that they disliked about modern America. Although some of their claims were rather extreme and based largely on anecdote and hyperbole, they captured media and congressional attention, prompting a movement to curtail the discretion of teachers and school officials in identifying children with ADHD and raising difficult questions about the extent to which schools properly met the needs and abilities of children.

### "Forced Drugging" in the Nation's Schools

One of the first disagreements over Ritalin in the nation's schools erupted over the question of how far school officials could go in encouraging parents to have their children examined for ADHD and, if ADHD was diagnosed, in compelling parents to medicate their children as a condition of school attendance. In 1991, the parents of Casey Jesson, a 12-year-old boy who had been diagnosed with ADHD, won a landmark victory in federal court.[96] In 1985, Casey began taking Ritalin to control his disruptive behavior, but his parents took him off the drug 2 years later, arguing that while on it, he had acted like a "zombie" and had had little appetite, insomnia, and facial twitches. Officials at the Derry Cooperative School District in New Hampshire eventually gave the Jessons an ultimatum: medicate their son or withdraw him from the public school system. The judge in the Derry case admitted that "Casey J. was a disruptive influence not only to himself but to his teachers, classmates and his long suffering parents," and he noted that the school district had "acted with the patience of Job," repeatedly shuffling Casey between special education classes and the mainstream classroom because of his behavioral problems.[97] But still, he ruled in favor of the Jessons. The school, the judge argued, could not insist on medication as a condition for Casey to attend regular classes, and he held that the district had not tried hard enough to meet the individualized needs of a child whose disability should be accommodated instead of automatically medicated.[98]

Soon parents in several states brought lawsuits contesting the "forced drugging"—as Ritalin's critics called the practice—of their children. Not every case worked out as well for the parents as the Jesson case had.[99] In 2000, a family court judge in Albany, New York, ordered the parents of 7-year-old Kyle Carroll to put their son back on ADHD medication or else face charges of educational neglect and loss of parental custody. The Carrolls had given Ritalin to their son after he was diagnosed at the urging of school officials, but they sought to take him off the medication after he began experiencing insomnia and loss of appetite. School officials protested and brought legal action against the Carrolls.[100] Siding with the school district, Kyle Carroll's court appointed guardian adamantly argued at trial, "The child was diagnosed with ADHD, not by the school but by a psychologist, and a medical doctor prescribed Ritalin based on the recommendations of the psychologist." Thus, it was not for the parents to decide "unilaterally . . .

because of their own beliefs" to take their son off the drugs.[101] Parents' groups, however, were outraged. Said one parent advocate, "It is terribly damaging for children for the state to rush in willy-nilly and substitute its judgment for parents in those situations."[102]

A few years later, the story of Patricia Weathers made national news. Testifying before Congress in 2002, Weathers, founder of the parent group Ablechild, recounted how school officials in her hometown of Millbrook, New York, pressured her to place her son on Ritalin.[103] After he became withdrawn and agitated, he was diagnosed with social anxiety disorder and placed on the antidepressant Paxil in addition to Ritalin. Soon he began to hallucinate and hear voices, prompting Weathers to take her son off his medications. When Weathers resisted school entreaties to try alternative drugs, her son was dismissed from class, and school officials threatened to charge Weathers with medical neglect and remove her son from her custody.[104] Almost overnight, the Weathers story became a rallying cry among socially conservative, pro-family groups. Schlafly, for instance, argued in the newsletter for her organization, the Eagle Forum, that compulsory medication was an incursion into the autonomy of the family and the authority of parents. That this heavy-handed state action was sometimes carried out with the help of "activist judges" further fueled her outrage.[105] Academic observers also were troubled by the intrusiveness of school officials. Said one legal commentator, "custodial parents are more likely than the state or its agents faithfully to discover and pursue the child's welfare." Therefore, "the majority ought not substitute its educational judgment for that of the child's custodial parents merely because it disagrees with their reasonable conception of the child's emotional good."[106]

Other isolated accounts of "forced drugging" made newspaper headlines. In fact, the *New York Post* ran an entire series on the issue of forced drugging with a great deal of attention paid to the Carroll and Weathers cases.[107] Nevertheless, it was not clear how widespread the "forced drugging" of children was, and though there was some evidence of isolated incidences, there was no proof that it was common practice.[108] But that did not stop Congress and state governments from jumping on the bandwagon, especially once antipsychiatry parents' groups and conservative organizations mobilized. Several states moved to limit the ability of teachers and other school officials to insist on placing children on psychotropic medications. In November 1999, the Colorado Board of Education passed a resolution urging teachers to use "proven academic and/or classroom management solutions"—that is, traditional forms of discipline—to deal with problem students rather than encouraging parents to place their children on medication.[109] Conservative proponents of the Colorado measure stated that they were reacting both to parents' complaints about teachers insisting on medication and to reports that Eric Harris, one of the gunmen in the Columbine High School shootings in Littleton, Colorado, earlier that year, had been taking the antidepressant Luvox at the time of the massacre.[110] Opponents of the measure objected to the manner in which the resolution, though voluntary, hamstrung teachers. Said one representative of a mental health advocacy organization, "If a child has hearing or vision problems that the teacher identifies, we would expect the teacher to talk to the parents. The same thing for mental health."[111] However, Patti Johnson, the board member who sponsored the resolution, defended the measure. "The resolution does not stop teachers from communicating with parents," she emphasized. "What it does do is stop teachers from giving parents an ultimatum."[112] The Texas State Board of Education followed suit the next year, enacting a resolution that recommended that teachers and parents explore disciplinary measures and behavioral forms of treatment for ADHD before trying medication.[113]

The movement gathered steam, and within a few years, many states had copied Colorado's and Texas's examples, passing even more stringent laws that limited what teachers could say to parents about their children's behavioral troubles.[114] In the summer of 2001, Minnesota became the first state to prevent school or child protection services officials from telling parents that they must treat their children's ADHD with drugs. A few months later, Connecticut went even further, barring teachers and school administrators from discussing any sort of drug treatment with parents. By 2003, 15 states had passed or were considering passing similar laws restricting the ability of school official and teachers to recommend or compel medication for a student's behavioral or academic troubles.[115]

With the controversy over compulsory medication intensifying at the state level, the fight entered national politics.[116] In 2003, Representative Max Burns (R-GA) introduced the Child Medication Safety Act, a bill dedicated to "protecting children and their parents from being coerced into administering psychotropic medication in order to attend school."[117] The bill required states to create procedures that would prevent school officials from compelling a child to take medication as a condition of attending class. A formidable coalition of advocacy and professional groups that included CHADD, the American Academy of

Child and Adolescent Psychiatry, the National Alliance for the Mentally Ill, and the National Mental Health Association lined up against the bill, fearing that it would undermine the "vital role that teachers play in providing observations to diagnosing professionals."[118] The showdown pitted opposition groups such as the CCHR and Ablechild, which questioned the very validity of ADHD, against the mainstream medical establishment, a contrast that ADHD supporters highlighted. "Just remember," said a CHADD spokesperson, "that the Citizens Commission for Human Rights is behind the bill." Pointing out the extreme position of the measure, he noted that the CCHR was affiliated with the Church of Scientology, which "is opposed to children being on any psychiatric medications."[119]

The Child Medication Safety Act sailed through the House of Representatives but stalled in the Senate. There a group of liberal senators led by Edward Kennedy (D-MA) struck a compromise that pared back the bill, which then received bipartisan support in both houses.[120] In explaining its rationale, the House report tried to convey Congress's middle-of-the-road approach. It explained that lawmakers had been made aware of incidents where local educational agency officials had required parents to place children on psychotropic medication in order to attend school or receive services. This they found troubling since "school officials should not presume to know what medication a child needs, or if the child even needs medication." However, noting "the importance of open and effective communication between the parent and school officials (including teachers) regarding the needs of the child as a whole," lawmakers reiterated that they did not intend for their measure to gag teachers either.[121] Thus, the law made clear that it was not intended "to create a Federal prohibition against teachers and other school personnel consulting or sharing classroom-based observations with parents or guardians."[122] The compromise provisions were rolled into the 2004 amendments to the Individuals with Disabilities Education Act, but this meant that their restrictions on school officials extended only to special education students covered by IDEA.

Disappointed, anti-Ritalin forces vowed to try again. Conservative activist Phyllis Schlafly argued that broader protections for all schoolchildren were sorely need in light of the recommendations of President George W. Bush's New Freedom Commission on Mental Health.[123] In a report released in 2003, the New Freedom Commission urged the creation of a comprehensive mental health screening process in the nation's schools.[124] As harmless as it sounded, the screening process,

Schlafly contended, was "part of a larger plan to get more and more people labeled and in the psychiatric system or, as some say, to move children into the psychotherapeutic state . . . That means prescribing more expensive patented antidepressants and psychostimulant drugs such as Ritalin."[125] In response to fears of widespread compulsory medication following the implementation of universal mental health screening, in 2005 Representative John Kline (R-MN) reintroduced the Child Medication Safety Act in the House, this time extending to all children, not just disabled ones, the protections that had become part of the IDEA. At the same time, Representative Ron Paul (R-TX) submitted the Parental Consent Act of 2005, which banned federal funds from being used to create universal or mandatory health screening programs. The bill also barred funds from going to local educational agencies that charged parents who refused a mental health screening for their children with child abuse or educational neglect. Neither bill passed Congress.[126] Thus, while it is not clear that any of these bills would change how most school officials behave (simply because it is not clear how often "forced drugging" occurs), the episode illustrates the deep distrust that some conservatives had for psychiatry, viewing it (as Szasz and labeling theorists had) as an agent of state control over individuals and families.

*Progressive Pedagogy and "Drill-and-Kill" Testing*

In the eyes of some conservative critics of ADHD, the problem of over-medication was not limited to the issue of "forced drugging," but was related instead to recent trends in the educational system, including the demise of traditional pedagogical practices and discipline in the classroom. Summarizing this position, Patti Johnson compared the 1950s to the 1990s. In the 1950s, she argued, "The traditional classroom was expected to be a quiet, well-ordered environment. Desks were arranged so that all students could make eye contact with the teacher, see the demonstrations and read instructions. Students were not permitted to distract or disrupt others. The teacher was presumed to know more than the children, and so gave direct, group instruction." Unfortunately, "progressive educators undermined this approach." In the classroom of today, "desks are arranged in groups. Students cannot see the teacher and so students distract one another . . . Children are passed on to the next grade without learning to read. Discipline is sometimes lax and supervision is casual."[127] Freed from strict discipline and close supervision, children are inattentive and out of control.

Yet rather than enforce discipline, conservatives argued, parents, teachers, and school officials choose to "drug children into compliance." In a 1999 article for the Heritage Foundation's journal, *Policy Review*, Mary Eberstadt summarized this viewpoint. She faulted today's authority figures for being too lazy and too worried about offending children's budding sense of self-esteem to teach children proper behavior. They relied on Ritalin instead of traditional techniques of controlling children. "One day at a time," Eberstadt asserted, "the drug continues to make children do what their parents and teachers either will not or cannot get them to do without it: Sit down, shut up, keep still, and pay attention."[128] Bolstering these claims, critics characterized children taking Ritalin as "zombie-like" and "docile, placid, and conforming."[129]

Other critics made a slightly different claim, arguing that rather than being too lax and too unstructured, schools were too regimented and monotonous.[130] The nature of the curriculum and the demands made on students' attention were beyond the capacities of most children, these critics asserted, and the situation would worsen with the enactment of the No Child Left Behind Act in 2001.[131] No Child Left Behind emerged from the emphasis on standards and accountability following the Department of Education's release in 1983 of *A Nation at Risk*, a landmark report that documented widespread underachievement among American students.[132] In response, during the late 1980s and early 1990s, the federal government encouraged states to toughen the curriculum and create a system for holding students and teachers accountable for meeting high academic standards. Several states implemented high-stakes standardized testing. These tests not only measured student progress but were also used as a benchmark for holding teachers and school districts responsible for students' learning. In states using high-stakes tests, a student's ability to graduate or move on to the next grade, teachers' salaries and bonuses, and school funding levels and autonomy were all tied to how students performed on standardized tests. The policy changes associated with the accountability movement culminated in the enactment of the No Child Left Behind Act, which required all states to erect a system of testing in reading and math and attached penalties to schools that did not meet state and federal performance goals and reporting requirements.[133]

Psychologist Leonard Sax argued that the shift toward high-stakes testing encouraged teachers to use a "drill-and-kill" approach to learning that bored students.[134] Teachers today, Sax argued, spend more time teaching basic skills like reading and mathematics than they do exploring electives like social studies, music, and art—courses that break up the monotony of the school day. Students lose interest in school, and parents and educators suspect ADHD or some other learning deficit.[135] The situation is made worse, critics like Schlafly and Johnson argued, when outlets for physical energy like recess are eliminated in order for teachers to spend more time "teaching to the test."[136] In this environment, little wonder that children, especially rambunctious boys, give up on schoolwork, begin to fidget and daydream, and become disruptive. Many children, critics assert, simply do not have the temperament to sit still and concentrate for long periods of time.[137] Thus, rates of ADHD diagnosis increased during the 1990s not because of new psychiatric and neuroscience knowledge but because more demands were placed on children than in the past. These allegations are difficult to substantiate, but what is clear is that there is little indication that this situation will change soon. Instead, in the wake of No Child Left Behind, students today are compelled to spend more time than ever in the classroom at their desks, their heads buried in practice drills for tests.[138]

## An Intolerance for Boys?

Some conservative commentators saw boys as bearing the brunt of the increasing regimentation and moral permissiveness of the nation's public schools. Without the structure provided by authoritarian discipline or outlets for their naturally high spirits, Johnson claimed, boys fared poorly.[139] In addition, pointing to statistics showing that boys were four times more likely to be diagnosed with ADHD than girls, conservative critics viewed the disorder as a sign of America's growing intolerance for "male" traits, such as aggression, recklessness, and intrepidness. Rather than openly disparaging male traits, modern society, they argued, preferred to pathologize undesirable characteristics and then eradicate them using medication.[140] ADHD, therefore, served as a convenient staging ground for conservative attacks on liberal feminism and society's supposed neglect of boys.[141]

Under the surface of discussions of ADHD's symptoms, some conservatives saw an insidious plot to "feminize" men starting at a young age. Columnist Thomas Sowell observed, "The motto used to be: 'Boys will be boys.' Today, the motto seems to be: 'Boys will be medicated.'" He called the increase in ADHD diagnosis part of a vast social conspiracy to alter natural male traits through "repression, re-education, and Ritalin."[142] Similarly, conservative intellectual Francis Fukuyama observed "a disconcerting symmetry between Prozac and Ritalin." While Prozac gave "depressed women lacking in self-esteem . . . the alpha-male feeling that comes with high serotonin levels," Ritalin targeted "young boys who do not want to sit still in class because nature never designed them to behave that way." The two drugs working in concert, Fukuyama predicted, would lead to "that androgynous median personality, self-satisfied and socially compliant, that is the current politically correct outcome in American society."[143] To some conservatives, therefore, ADHD was merely an excuse concocted by liberals to justify efforts to socially reengineer young boys to fit the feminist ideal of behavior. If boys could not be taught to be compliant, cooperative, and quiet, then Ritalin would make them so.[144]

The backlash against the diagnosis of ADHD in boys was only a small part of a larger political movement that sought to balance, perhaps even counter, gains made by feminist education reformers, who had argued in the 1970s and 1980s that girls were being shortchanged by the American school system.[145] Citing evidence that girls lagged boys in academic performance as they reached advanced grades, feminist reformers had called for changes in curricula and teaching methods that would make the classroom more amenable to girls.[146] In reaction, critics who regarded the high rates of ADHD diagnosis among boys as the result of overidentification drew from the research of a handful of social scientists studying the psychology of boyhood. Citing the works of Dan Kindlon, Michael Thomson, William Pollack, and Michael Gurian, boy-oriented reformers called for renewed attention to the attributes of boys and the problems boys faced in modern America.[147] In the late 1990s, a rash of violent school shootings threw the national spotlight on data showing that boys performed more poorly in school than girls and were more likely than girls to drop out of high school and college, commit suicide, or suffer from emotional disturbances, learning disabilities, and of course behavioral disorders such as ADHD. Media reports began questioning whether "Boys Lost Out to Girl Power," or whether society's demands and expectations had created "The Debilitating Malady Called Boyhood" by failing to value or respond to the unique characteristics of boys.[148] Using a vivid metaphor, one child specialist reflecting on the current social climate toward boys noted, "There is now an attempt to pathologize what was once considered the normal range of behavior of boys. Today, Tom Sawyer and Huckleberry Finn surely would have been diagnosed with both conduct disorder and ADHD."[149] Not all of the boy advocates were anti-Ritalin critics, but the prevalence of ADHD among male schoolchildren was an indication to these advocates that something was amiss.

In a 2005 article published in the conservative magazine *National Review*, George Gilder summed up the thoughts of some conservative intellectuals when he claimed that boys were underachieving because schools did not meet their needs or speak to their interests. He argued that young men were intentionally shunning education because schools, especially universities, were so feminized that no "self-respecting boy" would want to attend them.[150] Though Gilder lacked empirical support for his claims, he found a receptive audience as advocates for boys sought to redesign schools around the needs of boys, countering what they viewed as a feminist agenda that had swung too far toward the needs of girls. Advocates pushed for single-sex schools or classes, all-boy activities like scouting, and more awareness on the part of teachers for the ways that boys learn differently from girls. They recommended that teachers provide more opportunities for recess and spend more time reading adventure or sports stories or engaging in physical activities, all of which tend to interest boys more than girls.[151] Other critics called for more structure and discipline in the classroom as well as the return of the authoritarian teacher and competitive rather than cooperative learning.[152] The push for these sorts of "boy-oriented" initiatives extended beyond a concern for ADHD alone; these measures represented the extent to which some critics of education feared that the nation's schools had become so vigilant about achievement among girls that they had become indifferent, if not hostile, toward boys and their needs.[153]

But beyond generating perhaps some public awareness of the unique attributes of boys, it is hard to discern what effect if any this boy-centered intellectual movement and the much narrower conservative attack on ADHD and feminism have had on the nation's educational system.[154] Despite the documented problems of boys, there was little evidence that boys were systematically disadvantaged in school. In fact, some experts argued, it was not the case that boys were doing worse in school relative to their achievement in the past, but that girls were narrowing the gap with boys.[155] Moreover, many of the reforms that advocates for boys urged on schools sounded reminiscent of turn-of-the-century fears that urbanization and the rise of white-collar work would lead to the feminization of young boys. In other words, they sounded like reactions against the dislocations of modern life.[156]

Finally, even though conservative critics of ADHD, public education, and feminism raised important questions about the extent to which our nation's schools met the needs of children, boys and girls, their attack on the validity of the disorder is itself an extreme claim among conservatives. Indeed, some prominent conservatives, even those who are rather critical of both public education and feminism, flat-out rejected any link between the school environment and ADHD in boys. For example, the most cogent expression of the argument that schools and society have become hostile toward boys is Christina Hoff Sommers's book, *The War against Boys*, which was widely cited by conservative skeptics of the ADHD phenomenon.[157] But nowhere in her book does Sommers cite ADHD as part of the feminist conspiracy against boys. "Originally I was going to have a chapter on it," Sommers explained in an interview. "It seemed to fit the thesis." She changed her mind, however, after reading the medical literature and meeting boys diagnosed with ADHD.[158] Similarly, psychiatrist and research fellow at the conservative think tank the American Enterprise Institute Sally Satel dismissed objections that ADHD was being overdiagnosed. Satel observed that, at the same time ADHD was likely being overdiagnosed in middle-class communities, it was no doubt being underdiagnosed among poor and working-class children. She further argued that awareness of the disorder meant that today "children suffering from ADHD are much less likely to slip through the cracks."[159] Not surprisingly, then, Sommers and Satel left ADHD out of their 2005 book, *One Nation under Therapy*, an indictment of the contemporary tendency to medicalize common problems of daily life and treat them with pharmaceutical drugs or psychotherapy.[160] Dismissing claims that ADHD was a sham disorder and that Ritalin was a way for parents and teachers to shirk their disciplinary responsibilities, Satel saw the issue differently. She pointed out that Ritalin could enforce responsibility rather than undermine it: "Too many psychologists and psychiatrists focus on allowing patients to justify to themselves their troubling behavior," she explained. "By treating ADHD, you remove an opportunity to explain away bad behavior."[161]

## The Parents' Dilemma

It is easy for casual observers of the growth in Ritalin use to fault parents. As one physician explained to a reporter, "I think parents are genuinely trying to get help for their children. But when they found out that they could get special services and accommodations by getting the diagnosis, they flocked to their physicians. Word spread, and along the way, you also got Ritalin."[162] Another physician concurred, attributing much of the growth of ADHD to the "increasing power and passion on the part of parents, who felt like their children had fallen between the cracks."[163] One journalist went so far as to scold parents for engaging in "academic doping" in order to turn their children into "superstars."[164]

Yet given the polarizing and contentious debates concerning the validity of ADHD and the appropriateness of stimulant therapy, one cannot help but resist these rather simplistic characterizations of the academic and social problems that children with ADHD grapple with and of the reasons why parents place their children on stimulants. The criticism also oversimplifies how children with ADHD are diagnosed. When reading the comments of critics such as Breggin, Schlafly, Johnson, and Fukuyama, one would think that any child can be diagnosed with ADHD and that it is almost entirely environmental, the result of everything from social intolerance for childhood behaviors to "forced drugging," incompetent teachers, progressive pedagogy, drill-and-kill testing, even the arrangement of desks in the classroom or a feminist plot against boys. However, it is important to keep in mind that children diagnosed with ADHD are quite different from one another. Some are diagnosed according to a strict adherence to DSM criteria, as the American Academy of Pediatrics urged, but many are not, for all the reasons discussed in Chapter 5.

One would also believe, after listening to the extreme voices in the debate, that ADHD is something that could be easily remedied if only parents and teachers would devote a little more time (and a bit more spanking) to wayward children. But it would be a mistake to believe that the vast majority of parents are rushing to get their children diagnosed with ADHD and on stimulants. In fact, sociological studies of parents find that most are hesitant to accept the ADHD label or to use stimulants. In one such study, Claudia Malacrida found that how mothers of children with ADHD responded to the disorder's label depended on how they were treated by the authority figures that determined their children's well-being (teachers, school officials, and physicians). When they despaired over their children's poor academic performance and social skills, the mothers were open to the idea that their children had ADHD. However, because their children tended to respond well to teachers who were sympathetic to ADHD but then struggled academically in years when they had unsympathetic teachers, the mothers came to doubt the medical validity of ADHD.[165]

Moreover, even if the clinical research found that stimulants were generally safe and effective, media stories of lax FDA enforcement of pharmaceutical safety, the withdrawal of several popular prescription drugs from the market, the controversy over the off-label use of psychotropic drugs on toddlers and preschoolers, and the aggressive marketing tactics of pharmaceutical companies cannot help but contribute to doubts that parents have about medicating their children. Indeed, many of Malacrida's mothers became concerned after they researched their children's condition on the Internet and found critics' accounts of rampant misdiagnosing of ADHD and the rare but devastating side effects of Ritalin. Some stopped using Ritalin; others continued, but with mixed feelings.[166]

Similarly, in his book recounting his experiences working with hyperactive or inattentive children and their families, behavioral pediatrician Lawrence Diller noted that a few parents would immediately seek an ADHD diagnosis and medication for their academically weak child. But most of the parents he met were nothing like this. More often than not, they were confused and frustrated by their child's behavior, worried about his or her future, and reluctant to place their child on medication. Many gave in despite their doubts because they were no longer able to control their child's behavior, and they were scared that he or she was in imminent danger of being expelled from school.[167] Likewise, studies of parents found that many felt worn down by their child's demands, hurt by the social rejection their child encountered from peers, and isolated by the reproach they felt from teachers and mothers appalled by their child's often boorish behavior. Yet the parents still were reluctant to label their child with ADHD.[168]

This is not to say that a diagnosis and medication did not bring a sense of relief to many parents. Many of Malacrida's mothers regarded medication as a godsend because it resulted in dramatic improvements in their children's disposition. But as Malacrida explained, this relief was often short-lived. She wrote, "When mothers were happy with the label, it was because it provided hope that their children would receive assistance, because it provided their children an opportunity to be seen not as bad children but as struggling children, and finally because mothers hoped that they could learn to understand their children better."[169] That sense of relief, however, quickly faded once it became clear that the educational services, the multimodal treatment, and the understanding from educators and physicians that mothers thought a diagnosis of ADHD would bring were not necessarily forthcoming.[170] Medicating children, in other words, is not a decision that parents entered into lightly; it was a step they took because they had run out of options and they saw that the stimulants worked.

## Conclusion

At the heart of the controversy over ADHD were questions of boundary drawing. Children exhibit symptoms of inattentiveness, hyperactivity, and impulsiveness along a continuum. Despite the fact that scientific research can inform our choices, where the boundary between ADHD and typical childhood behavior is located is ultimately a political and social choice, not a scientific one. No amount of clinical research, therefore, can resolve this question for us. Moreover, to the extent that the boundary between sickness and health is, in the case of mental disorders such as ADHD, demarcated without the ability to reference objective clinical signs or indicators of illness, debates about underdiagnosis or overdiagnosis invariably tap into society's ambivalence about mental disorders. The DSM was designed to identify children with the severest symptoms, those with the lowest levels of functional ability. Yet the DSM is not applied in a vacuum. As Chapters 4 and 5 indicate, social, political, and economic forces impinge on where physicians, educators, program administrators, and others decide to locate the boundaries of medical dysfunction. Criticisms of ADHD are criticisms both of the limits of clinical knowledge and of the extra-clinical forces that influence diagnostic decision making.

ADHD, of course, is not alone; the diagnoses of all mental disorders are subject to influences outside of clinical medicine. ADHD, however, is unique in the extent to which it elicits intense reactions from people. Because the symptoms of ADHD are often most evident in the school setting, where adults make sometimes tremendous demands on children, some critics worry that the identification of children with the disorder is driven more by the wants and expectations of teachers, parents, and school administrators than by the needs of the students. More important, because ADHD can be treated with pharmaceutical drugs, other critics worry (for good reason) about the influence of corporate profit-seeking motives on the diagnosis of children. ADHD is among the most visible and controversial mental disorders, in short because it is a vehicle through which many controversial social and political trends can be criticized.

In the middle of this confusion are the parents of children with ADHD. They must decide whether to accept the label of the disorder, and they must choose which of the many forms of treatment and school-based interventions to pursue: behavioral therapy alone, medication alone, medication in combination with behavioral therapy, which medication, which kinds of behavioral therapy. The path to choose is far from evident, and choices are constrained by health-care financing arrangements and the attitudes of teachers and physicians toward their children's ADHD. In addition, critics like Breggin and Schlafly write for a broad audience with colorful anecdotes and pithy phrases, and they publish their work in places that are easily accessible to the general public. Meanwhile, most researchers write for an expert audience in specialized journals and in language filled with clinical and scientific jargon that lay readers might find difficult to comprehend. As a result, even with the advances in our understanding of the nature of ADHD and especially in our knowledge of effective treatments brought about by extensive research (including the Multimodal Treatment Study of Children with ADHD and numerous carefully designed medication trials), parents often have easier access to the vocal, and sometimes extreme, views of critics of stimulant treatment via the Internet and news reports than to the research published in scientific journals. It is little surprise, then, that despite the growth of scientific knowledge of ADHD and stimulants, parents are swayed by the extremists and unsure about which treatment to pursue; the misinformation that fills the public debate over ADHD only serves to heighten parents' fear that they will choose the wrong path. Thus, even if parents decide to medicate their child, it is a decision that can be fraught with guilt and anxiety.[171] Although other mental disorders were difficult to diagnose with accuracy, although rates of childhood depression and other disorders were also on the rise, and although the growing pediatric use of psychotropic drugs was not limited to stimulants, no other disorder touches upon so many vexing social and political questions, a situation that amplifies the ambivalence that parents feel about medicating their children.

# CHAPTER SEVEN

# Current Questions about Stimulant Treatment for ADHD

Adult ADHD continues to seize the public imagination. The media present the diagnosis in widely discrepant but equally unrealistic tones. Diagnosis of adult ADD is not a medical attempt to prevent boys from being boys. We hope that increased diagnosis will not lead to rampant dissemination of stimulants and drug abuse. Nor will diagnosis and treatment prove to be a simple fix for the major life problems of a large segment of the population. As the media flood our awareness with these images, will there be room for the quiet work of research and skill development? Can we cope with the task of undoing unrealistic claims, but still leave the door open to treatment for those who would benefit?

—MARGARET WEISS, LILY TROKENBERG HECHTMAN, AND
GABRIELLE WEIS, *ADHD IN ADULTHOOD,* 1999

John . . . has been prescribed Ritalin since he was diagnosed with ADHD in the sixth grade. Last week he was
approached by his roommate who was on his way to
the library to write a paper and said he needed a
Ritalin to focus. With the same nonchalance that
someone might give an Advil to a friend with a
headache, John gave his roommate a 10 milligram
Ritalin from the container he keeps in his desk drawer.
"Good luck with the paper," he told him.

—*THE COLLEGIAN* (UNIVERSITY OF RICHMOND STUDENT
NEWSPAPER), FEBRUARY 9, 2006

The increase in diagnoses of ADHD and use of stimulant medications among children, especially in the 1990s, led to questions among parents, practitioners, researchers, and others about longer-term implications of medication use and increased availability of the drugs—to what extent are diversion and illicit use of stimulants widespread problems, and are children who use stimulants to manage ADHD symptoms at risk for abuse of other drugs? In part, these concerns echo the backlash against ADHD described in Chapter 6, yet they also represent important questions that should be asked as part of the decisionmaking process in prescribing any form of treatment for any disorder. In addition, recognition that children and adolescents with ADHD may grow into adults with ADHD and an increase in the number of adults who were diagnosed with ADHD for the first time have raised questions about the effectiveness of medications for adults with ADHD.

This chapter reviews the scientific research on these three issues related to the use and abuse of stimulant medication. First, what do we know about the extent of illicit stimulant use? How prevalent is this potential problem, particularly among adolescents and young adults, and are there links between nonmedical use of prescription stimulants and abuse of other drugs? Second, does treatment of ADHD with stimulants increase the risk of substance abuse among children and adolescents? A related question is whether ADHD is associated with substance abuse. Third, are stimulant medications effective for managing ADHD in adulthood? An important corollary to this question is whether ADHD symptoms in childhood, adolescence, and adulthood are the same. These three issues are considered together because they represent current questions about stimulant treatment for ADHD and as such represent significant areas of public concern in the 2000s. These questions are of interest to parents and policy makers as well as clinicians and researchers and have increased in salience as the number of prescriptions for stimulants for children, adolescents, and adults has increased. We take stock of what research evidence has to say about them in this chapter.

## Rates of Illicit Use of Prescription Stimulants

A recent headline in our own university's student newspaper claims that "Students Self-Medicate."[1] The article specifically reports on illicit stimulant use on campus and presents interviews with two college students. John was diagnosed with ADHD in the sixth grade and has been treated with stimulant medication since that time, and Kevin said that he reported ADHD symptoms during a brief meeting with a physician and received a prescription for stimulant medication. Though not stated, the article implies that Kevin received his prescription relatively recently. Both students talk about giving their medication to friends, usually to help them study, stay up late to finish a paper, or otherwise focus on their academic work. They also report an increase in the number of students they have seen who take their friends' prescription medications for a variety of reasons. John describes his willingness to dispense his medication, saying, "I don't see any moral problems with helping my friends. It's not like [Ritalin] is bad for anyone. Most people could probably get a prescription on their own anyway."[2]

The issues of diversion and illicit, nonmedical use of psychotropic medication are not limited to medication for ADHD, and news reports have been quick to paint these misuses as significant problems for young adults. According to a recent *New York Times* article,[3] many young adults describe a clear difference in the use of medications without a prescription and the use or abuse of illegal drugs such as marijuana. Specifically, "The goal for many young adults is not to get high but to feel better—less depressed, less stressed out, more focused, better rested."[4] For some (like John, the student described above), there is an assumption that medications such as stimulants must be safe for everyone given how many people they know have a prescription for them. Similarly, anecdotal evidence suggests that some young adults draw a clear line between drugs they perceive to be harmful (illegal drugs such as cocaine and heroin as well as legal drugs such as prescription painkillers) and drugs they perceive to be helpful (stimulants such as methylphenidate and antidepressants such as SSRIs). They conclude, then, that these latter medications would help them, too, in managing the stresses and strains of everyday life.

The extent of stimulant misuse and the degree to which diversion of stimulants differs from diversion of other psychotropic medications and from the abuse of illicit drugs are empirical questions. Nevertheless, relatively few studies have addressed the prevalence of stimulant misuse among adolescents and young adults. There are two general types of studies examining such illicit stimulant use. The first involves large-scale population-based epidemiological studies. Two such studies are the Monitoring the Future (MTF) Study[5] and the National Survey on Drug Use and Health (NSDUH), conducted by the Substance Abuse and Mental Health Services Administration (SAMHSA).[6] The MTF study is an annual survey assessing substance use among representative samples of eighth-, tenth-, and twelfth-grade students as well as college students. The MTF study is conducted by researchers at the University of Michigan and funded by the National Institute on Drug Abuse. In 2004, more than 56,000 participants were included in the assessment. The NSDUH involves an annual interview assessment of a representative sample of the noninstitutionalized U.S. population age 12 years and older. The questionnaires assess use of drugs, alcohol, and tobacco and mental health problems. More than 67,000 NSDUH interviews were conducted in 2003.

The second type of study includes smaller-scale assessments of particular samples of high school or college students. Such studies have been conducted at single colleges and universities or school districts across the United States. These investigations document rates of drug use and also allow for questions about motives for use. Together, these two types of studies provide evidence to assess the prevalence of stimulant misuse in the United States and to suggest some preliminary conclusions.

### Evidence from National Epidemiological Surveys

We turn first to the evidence from national epidemiological surveys. The general conclusion from the MTF study about Ritalin (methylphenidate) use without a prescription suggests that Ritalin use has been relatively stable or perhaps declining slightly from 2001 to 2004. Because of the significant increase in rates of Ritalin use in the 1990s, a new specific question about Ritalin use was added to the survey in 2001. Figure 7.1 shows the percentage of respondents in each age-group who reported using Ritalin without a doctor's prescription in 2002, 2003, and 2004. In terms of frequency of use in the past year, just under half to half of eighth-, tenth-, and twelfth-grade respondents who reported misusing Ritalin indicated that they took the drug on only one or two occasions. Male and female respondents reported roughly the same prevalence of illicit Ritalin use in eighth and tenth grade, with male students reporting slightly more (2.6% vs. 2.4% in eighth grade and 3.6% vs. 3.0% in tenth grade). This gender difference increases in twelfth grade (6.0% for males vs. 4.0% for females) and more than doubles by college age (3.7% for males vs. 1.6% for females). Male students also account for more of the frequent users. Consistent with the reports for most other types of drugs, students with plans to attend college had lower rates of Ritalin misuse than students with no college plans. Interestingly, however, when college students were compared with same-age peers not enrolled in college, there was a higher prevalence of misuse among those attending college. This latter finding perhaps speaks to college students' use of Ritalin to stay awake longer to complete academic work.

In contrast to the MTF study, which assesses Ritalin misuse in the past year, the NSDUH survey asks participants about lifetime use

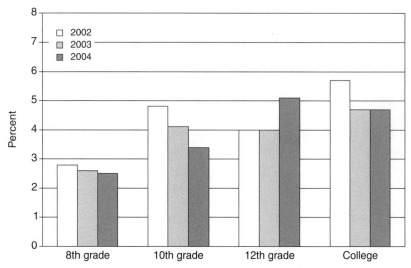

*Figure 7.1* Prevalence of Ritalin misuse in the past year, Monitoring the Future Study

("Have you ever . . ."). These lifetime rates of illicit Ritalin use are expected to be higher than rates in the past year, but they are actually fairly consistent or somewhat less. Figure 7.2 presents the rates of reported Ritalin misuse for all respondents and for specific age-groups. These percentages from 2002 and 2003 suggest that 4.2 million to nearly 4.5 million people over the age of 12 have used prescription stimulants without a prescription at some point in their lifetimes. As shown in Figure 7.2, the 18-to-25 age-group is responsible for the highest rates of Ritalin misuse. From 2002 to 2003 the overall rates of misuse are consistent, except for a statistically significant decrease for the 26-and-older age-group. When researchers examined NSDUH data over a longer span of time, they showed that from 1999 to 2003, the rates of misuse were consistent except for a gradual increase over time in the 18-to-25 age-group.[7]

One limitation of these data is that they do not distinguish between individuals who simply experiment with a stimulant by using it once and individuals who regularly misuse prescription stimulants. A recent secondary analysis of NSDUH data from 2002 provides some of the first evidence for the degree to which the latter may be a problem.[8] Larry Kroutil and colleagues estimated that 1.6 million Americans

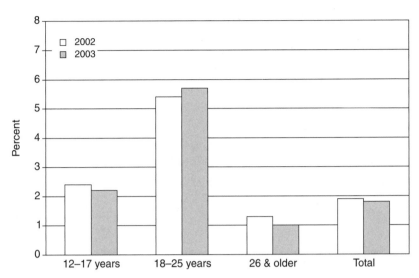

*Figure 7.2* Lifetime prevalence of Ritalin misuse, National Survey on Drug Use and Health

misused a prescription stimulant other than methamphetamine (which is commonly produced illegally as a "street" drug) in the past year. This number includes 800,000 people who misused a stimulant with specific indications for treating ADHD. Most of the individuals (60% of the nonmethamphetamine-stimulant misusers and 80% of the ADHD-stimulant misusers) were adolescents and young adults between 12 and 25 years of age, and in fact, the odds of misuse in both the 12–17 and 18–25 age-groups were more than 10 times greater than the odds of misuse among older individuals. Perhaps most important in Kroutil and colleagues' analysis were the findings about substance abuse and dependence related to prescription stimulants. Approximately 10% of the 12- to 25-year-old adolescents and young adults who misused stimulants other than methamphetamine in the past year (an estimated 75,000 people) reported problems consistent with symptoms of substance abuse or dependence. It is not known from these data, but it is likely that many of these individuals have histories of other drug misuse and other conduct problems. A further analysis of these 2002 data showed that being white and attending college (or being a college graduate) were the demographic factors associated with nonmedical use of prescription stimulants in the past year.[9] Psychological factors—including high levels of distress and enjoying risk taking (sensation seeking)— selling drugs in the past year, binge drinking, and using marijuana and other illegal drugs all increased the likelihood of illicit stimulant use among 18- to 25-year-olds.[10]

Taken together, these epidemiological surveys suggest some important trends in the illicit use of Ritalin, the most commonly prescribed medication for ADHD. These trends include relatively stable rates of reported misuse over the last several years, higher rates of use during college than at other times during the life span, and greater prevalence among men than women. These data assess rates only of illicit methylphenidate use. The NSDUH study also includes questions about other stimulants used in the treatment and management of ADHD. If Dexedrine and dextroamphetamine are included, lifetime rates of illicit prescription stimulant use increase by 1% to 2%.

In addition, in evaluating the extent of stimulant misuse among high school and college students, it is helpful to place these rates in the context of information about the use of other drugs among these same age-groups. Alcohol and marijuana provide key contrasts. According to NSDUH data from the 2003 survey, adolescents in the 12- to 17-year-old age-group report marijuana use at much higher rates than use of prescription stimulants—nearly 20% acknowledge use at some point in their lifetime, with 15% indicating use in the past year and 8% reporting use in the past month. These rates are considerably higher for 18- to 25-year-old young adults—54% lifetime use, nearly 29% past-year use, and 17% past-month use. As expected, alcohol use is even more common, with nearly 43% of 12- to 17-year-olds and more than 87% of 18- to 25-year-olds reporting use of alcohol in their lifetime. Perhaps more telling are the rates of binge drinking (defined as five or more drinks on one occasion within the past month) and heavy drinking (defined as five or more drinks on the same occasion at least 5 days in the past month), which indicate more significant alcohol use. Binge drinking is reported by more than 10% of adolescents and nearly 42% of young adults. Heavy drinking rates are nearly 3% and more than 15% for these age-groups, respectively. In interpreting rates of stimulant misuse, these substantially higher levels of alcohol and marijuana use provide an important context. Depending on one's perspective, then, rates of stimulant misuse hovering around 5% or less may seem problematic or may seem relatively low given rates of use of other drugs, particularly among adolescents and young adults.

*Evidence from Smaller-Scale Investigations*

The smaller-scale empirical studies investigating illicit use of methylphenidate and other stimulants used to treat ADHD among young adults have found wide variability in the prevalence of stimulant misuse. Figure 7.3 presents rates of prescription-stimulant misuse across six studies of college students, described in detail below. In one of the first studies of stimulant misuse among college students, researchers distributed surveys to all students at a small liberal arts college in the Northeast.[11] More than half of the respondents indicated knowing a fellow student who had taken Ritalin "for fun," and more than 16% reported taking Ritalin themselves for nonmedical purposes, including more than 12% who reported taking the drug intranasally. In addition, approximately 30% of respondents indicated that they believe Ritalin is a drug of abuse on their campus. Consistent with the drop in reported Ritalin use after age 25 in the NSDUH, the reported recreational use of Ritalin was higher among traditional-age students than those age 24 or older.

At another small liberal arts college in the northeast, 150 students were surveyed about their use of Adderall, methylphenidate, or dex-

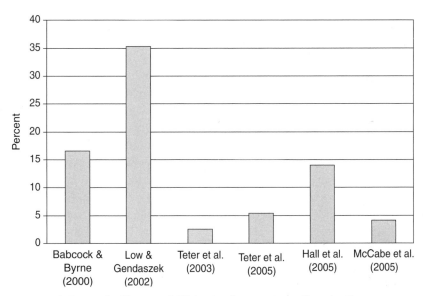

*Figure 7.3* Rates of self-reported illicit stimulant use in studies of college students, lifetime use (Babock & Byrne; Hall et al.) or in the past year (all others).

troamphetamine without a prescription.[12] More than a third of the students (35.3%) reported such misuse in the past 12 months, with 10% of those indicating that they used the drugs monthly. A similar study in a larger midwestern university found that nearly 14% of respondents acknowledged illicit use of stimulant medication.[13] Students reported that they used stimulants to help with their academics (27% used stimulants during finals week and 15% indicated using stimulants before a test) and for recreation (12% used stimulants when they "party"). Aside from their reports of their own use, students perceived stimulant use to be a problem for their classmates. More than 20% believed stimulants were abused on their campus, and more than 43% knew students on campus who misused stimulants.

Lower rates of illicit use are found in some studies. In one survey of 2,250 students at the University of Michigan, approximately 3% of students reported using methylphenidate in the past year without a prescription—a rate more consistent with the MTF and NSDUH epidemiological surveys than those found by the first two studies.[14] These students were compared to students who used stimulant medication in the past year *with* a prescription and to students who reported no stimulant use in the past year on a variety of demographic variables and drug use behaviors. Interestingly, on most comparisons, the group with illicit stimulant use differed from the other two groups, but the group who had a prescription for a stimulant and the group who had not used stimulants at all did not differ from each other. The students who reported illicit methylphenidate use also reported greater alcohol consumption, more significant consequences from alcohol or drug use, and lower grade point averages than the other two groups. In addition, a greater percentage of illicit-stimulant users reported earlier marijuana and alcohol use, use of marijuana and ecstasy in the past year, and cigarette smoking in the past month. One illustrative example is that 100% of illicit methylphenidate users said that they used marijuana in the past year compared with 50% of prescription-stimulant users and 30% of nonusers. In addition, two of the strongest predictors of illicit methylphenidate use were hours of weekly party behavior and number of sexual partners in the past year. The findings from this study do not provide any evidence for a causal role of illicit methylphenidate use in other risky behaviors or drug use. However, just as the use of other illicit drugs is associated with risky behavior among college students, such as frequent partying behavior and numerous sexual partners, illicit stimulant use appears to fit a similar pattern of associated behaviors.

Some evidence for the hypothesis that ready access to stimulants is associated with illicit use was suggested by examining the pattern of stimulant use in various residence halls in the report by Christian Teter and colleagues.[15] Specifically, in a number of residence halls where no students reported using stimulants with a prescription, there was also no report of illicit use. In contrast, in 75% of the residence halls where students used stimulants with a prescription, there was also illicit methylphenidate use. These findings raise the question of who is diverting their prescription medication. As part of a longitudinal study following children diagnosed with ADHD, Timothy Wilens and colleagues asked seven simple self-report questions of their young adult sample to assess diversion and misuse of medication for ADHD.[16] Approximately 11% reported selling their medication, 22% reported misusing their medication, and 10% reported using their medication to get high. These medications were not limited to stimulants, though the vast majority of the young adults (96%) were prescribed stimulants, and nearly one-third were prescribed selective serotonin reuptake inhibitors (SSRIs). Interestingly, all of the young adults who reported selling their medication had a comorbid diagnosis of either conduct disorder (CD) or substance use disorder (SUD). This finding suggests that physicians need to be especially careful about monitoring the appropriate use of prescribed medication for young adults with comorbid CD or SUD.[17]

Rates of illicit stimulant use tell us nothing about why students might use these drugs without a prescription. An additional study conducted by the same research group at the University of Michigan focused on the motives for illicit use of stimulants.[18] In the sample of more than 9,000 undergraduate students, 5.4% reported illicit use of prescription stimulants in the past year, and 8.1% reported use in their lifetime. Unlike the earlier study, men reported higher lifetime rates of use than women—a finding that is consistent with national surveys. Students were asked to choose from a list of motives their reasons for using stimulants without a prescription. The primary motives were to help with concentration, to increase alertness, and to get high. Similar to findings in the earlier study, a higher frequency of students reporting illicit use of stimulants also acknowledged alcohol and cigarette use in the past month, binge drinking in the past 2 weeks, and cocaine use in the past year as compared to nonusers. Notably, the higher rates of alcohol and other drug use among the illicit stimulant users did not depend on the motive for using stimulants. Thus, using stimulants to get high is not more likely to be associated with use of alcohol and other drugs than is using stimulants to help with concentration. As Teter and colleagues noted,[19] this finding does not fit with the anecdotal reports of students and young adults interviewed for news articles who indicate that they or their friends use small doses of stimulants to study or help with academic work but do not engage in other risky behaviors.

The rates of reported prescription stimulant misuse vary widely in these studies of single institutions, and indeed, characteristics of colleges appear to reliably predict rates of stimulant misuse.[20] A representative sample of more than 10,000 students from 119 four-year colleges across the United States allowed for a systematic investigation of rates of reported stimulant use (Ritalin, Dexedrine, or Adderall) as a function of school characteristics. The average prevalence of nonmedical prescription stimulant use was 4.1% in the past year and 6.9% when lifetime use was considered. These overall rates are consistent with other national surveys. Most interesting, though, was the considerable variation across schools—from 0% to 25% of students at individual colleges reported nonmedical stimulant use in the past year. Similar to other studies, individual characteristics such as being male, white, a member of a fraternity or sorority, and earning a low grade point average predicted greater use. At the level of institution characteristics, rates were higher at schools in the Northeast and at schools with highly competitive admission standards. This geographical predictor is consistent with findings from the single-institution studies described above, in which the highest rates were reported at schools in the Northeast.[21]

Hypotheses about why students misuse stimulant medications focus on stimulant use as a way to gain other desired reinforcement, such as social interactions, studying, or work, or to avoid unpleasant consequences, such as a negative mood that accompanies fatigue or sleep deprivation.[22] The college environment may be particularly well suited for encouraging the misuse of stimulants.[23] College students frequently feel pressure to delay sleep and function on limited sleep—for social and entertainment reasons and for academic reasons ("to pull an all-nighter"). The fact that stimulants may help students put off their need for sleep may foster experimentation with these drugs on college campuses. In addition, especially in selective, competitive environments, students may perceive the use of prescription stimulants as a way to gain a slight advantage over others, allowing them to concentrate better and maintain focus longer.[24] Although more carefully designed long-term studies are needed, preliminary evidence suggests that illicit use of prescription stimulants is more of a problem in college students than in other age-groups or in same-age peers who do not attend college.

Few studies have investigated whether stimulant misuse begins earlier than college age, though epidemiological studies suggest that it does. One research group conducted an Internet-based survey of more than 1,500 students in the sixth through eleventh grades of a single school district in Michigan.[25] Approximately 4.5% of the sample reported using stimulants illicitly. Interestingly, more than 23% of students who indicated that they had a prescription for stimulant medication acknowledged that they had been asked to sell, give away, or trade their medication. The use of alcohol, tobacco, and other drugs by students who used prescribed stimulants for treatment of ADHD was similar to that by students who did not report any stimulant use—either prescribed or illicit. However, students who reported using stimulants both as prescribed and illicitly had profiles of alcohol, tobacco, and other drug use that were similar to the profiles of students who reported only illicit stimulant use and were characterized by much greater use of these substances than the former two groups.

In sum, news reports and anecdotal evidence suggest that illicit, nonmedical use of stimulants is a serious and growing problem, particularly in late adolescence and early adulthood. It is unclear, however, how well these reports reflect rates of stimulant misuse in the general population. Conclusions from epidemiological surveys and surveys of college students indicate that overall levels of use may be below 5% and may be associated primarily with experimentation except among a smaller number of students who may have histories of conduct problems and other risky behaviors. For example, nearly half of the 5% of students (48%) who reported using stimulants in the past year in one study reported using the drugs only once or twice.[26] In addition, in evaluating the level of stimulant misuse on college campuses, it is important to consider students' abuse of other substances. To provide some comparison, the 2003 NSDUH survey showed that among 18- to 22-year-old full-time college students, nearly 65% reported using alcohol in the past month, with just under half (44%) reporting binge drinking and more than 17% reporting heavy drinking (defined as binge drinking on 5 or more days in the past month).

Nevertheless, considerable variability exists in the extent of prescription-stimulant misuse, particularly across different college environments. One difficulty in comparing rates of stimulant misuse across studies is that the assessments differ in important ways. There are at least three methodological challenges that make comparisons across studies difficult. First, some studies ask specifically about Ritalin use; others ask about any prescription stimulants; still others provide a list of several of the most common brand names. Unlike other types of illicit drugs in which there is one or only a few different formulations (marijuana or cocaine), the many different kinds and preparations of stimulants commonly prescribed for ADHD make it difficult for researchers to design questions that index all of the medications they want to study.[27] Second, studies ask about different time frames of reference, making comparison of rates somewhat difficult, and often no information about frequency of use is gathered. For example, some studies ask about lifetime use, and others ask only about use in the past year. Similarly, when students are simply asked whether they have ever used stimulants within a given time frame, but they are not asked about the frequency of use, rates may be inflated by including students who have tried the medication only once. This kind of experimental use is likely to be common on college campuses, especially when students hear from peers or friends that it will help them concentrate on studying or finish a paper, and when students have the view that prescription stimulants are perfectly safe. Students whose use is experimental should be clearly distinguished, however, from the smaller number of students whose misuse leads to abuse or dependence. Third, the definition of nonmedical or illicit use of prescription stimulants may not be clear to some participants. Sometimes it is described solely as using the drug when you do not have a prescription for it. Other times, a more inclusive definition of nonmedical use includes using medication that is prescribed for the person in a way that the doctor did not prescribe it, such as using more of the medication.

The findings of existing survey research, particularly those investigations that ask about motives, suggest important avenues for preventive interventions. First, if anecdotal evidence is accurate, at least some students underestimate the potential dangers of prescription-stimulant use. The belief that if these medications are prescribed by doctors for their peers then they must be safe for everyone is clearly a problem. It may be that the increased use of stimulants among college students to treat ADHD has had the effect of destigmatizing the use of stimulants—even illicit use.[28] A related belief among some students is that taking a prescription stimulant illicitly is dramatically different from taking other illicit drugs. It is not uncommon to hear students say that they would never take an illegal drug like cocaine but there is no problem taking a friend's Ritalin to help with concentration. These inaccurate beliefs suggest that education about the potential dangers of using stimulants (or any other medication for that matter) without a prescription and the abuse potential of stimulants may be an important preventive intervention. College counseling and health centers, first-year student orientation, and residence hall programs may be obvious places for such intervention to occur.

Second, the specific relationship between misuse of prescription stimulants and use or abuse of other drugs is unclear. Although some students report a clear distinction between the two, other evidence suggests a correlation between illicit methylphenidate use (but not use of stimulants with a prescription) and both use of other drugs and risky behaviors that are associated with illicit drug use, such as frequent partying and having more sex partners.[29] Perhaps more important is the finding that the alcohol and other drug use behaviors of students who use prescription stimulants illicitly are higher than those of nonstimulant users *regardless* of why they use stimulants. In other words, those who reported using prescription stimulants to help with concentration and those who reported that they use prescription stimulants to get high used comparable rates of other drugs.[30] This finding directly contradicts the argument above that students may use prescription stimulants for academic reasons but refrain from use of other drugs and other risky behaviors. A similar concern is that if students are using prescription stimulants to help them "party harder" and this leads to other risky behaviors such as binge drinking, nonmedical use of stimulants may simply contribute to other significant problem behavior for college students aside from whatever risk is incurred simply from using the stimulant medication. Overall, then, comprehensive drug education programs and preventive interventions for college students aimed at preventing abuse of alcohol and other drugs might do well to include prescription stimulants as well.

## Use of Stimulants and Abuse of Other Drugs

In addition to public concern about the potential for illicit use that might accompany the significant increase in prescriptions for stimulant medication in the treatment of ADHD is concern that children who use these medications are more likely to abuse other substances in adolescence and adulthood. In part, this latter concern is fueled by some evidence that the prescription stimulants most commonly used to treat ADHD have the potential for abuse. The abuse potential of medications is gauged through various types of studies that assess the drug's chemical, pharmacological, and behavioral properties.[31] At the chemical level, methylphenidate is known to be structurally similar to other stimulants that are abused, such as cocaine and amphetamine. Pharmacologically, methylphenidate is also similar to cocaine in that both block the dopamine transporter.[32] Behavioral effects are assessed by examining the drug's reinforcing effects and subjective effects and by using drug discrimination procedures (studies that test whether animals perceive a substance such as methylphenidate to be like or unlike a drug to which they have been trained to respond, such as cocaine). In a comprehensive review of 60 studies examining the behavioral pharmacological profile of methylphenidate, Scott Kollins and colleagues concluded that 80% of the studies show methylphenidate to be similar to cocaine and other abused stimulants.[33] Nevertheless, they suggested that the research to date is unable to explain the fact that in actual rates of abuse, methylphenidate is abused much less than cocaine and amphetamine. There may be several reasons for this discrepancy. First, some pharmacological differences may be responsible. For example, methylphenidate clears the brain at a much slower rate than does cocaine and thus may not be associated with drug craving and frequent self-administration.[34] Second, drug abuse is characterized by significant impairment in major life domains, but most reports of illicit methylphenidate use focus on its mild stimulant effects (just as Kevin and John describe above, such as to stay awake for studying). Thus, methylphenidate may rarely lead to significant impairment and abuse as defined by the fourth edition of the American Psychiatric Association's *Diagnostic and Statistical Manual of Mental Disorders* (DSM-IV).

Questions about the use of stimulants and the abuse of other drugs are complicated by findings about the association between ADHD and substance use and abuse. Existing research on the degree to which ADHD in childhood places adolescents at risk for substance use and abuse has yielded inconsistent conclusions. For example, as compared to a control group of adolescents without ADHD, some studies find no increased risk for substance use disorder for a group of adolescents with childhood ADHD.[35] Others find higher rates of drug dependence in adolescence among those with a history of hyperactivity[36] or more rapid escalation from abuse to dependence.[37] Still others find that if serious behavior problems, such as conduct disorder, are taken into account, the apparently increased risk for substance use and abuse attributed to ADHD disappears.[38]

In one well-controlled study, adolescents with and without a history of childhood ADHD did not differ in whether they had tried alcohol, cigarettes, or marijuana,[39] but use of at least one illicit drug other than marijuana was reported more frequently by adolescents with an ADHD history. In contrast, levels of substance use more clearly differentiated the two groups. The adolescents who had been diagnosed with ADHD in childhood reported indicators of more frequent use and higher levels of substance use, including smoking daily and the number of times the adolescent had been drunk or had used marijuana in the past 6 months. These effects were clarified even further when the adolescents' current ADHD diagnosis and development of serious behavior problems, such as conduct disorder, were taken into account. Those adolescents who had a persistent diagnosis of ADHD since childhood and who had developed serious behavior problems by adolescence were the most likely to report use of alcohol, marijuana, cigarettes, and other illicit drugs. Thus, there is some evidence that ADHD, especially when it co-occurs with serious aggression and other behavior problems, increases the risk that children will try alcohol and other drugs, use them more frequently, and begin using them at an earlier age.[40] Recent analysis of the children with ADHD in the MTA study (see Chapter 2) supports these conclusions. At the age of 11 to 13 years, most children with ADHD in the study were not experimenting with alcohol, tobacco, or other drugs.[41] Nevertheless, roughly 17% of the MTA children compared to only 8% of the non-ADHD comparison group reported having used alcohol, tobacco, or another illicit drug. Consistent with what we would expect for children at this age, substance use was relatively low, but reliable group differences suggest "precocious use" by the children with ADHD.[42] Alcohol and cigarettes were the most commonly reported substances among the MTA children. When delinquency was also considered, the difference between the MTA and the comparison group emerged only for youth without at least moderate levels of delinquency.

Because ADHD appears to increase risk for substance use disorders and because many children with ADHD are treated with stimulant medication at some point, it is a foregone conclusion that some children who are treated with stimulants for their ADHD will develop substance use disorders.[43] The real question, then, is whether treatment with stimulants changes the level of risk attributed to ADHD in any way. Concern about use of stimulant medication as a treatment for ADHD centers on the worry that children who take stimulants are predisposed to higher levels of substance use and abuse in adolescence and adulthood.[44] In part, this concern stems from the possibility that use of stimulants may result in increased sensitization to later exposure to stimulants. Specifically, the behavioral sensitization process occurs when intermittent exposure to stimulants leads to a progressively greater response to the effects of the medication.[45] This sensitization hypothesis is based largely on research with animals that shows stimulant exposure leading to increased self-administration of stimulants. Because methylphenidate is very similar to cocaine and amphetamine in its pharmacological properties, animal studies of exposure to cocaine and amphetamines may apply. Specifically, rats that are pre-exposed to either cocaine or amphetamines more quickly learn to self-administer these drugs than rats that are not pre-exposed.[46]

In one recent study that demonstrates a similar phenomenon,[47] rats first learned to self-administer cocaine by pushing on a lever. Then the lever-pushing behavior was extinguished by making only saline and not cocaine available. After this extinction phase, the animals were given a dose of one of several drugs to test whether the earlier exposure to cocaine would make them more likely to seek drugs. In other words, would the rats push the lever that had previously given them cocaine? Animals who were given doses of methylphenidate, cocaine, or caffeine produced comparable responses—responses that were higher than during the phase of the study when only saline was available. Thus, methylphenidate was capable of reinstating the drug-seeking behavior. Only amphetamine produced greater responses. Similar findings in humans would suggest that children treated with stimulants might find them more reinforcing as adults and should prefer nicotine, cocaine, and other stimulants in later adolescence and adulthood.[48] Nevertheless, it is difficult to apply these animal models to humans, and arguments suggest that there is little evidence of this kind of sensitization in humans,[49] in part because of the very different ways that stimulants are prescribed to and used by children treated with ADHD compared to the intermittent high doses given to rats in animal studies.

Russell Barkley and colleagues examined the stimulant-sensitization hypothesis by following two groups who had been diagnosed as hyperactive in childhood—those who had and those who had not been treated with stimulants.[50] In adolescence, the two groups did not differ in their frequency of having tried any of 10 specific drugs. To test specifically the sensitization hypothesis, cocaine use and amphetamine use were combined, and adolescents who had and had not been treated with stimulant medication did not differ in their use of these drugs.

These findings extended into young adulthood as well, with 1 exception. The slightly increased use of cocaine among the adults who had been treated with stimulants disappeared once lifetime conduct disorder symptoms were taken into account, suggesting that the link between stimulant therapy and later cocaine use was explained by the link between behavior problems and drug use. Furthermore, treatment with stimulant medication was not associated with diagnoses of drug abuse or dependence. In sum, this study provided no clear evidence that stimulant medication in childhood as a treatment for ADHD is associated with increased risk for lifetime drug use, abuse, or dependence.[51]

Barkley and colleagues indicated that their findings are consistent with 11 of the 12 existing studies on stimulant treatment and drug use.[52] In one study (by Nadine Lambert and colleagues)[53] support was found for the stimulant-sensitization hypothesis. Children treated with stimulant medication began regular smoking at an earlier age and reported increased rates of daily smoking in adulthood compared to children who did not receive stimulant treatment. Cocaine dependence in adulthood was also more likely among children who had received stimulant treatment for more than 1 year than among children who did not use stimulants or those who had only limited treatment with stimulants. Several aspects of the Lambert study may be responsible for the findings that differ from most other studies.[54] First, Lambert included children without ADHD in the sample; thus, most of the children who did not receive stimulant treatment did not have a diagnosis of ADHD or had mild symptoms. Second, it is clear that lifetime symptoms of serious conduct problems must be controlled when evaluating the risk of substance use associated with ADHD. The Lambert study controlled only for childhood conduct problems.

Another frequently heard concern about the use of stimulant medication to treat ADHD in children is that it might serve as a "gateway" drug that leads to the use of potentially more dangerous drugs.[55] Despite this often-heard concern, there is limited scientific evidence to assess its accuracy. Joseph Biederman and colleagues compared three groups of adolescents in a 4-year follow-up study—boys with ADHD who were treated with pharmacotherapy (primarily stimulants, but other medications as well), boys with ADHD who were not medicated, and boys with no history of ADHD.[56] Not surprisingly, the unmedicated group with ADHD had significantly higher rates of any substance use disorder (including alcohol, marijuana, hallucinogen, cocaine, and stimulant abuse or dependence) than the adolescents without

ADHD. However, direct comparisons of the medicated and unmedicated groups with ADHD revealed a protective effect of medication for the development of later substance use disorders. In other words, boys who received medication for their ADHD had significantly *lower* rates of substance use disorder 4 years later than boys whose ADHD was not treated with medication. The protective effect of stimulant treatment appears to be robust across several studies,[57] and youths with ADHD who receive treatment with stimulants are approximately twice as likely *not* to develop a substance use disorder than youths with ADHD who are not treated with stimulant medication.[58]

A potential difficulty with studies like this, however, is that typically researchers must rely on naturally occurring groups—some children and adolescents receive pharmacotherapy to treat the symptoms of their ADHD and others do not—and comparisons of these groups give researchers some indication of whether treatment with stimulants raises the risk for problems with substance use. Unfortunately, though, the reasons that parents and physicians decide whether or not to treat particular children with medication may be associated with differential risk for substance use disorders. For example, children who are treated with stimulants and children who are treated with stimulants for longer periods of time often have more severe symptoms and behavioral impairments. Severity of symptoms is associated with worse outcomes. Given that more severe ADHD is associated with increased likelihood of developing serious conduct problems, and conduct problems, in turn, predict substance use disorders, the comparison of naturally occurring medicated and nonmedicated groups is problematic.[59]

Jan Loney and colleagues were able to overcome this design problem working with a particular sample of clinic-referred children.[60] It happened that there were three psychiatrists working in the clinic who had very different treatment preferences. Two recommended treatment with stimulants for nearly two-thirds of their patients, but the third recommended treatment with stimulants for only 3% of his patients. When parents called the clinic to schedule an assessment, they were randomly assigned to a particular psychiatrist based on availability. The boys who were treated by these psychiatrists did not differ on a number of important characteristics, including age, IQ, socioeconomic status, parent and teacher ratings of ADHD symptoms, and forms of psychosocial treatments they experienced. When the boys were followed up in young adulthood, they were asked about their use of 11 legal and illegal drugs. The boys who had received stimulant treatment for ADHD in childhood were significantly *less* involved with 4 of the 11 substances (tobacco, nonmedical stimulants, glue, and opiates) than were the boys who had not received stimulant medication in childhood. Medicated boys also had fewer diagnoses of alcoholism but did not differ from unmedicated boys in diagnoses of drug abuse disorders. Overall, then, treatment with stimulant medication did not increase risk for drug use and abuse among boys with ADHD, and in fact, stimulant medication in childhood showed a protective effect against some types of later drug use. In the follow-up of the MTA study described earlier, there was no evidence for either a positive or negative effect of medication on substance use, yet children were still young, and an association between medication and substance use might emerge in adolescence or adulthood.[61]

We have no definitive evidence for why treatment with stimulants in childhood might serve as a buffer against later substance abuse problems in adolescents and young adults with ADHD. At least two possibilities deserve comment.[62] First, youth and adults who suffer from ADHD symptoms and who have not found effective treatments for their inattention and impulsiveness may attempt to self-medicate. Thus, the greater use of particular substances may reflect their own attempts to find relief from their symptoms. According to the self-medication hypothesis, specific drugs are selected because of their psychopharmacological effects and the individual's particular emotional state and needs.[63] ADHD interferes with individuals' ability to regulate their emotions, assess cause-effect relationships thoroughly, and inhibit impulses. Lambert has suggested that self-medication results, in part, from difficulty controlling impulses to abuse substances, namely substances with stimulating properties.[64] Second, for most individuals, ADHD symptoms do not simply disappear with age, and, over time, youths who do not receive effective treatments are likely to experience continued distress. Their cognitive, emotional, social, and occupational impairments may build over time as their persistent difficulties are exacerbated. These continued symptoms and risk factors may place unmedicated individuals at increased risk for substance abuse. For example, as described in Chapter 2, untreated ADHD symptoms lead to rejection by peers, and rejection by conventional peers increases the likelihood that children and adolescents affiliate with deviant peers.[65] In turn, associating with deviant peers and friends is one of the strongest predictors of adolescent substance abuse.[66]

## ADHD and Stimulants in Adulthood

Over the past two decades, more and more adults have sought evaluation and treatment for ADHD. This increase is likely due to several factors—media attention on ADHD in adulthood, evidence for the chronicity of ADHD, and recognition of the disorder in adults who present with other comorbid conditions, such as depression or anxiety.[67] Use of medication to treat ADHD by adults has also increased dramatically. Susan Okie analyzed data on prescriptions for eight different medications commonly used to treat ADHD (as well as other conditions) and reported a 90% increase in prescriptions for individuals 19 years of age or older between 2002 and 2005.[68] Into the 1970s, the widely held assumption about ADHD was that children grow out of it. The 1980 edition of the DSM-III recognized the persistence of ADHD into adulthood, and it is now clear that as many as half to 80% of children continue to meet diagnostic criteria for ADHD in adolescence and beyond.[69] Although there is no adult-onset ADHD and the diagnosis requires evidence of ADHD symptoms prior to age 7, many adults are not diagnosed until adulthood.[70] For example, children who have primary symptoms of inattention rather than hyperactivity and disruptive behavior are more likely to have those symptoms overlooked until they are older and school demands increase. A host of other reasons (including variability in how tolerant people are of symptoms) contribute to the lack of identifying ADHD until adolescence or adulthood for some.[71] Nevertheless, estimates of the prevalence of ADHD in adulthood range from 2% to 7%, with 4% as a generally accepted rate.[72] In the largest study to date, the prevalence of ADHD among 18- to 44-year-old adults was estimated to be 4.4%.[73]

There are several controversies regarding the diagnosis and treatment of ADHD in adulthood.[74] With regard to diagnosis, the primary question is whether the existing DSM-IV criteria are appropriate for adults. The core symptoms of ADHD—hyperactivity, impulsivity, and inattention—change in severity and in the form in which they are manifest by adulthood. In part, these changes in the way symptoms present are due to the changing tasks and demands adults face as compared to children.[75] No longer are failing to complete homework and an inability to sit still in the classroom primary concerns. Instead, adults face challenges in their occupational life, in their marital and parenting relationships, and in other obligations—paying bills on time, for example.

It is well accepted that hyperactivity declines across late childhood and adolescence so that by adulthood, this is not usually a primary complaint. If adults report hyperactivity, it is more likely to be manifested in feelings of restlessness or tension[76] than in the more obvious behavioral hyperactivity (excessive running about or climbing) associated with ADHD in childhood. Some adults are able to cope with this restlessness adaptively by choosing a job that requires much physical activity, for example. For others, wanting to be busy constantly, moving quickly from one activity to another, and having difficulty sitting for long periods of time cause tension in social relationships and hinder their occupational functioning.[77]

Unlike hyperactivity, impulsivity is often a lifelong symptom of ADHD and is related to having a low frustration tolerance.[78] Margaret Weiss and colleagues have provided an excellent description of manifestations of impulsivity in adulthood:

> Unfortunately, in adulthood this trait may have more serious consequences. Quitting a job on the spur of the moment without having an alternative, ending a relationship that is treasured, losing one's temper with a child, and driving too fast or driving through red lights are only a few serious examples of impulsive dysfunctions in some adults.[79]

Similarly, attention difficulties are typically a significant problem in adulthood unless adults have modified their lifestyles to such an extent that they are rarely in situations that require sustained attention. Inattentiveness is frequently experienced as distractibility.[80] Other common complaints of adults with ADHD that are associated with inattention (though not diagnostic symptoms) include disorganization, lack of follow-through, difficulty managing time, forgetfulness, and procrastination.[81] Impulsivity, fidgetiness, and impatience are less frequently acknowledged as primary complaints for adults.[82]

A problem with diagnosing ADHD in adulthood is that the DSM-IV criteria, though intended to apply to children as well as adults, are based on field trials with children and adolescents from age 4 to age 16 years, and the applicability of some criteria to adults is questionable. In addition, there is a question about whether the number of criteria that must be met should be the same for adults and children or should be lower for adults.[83] Using the same criteria when behavioral symptoms decline with age may result in adults who "outgrow the diagnostic criteria while not actually outgrowing their disorder."[84] As a result, a number of rating scales and suggested diagnostic criteria have been developed specifically for the assessment of ADHD in adulthood. These scales focus on the more typical manifestations of the core symptoms of ADHD in adults and on the many areas of daily functioning in which adults with ADHD are likely to experience impairment, such as work and marital or romantic relationships.[85] Some of these rating scales include adult norms that allow for an assessment of the degree to which an individual deviates from similar-age adults without ADHD.[86] As described in Chapter 2, establishing that an individual's symptoms exceed the level that would be expected for others of the same age—developmental deviance—is necessary for an ADHD diagnosis. Caution should be exercised in relying solely on rating scales for diagnosis, as a number of individuals with psychiatric diagnoses other than ADHD receive positive screening scores on some rating scales.[87]

Unlike with most psychiatric disorders that exist across the life span, research on ADHD in adulthood lags far behind research on the disorder in childhood. This is clearly true in research on effective treatments for ADHD. For example, in a comprehensive review of pharmacological treatments for ADHD more than a decade ago, Thomas Spencer and colleagues found 140 controlled studies of stimulant medication for children and only 9 studies of stimulants for managing ADHD in adults.[88] Early studies of methylphenidate treatment among adults with ADHD[89] showed less robust responses (average response rate of 50%) than is typical for children and adolescents (a response rate of approximately 70%).[90] Several characteristics of the samples and dosages used in these early studies may be responsible for their lower response rates. First, the dose used was much lower than is typical in the treatment of children with ADHD. Second, many of the participants in these early studies would not meet the more strict diagnostic criteria used today.[91]

Nearly 10 years later, Spencer and colleagues conducted a rigorous placebo-controlled, double-blind (that is, neither experimenters nor participants knew when they received active drug versus placebo), crossover (that is, participants received either active drug or placebo for three weeks, and then, following a washout period, received three weeks of treatment with the other substance) study comparing methylphenidate and placebo.[92] Participants met strict diagnostic criteria for ADHD, and doses of methylphenidate by the end of treatment were at levels more consistent with effective doses in children and adolescents. Overall, 78% of participants showed clinically significant improvement in their ADHD symptoms with methylphenidate treatment versus 4% during placebo weeks. This robust response is promising and suggests that methylphenidate can be as effective in managing ADHD in adulthood as in childhood and adolescence. The effectiveness of methylphenidate in reducing ADHD symptoms in adults has been further confirmed by pooling results of six rigorous studies.[93] Stimulants other than methylphenidate that are often prescribed for children (such as amphetamines) have not received as much attention in adults; however, the limited evidence suggests that Adderall, which is a mixed amphetamine salts compound, may be effective and tolerated well in adults. Specifically, in a double-bind, placebo-controlled, crossover study, treatment with Adderall was associated with a significant reduction in ADHD symptoms for 70% of the sample, compared with 7% on placebo.[94] Also showing promising effects for managing ADHD in adulthood is the nonstimulant atomoxetine (Strattera), which is a norepinephrine reuptake inhibitor.[95]

Because of the strong associations between adults with ADHD and substance use, careful evaluation of ongoing substance abuse is important before beginning treatment with medication. Some recommend that treatment for the substance use disorder should proceed first, and medication treatment for ADHD commence only after a period of abstinence.[96] Use of atomoxetine may also be especially appropriate when substance use is a concern because it does not have abuse potential and is not a Schedule II drug.[97] Substantial co-occurrence with other psychiatric disorders, such as anxiety and depression, often accompanies ADHD in adulthood. These comorbid conditions, failure to respond to the first-line stimulants, or active drug abuse history are reasons to consider treatment with antidepressant medication, including tricyclic antidepressants or bupropion (Wellbutrin), though these medications have been studied less extensively than stimulants.[98] Wilens and colleagues have suggested that the combination of medication and structured cognitive-behavioral therapy might be particularly effective in treating adult ADHD.[99] This is in part due to the fact that ADHD in adulthood may often be more complex than in childhood because of its long-term effects on the individual's development and the symptoms of co-occurring conditions that do not decrease with medication for ADHD symptoms.[100]

Given recent evidence for the effectiveness of stimulant medication for ADHD in adulthood, the concern about using medication to treat adults with ADHD is no longer based primarily on a question of whether it is an appropriate approach in terms of symptom reduction. Rather, critics are often skeptical because of claims that ADHD is not a "real" disorder in adults or that adults should be able to control symptoms of restlessness and difficulty focusing. In addition, there is a need to recognize the important new market that treatment of ADHD in adulthood has provided to pharmaceutical companies. Weiss and colleagues noted that for some critics, the symptoms of ADHD in adulthood "are understood in moral terms. A pill for laziness? A pill for messiness? A pill for lateness?"[101] Sociologist Peter Conrad and his colleague Deborah Potter contend that ADHD in adulthood represents an expansion of medical categories that resulted from a convergence of lay, professional, and media focus and interest in the 1990s. They raised concerns about the "medicalization of underperformance" that "allows" adults to reframe their poor performance at work, for example, as the result of a medical disorder rather than a personal shortcoming. In many ways, recent controversies about ADHD in adulthood are similar to those that emerged and grew several decades ago about ADHD in childhood. To the extend that some adults may self-refer for treatment and embrace a diagnosis of ADHD as a cause of behaviors that may have better alternative explanations, criticisms about the process of assessment and diagnosis are warranted. Nevertheless, these concerns should not diminish recognition of the distress and impairment that adults with untreated ADHD may experience.

## Conclusion

As with any drug, it is critically important to evaluate the abuse potential of prescription stimulants and the potential for prescription stimulant use to lead to problems with substance abuse. In addition, in the context of the rapid rise in prescriptions for stimulants, including for adults, and the increase in production of stimulants,[102] it is not surprising that concerns of diversion, illicit use, and abuse have surfaced in recent years. The research reviewed in this chapter suggests that illicit use of prescription stimulants occurs, particularly among college students, yet many may experiment with the medication once or only a few times. In addition, despite the significant increase in prescriptions for stimulants among children, adolescents, and adults in the past two decades, the levels of misuse among high school and college students (according to large-scale epidemiological surveys) have not increased dramatically in recent years. This fact calls into question the idea that stimulant diversion and abuse is due to the rise in stimulant prescriptions and increased production of stimulant medications beyond these factors making the medications more available. In addition, these findings should not take away from the well-established effectiveness of these medications as a treatment for ADHD across the life span.

With regard to concerns about stimulant treatment for ADHD leading to substance abuse, the available evidence does not support this conclusion. There appears to be a fairly complicated association between ADHD and substance abuse. The risk for substance use disorders does not appear to differ between youths with and without ADHD up to early adolescence. However, rates of substance use disorders increase for youths with ADHD in adolescence, and by adulthood individuals with ADHD have significantly higher rates of substance abuse and dependence compared to control groups.[103] Comorbid disorders (particularly conduct disorder), persistent ADHD symptoms, and other risk factors such as a family history of substance use disorders or involvement with deviant peers moderate or mediate the relation between ADHD and substance abuse. Nevertheless, in contrast to popular concern, treatment of ADHD with medication may actually protect children against later development of a substance use disorder. With additional, carefully controlled longitudinal studies that investigate the short- and long-term efficacy of various interventions to manage ADHD—both psychosocial and pharmacological—in children, adolescents, and adults and that identify factors that make certain treatment interventions more effective for certain individuals, it will be easier for parents, individuals with ADHD, and physicians to weigh the potential costs and benefits of various treatment components in a comprehensive treatment plan.

# CHAPTER EIGHT

# Conclusion

> The beliefs underlying the Ritalin wars (I am using
> "Ritalin" here as shorthand for the whole practice
> of diagnosing children and treating them with
> psychotropic drugs) have truly now become like a
> creed. They're only superficially about diagnosis and
> medication. For most people, they're more profoundly
> about a sense of menace bearing down upon the world
> of our children . . . There's a sense that childhood has,
> in many ways, been denatured, that youth has been
> stolen, that the range of human acceptability has been
> narrowed for our kids to a point that it has become
> soul-crushingly inhuman. I share all these feelings . . .
> But where I differ (now) from those eager to pile onto
> the anti-ADHD bandwagon is that I'm not willing—
> anymore—to sacrifice real children and their parents
> on the altar of ideology.
>
> —JUDITH WARNER, *NEW YORK TIMES*, NOVEMBER 15, 2007

The use of stimulant medication for the management and treatment of ADHD has vocal supporters and critics alike, and as the previous chapters describe, the history of the diagnosis and treatment of the disorder reveals numerous controversies. Today, however, the controversy is not focused as much on whether or not ADHD is a "real" disorder. It is largely recognized as such.[1] There are several reasons for this change. During the 1990s, in particular, greater recognition of the biological factors that contribute to ADHD led to wider acceptance of the disorder as having neurological underpinnings that interact significantly with children's school and home environments. Given this evidence, it has become increasingly difficult to argue that the disorder has been entirely socially constructed or is the invention of incompetent and overburdened parents and schools. This is not to say that social or environmental factors are irrelevant. Again, clinical descriptions and empirical research suggest that environmental factors play critical roles in how the symptoms of ADHD are expressed, in the impairments that result from those symptoms, and in the management and treatment of the disorder, and thus they interact with neurological and other biological influences. However, environmental factors—parenting styles, discipline practices, or diet, for example—are no longer widely considered to be the *primary* causes of ADHD, and it appears to be nonshared environmental influences (those that are not shared among siblings) that may be the most critical environmental factors.[2] In addition, along with the acceptance of ADHD as a developmental disability and longitudinal studies that followed individuals diagnosed in childhood over the course of their lives came this recognition: for many children, ADHD is a chronic condition that can result in significant impairment in many aspects of daily functioning.[3]

Two consensus statements summarize the acceptance of ADHD as a legitimate disorder and suggest that the mainstream scientific community does not doubt the validity of ADHD and the considerable impairments and challenges individuals with this disorder face in their everyday lives. The National Institutes of Health sponsored a consensus development conference on the diagnosis and treatment of ADHD in November 1998. The resulting statement was prepared by a nonadvocate panel and was based on presentations by scientific researchers, open discussion among the investigators and the panel, and closed deliberations among the panel members.[4] It summarizes the panel's views on the state of knowledge about the disorder at that time. This consensus statement recognized the controversies surrounding ADHD—particularly with regard to treatment with stimulant medication—and noted the need for additional research on the causes of ADHD and on diagnostic criteria, but it found support for the validity of the disorder.

Second, in January of 2002, the prominent researcher and clinician Russell Barkley organized an international consensus statement that was signed by more than 80 of the leading researchers studying ADHD, was widely circulated, and was published in *Clinical Child and Family Psychology Review*.[5] In describing the reasons for organizing this group of clinicians and researchers, Barkley noted his frustration with "superficial, biased, or sensational" accounts of the disorder: "conflicting views of ADHD described as if they were some sporting event, with two sides being presented on the issues as if there was nothing but controversy in the professional community over the existence of ADHD, its causes, or its treatment with medication, when nothing could be further from the truth."[6] Rather, Barkley was suggesting that there is, indeed, a consensus about our basic knowledge about ADHD.

Like the 1998 statement, the 2002 statement supports the validity of the disorder and expresses clearly that "the notion that ADHD does not exist is simply wrong."[7]

If controversies about ADHD continue, then, they are focused less on the existence of the disorder and more on some of the consequences of the disorder. For example, what are the policy implications and how extensive are they? What are the consequences of the increase in the use of stimulant medication in recent years? And how do ADHD and the use of stimulants fit with concerns about "cosmetic psychopharmacology"?

## From Science to Policy

Once we leave the realm of mainstream science, the consensus about ADHD begins to break down. There are, of course, extreme voices in the debate, the loudest of which has historically been the Church of Scientology.[8] Yet the enduring controversy about ADHD in the public arena reflects, not so much the validity of the science behind ADHD, but the discomfort about what happens when the science is translated into policies and rules that govern how children will be treated.[9]

For some, this calls into question what childhood is really about. Over the past 100 years, expectations of and roles for children have changed dramatically.[10] As a nation, noted Jerry Rushton, director of the pediatrics residency program at Indiana University School of Medicine, we have moved from child labor and minimal organized schooling to highly demanding parents and educational systems with upwards of 25 or even 30 students per teacher and 8- to 10-hour days for 5-year-olds.[11] So while expecting students to maintain sustained levels of concentration, adults also expect children to be impulsive, energetic, and raucous; we expect them to daydream, to blurt out what is on their minds, to leap before they look, and to think little of the consequences of their actions. In fact, for many adults, to be carefree and impetuous is still the essence of childhood before it is reined in by parental discipline, an adult's awareness of social obligations, and the demands of school. To them, the decision to medicate children—even children who are significantly more impulsive, energetic, and raucous than their peers, perhaps destructively so—seems a tragedy, a move that when applied to too many children could strip them of their "natural exuberance." But to see children suffer from academic failure, rejection by their peers, conflict with parents and teachers, and difficulty participating in many of the joys of childhood when effective treatments may be available is also a tragedy.

A diagnosis of ADHD is not simply a private medical finding; it carries with it a host of public ramifications. Will the child receive medication, or will more effective discipline strategies work? Will parents retain exclusive control over what prescription drugs their child ingests, or will school officials, judges, and child protection workers also have a say? Will an impoverished child with ADHD and his family receive extra government assistance, or will they have to get by on what the rest of the poor families live on, which could amount to no government assistance at all? Will a child struggling socially and academically in school receive special assistance and accommodations, or will he or she have to plod along with everyone else?

Moreover, although most scientists generally agree that there is a set of core conditions that can be characterized as a medical dysfunction called ADHD, there is little consensus among policy makers about how many children have this dysfunction. The conundrum is not the comparatively smaller group of children with ADHD symptoms so debilitating that virtually everyone would agree they need some sort of help—most likely a combination of drug and behavioral therapy. The real problem is the much larger number of children who have a "shadow" of the disorder, symptoms that are severe enough that the child's behavior irritates teachers, wears down his or her parents, alienates peers, and leads to his or her own unhappiness. Yet in the eyes of some, the "symptoms" are the sign not of a medical disorder but of behavior that adults find troublesome.[12] Of course, clinicians will emphasize that children with ADHD are not "bad kids." They have significant functional impairments that challenge the abilities of even the most dedicated parents and teachers. "I think the general public doesn't understand that we're not talking about kids who won't stay in the grocery cart," noted Marsha Rappley, a pediatric researcher familiar with ADHD.[13]

But herein lies the rub. Estimates of how prevalent ADHD is range from 3% to 5% of all school-age children to as high as 10%.[14] In the public debate, we are not always talking about the same children as those involved in empirical research studies. Because the diagnostic criteria are not consistently applied rigorously, the diagnosis encompasses children who most everyone would agree have a serious disorder *and* children where the decision is a judgment call, children who are extremely taxing to those around them but whose actions may not be the result of a neurological impairment. Clinician Lawrence Diller described the problem this way:

> When parents ask, "Does he have ADD?" often what they really want is to resolve the "can't" versus "won't" dilemma . . . ADD's implied neurological basis suggests "can't" (as does a learning disability) and thus diminishes the importance of willful conflicts with parents and teachers. "Won't" implies problems that are much more emotional or relational in nature—or if one thinks in terms of larger systems, problems for which parents and teachers are partly responsible.[15]

As a matter of policy, Americans are more willing to provide social assistance and accommodations to people who "can't" meet their social obligations, however willing they are, than to give the benefit of the doubt to those who "won't."[16] Thus, the conflict over the existence and prevalence of ADHD endures, despite all of the scientific evidence, because "[i]n reality, behavior is never 100 percent either 'can't' or 'won't.' "[17]

## The Ongoing Controversy

It seems virtually impossible to give a presentation on or even just talk about ADHD and stimulants without being asked if the drugs are overused in the United States. We assume that many readers of this book are curious about this too. As the previous chapters suggest, the answer is yes and no. In some geographic areas and among specific childhood populations, ADHD appears to be overdiagnosed and the drugs overused.[18] Yet several of the same research findings that identify this overuse also identify areas and populations in which ADHD is likely underdiagnosed and the drugs underused, with serious personal and public health consequences.[19]

This more complicated and nuanced reality of both over- and underuse of stimulants is rarely presented in the popular press, but it reflects three important factors. First, while a valid disorder,[20] ADHD is also—like many mental disorders—one that primary-care physicians routinely diagnose in a less than strictly thorough manner due to the intense economic and time constraints they face, as well as to their training (or lack thereof) in the area of mental disorders.[21] This reality is important because, as noted in previous chapters, primary-care physicians make the majority of ADHD diagnoses and stimulant drug prescriptions.[22] In addition, ADHD is categorized as a mental disorder, like schizophrenia and bipolar disorder, but this label does not fit the disorder well. It is not clear to clinicians, researchers, or the general public if ADHD is primarily a medical disorder, a behavioral problem manifesting mostly in schools, a mental illness, or an evolutionary disorder of human adaptation.[23] It is also not self-evident how hyperactive, inattentive, and/or impulsive a child has to be to warrant a diagnosis, because the benchmark of comparison for diagnosing a child is whatever is considered "normal" for his or her peer age-group.[24] In short, the diagnostic criteria are neither "normed" nor quantified. The ambiguity over ADHD's classification, and the manner in which ADHD is regularly diagnosed, contribute to significant variation in diagnostic and treatment styles by clinicians: actual diagnosis rates for the disorder range from as low as 2% to as high as 18% in different communities across the United States.[25] This variation results in a serious mismatch between the need for and provision of pharmacotherapy, with both "under-treatment" of ADHD[26] and the "overuse" of stimulants by many children who do not meet full ADHD diagnostic criteria (as well as some children who exhibit no symptoms of ADHD at all).[27]

A second factor that fuels the debate is that stimulants are heavily regulated Schedule II drugs, which are effective in helping individuals with *or* without ADHD.[28] In other words, they enhance most individuals' ability to sustain their level of concentration.[29] This is not the way the public understands medical interventions to operate. The general view of medicines is that they treat people with a chronic or acute episode of illness or a disorder, but that they would either have no effect or possibly be harmful to someone who did not have an illness or a disorder.[30] Consequently, when stimulants help those with ADHD *and* enhance the performance of individuals without the disorder, they invite skepticism about the appropriateness of stimulant use by millions of children.[31] Moreover, using a child's positive response to stimulant treatment as a diagnostic tool is neither legitimate nor valid. Yet the working plan for many clinicians is to first treat a child with stimulants; if his or her functioning improves, the positive change in his or her behaviors or symptoms is then used to support a diagnosis of ADHD. But behavioral response does not constitute proof of a disorder.[32] Cough and fever are symptoms of an underlying illness, but they are not diagnoses in themselves. "Although codeine suppresses cough and ibuprofen suppresses fever, treatment of symptoms is not the primary or only diagnostic and therapeutic approach," noted Lydia Furman, an associate professor of pediatrics at Case Western Reserve University School of Medicine. "Either cough or fever can be due to a concerning underlying condition or to a fleeting minor ailment, and evaluation will be based on the details of the child's history and physical examination."[33]

Finally, although the prevalence of ADHD is often considered to be stable across different countries, provided the same diagnostic criteria and methods are used,[34] in practice rates of diagnosis and prescription stimulant use are significantly higher in the United States than they are elsewhere.[35] Between 2003 and 2005, the per capita consumption of methylphenidate in the United States was approximately 6 times greater than that of Australia, 8 times greater than that of Spain, and 18 times greater than that of Chile.[36] This enormous variation in stimulant use suggests that the boundaries between "normal" and "abnormal" (or disordered) are strongly influenced by societal, cultural, and policy variations among different countries. The United States consumes the majority of the world's production of stimulants, with school-age children in America using as much as 3 times more psychiatric medication than children in the rest of the world combined.[37] In some European countries, only a child psychiatrist can prescribe a stimulant for a minor diagnosed with ADHD, while in other countries the drugs can be prescribed only if approved by three independent professionals.[38] These regulations are primarily cultural in nature and have precluded a similar growth in stimulant use in other developed countries.[39] So ADHD symptoms may be relatively consistent throughout the world, noted Brazilian psychiatrist Olavo Amaral, but there is little evidence for a universal biological threshold for diagnosing ADHD because the definition of such a threshold is the collective social duty of physicians, parents, and individual societies.[40]

## Are ADHD and Stimulants Unique?

These kinds of debates at the intersection of science and policy are perennial ones, and in many ways ADHD and the use of stimulant medications are not unique in terms of the issues they raise. With regard to concerns about cosmetic pharmacology, the fervor over drawing the line between treatment and enhancement also arose in the early 1980s with respect to human growth hormone.[41] The hormone was once reserved for use in very short children with proven hormone deficiencies in order to enhance their adult heights by a few inches. By the mid-1980s, however, researchers had developed a way to manufacture the hormone more quickly and cheaply, raising the prospect of administering it to children of normal height with no hormone deficiency. No doubt tall children could gain a cultural and athletic advantage over shorter children. But was administering the hormone to healthy children ethical?[42] The question crops up with respect to a number of medical advances that address conditions that, while not diseases in the traditional sense of the term, nonetheless are unpleasant for most people: treating the symptoms of aging with hormone replacement therapy, impotence with Viagra, and perceived unattractiveness with cosmetic surgery.[43] And now, most recently, the controversy has extended to medicating children with antipsychotic and antidepressant medications.[44]

The debate over pharmacological enhancement is likely to intensify as researchers discover ever safer and more effective forms of pharmacological treatments for a whole host of cognitive and psychiatric ills. New drugs to enhance memory and cognitive skills, originally designed for early-stage Alzheimer's patients, are being tested on healthy people and could find a large market among "the more than 70 million baby boomers who are tired of forgetting what they meant to buy at the shopping mall" and "students who think such drugs could gain them hundreds of points on their SATs."[45] ADHD and stimulant medication, then, have been the tip of the proverbial iceberg.

Is the significant increase in use of stimulant medication to treat ADHD in recent decades unique? This increase should not be viewed in isolation. Between 1987 and 1996, there was a nearly threefold increase in use of psychotropic medications, including stimulants (fourfold increase) and antidepressants (well over a threefold increase), among children and adolescents in the United States.[46] Antidepressant use among children and adolescents continued to increase significantly between 1997 and 2002.[47] This increase was particularly among adolescents and was due to the increase in use of SSRIs and other newer antidepressants (use of older tricyclic antidepressants decreased during this time). A recent study of prescriptions for antipsychotic medications also showed a significant increase in the number of prescriptions written for children and adolescents. According to records of visits to physicians, the estimated annual number of youths' office-based visits with a diagnosis of bipolar disorder increased from 25 (1994–1995) to 1,003 (2002–2003) visits per 100,000 population—a fortyfold increase; in 2002, approximately 1,400 per 100,000 children and adolescents received a prescription for antipsychotic medication compared to 275 per 100,000 between 1993 and 1995—a fivefold increase.[48] In contrast, the period 1987 to 1996 was characterized by a relatively constant level of antipsychotic medication use among children.[49] Thus, the increase in use of antipsychotic medication lagged 5 to 10 years behind the explosion in stimulant use. The bottom line, then, is that use of many psychotropic medications among U.S. children and adolescents— and not stimulants alone—has increased dramatically in recent years.

Several factors do, however, make the increase in diagnoses of ADHD and use of stimulants unique. First, the sheer number of children who use stimulant medication for the management of ADHD is much higher than the number of children taking antidepressant or antipsychotic medication, even if the rates of increase are similar. Second, the increase in use of antidepressant and antipsychotic medications is explained, in part, by the development of new types of medication that are used more frequently with children and adolescents than earlier, first-generation medications. For example, fluoxetine (Prozac) was first marketed in the United States in 1988, and other SSRIs soon followed. Newer atypical antipsychotic medications, also called second-generation antipsychotics, were first available in the early to mid-1990s. These new drugs had fewer of the significant side effects that had precluded the more widespread use of earlier antidepressant and antipsychotic medications among children and adolescents. In contrast, stimulants have been available and used since the 1950s.

Third, because ADHD has traditionally been viewed as a disorder of childhood, the increase in use of stimulants began with children and adolescents as numerous carefully controlled studies demonstrated their effectiveness in managing symptoms of ADHD. It is only recently that the number of prescriptions for stimulant medications given to adults has dramatically increased—as much as 90% between March 2002 and June 2005.[50] In contrast, when the newer antipsychotic and antidepressant medications were developed and marketed, they were approved for use among adults, and the increase in use began with adults and has much more recently trickled down to children and adolescents. This is not surprising given that major depressive disorders and disorders that might be treated with antipsychotic medication— such as schizophrenia and bipolar disorder—were not diagnosed in children and adolescents in significant numbers until recently, and in fact, none of the second-generation antipsychotic medications are approved by the FDA for use in children. In comparison to studies of the effectiveness of stimulants for managing ADHD, there are very few studies of the use of antipsychotic medications in youth, and the earliest controlled clinical trials demonstrating the effectiveness of SSRIs for depression in children were published in the late 1990s.[51]

## Future Directions

Given the overwhelming interest in ADHD in the scientific and medical communities, the media, and the general public, there is no doubt that the next decade will witness additional dramatic developments in both our knowledge and our perceptions of the disorder. From the clinical perspective, we anticipate important advances in at least three areas. First, although ADHD is already the most well-researched disorder in childhood, the body of scientific research continues to grow at a rapid pace. Particularly important developments are likely to take place within the next decade (and sooner) in our understanding of the neurological and especially the genetic bases of ADHD. These discoveries will likely further the understanding of the causes of the disorder. Molecular genetic research on ADHD is still in its infancy but growing rapidly with the identification of several candidate genes for the disorder, particularly dopamine receptor and transporter genes, and studies linking specific gene combinations and expressions with ADHD symptoms, behavior problems, and outcomes.[52] Likewise, the continued expansion of neuropsychology and especially neuroimaging research affords great possibility for understanding the causes and biological origins of ADHD, differences among subtypes of ADHD, and responses to particular treatments.[53]

Second, in the area of treatment, additional long-term studies and carefully controlled randomized clinical trials comparing various treatment alternatives and combinations of treatments are needed. As noted in Chapter 2, the MTA study was one of the most important developments in the area of treatment in the 1990s, and as that sample of children is followed into adolescence and adulthood, further understanding of long-term effects of various treatments will emerge. Interestingly, the most recent follow-up study of the MTA found that 3 years later the four treatment groups no longer differed on any of the primary outcome measures.[54] These findings have only added to the controversy over stimulant pharmacotherapy. Much attention is also being paid to disorders that commonly occur with ADHD and the ways in which co-occurrence affects the response to particular treatment interventions, such as the enhanced effectiveness of behavioral treatments in children with ADHD and anxiety disorders.[55] As evidenced by the growth in use of atomoxetine (Strattera, a nonstimulant treatment for ADHD), since its FDA approval in 2003 and the development of innovative delivery systems for stimulant medications, it is clear that continued advancement related to the pharmacological treatment of ADHD is on the horizon. These are particularly welcome developments, as concerns about illicit use of stimulant medication, particularly among college students, increase. Atomoxetine, for example, does not have abuse potential, and the delivery systems used for some of the sustained-release forms of stimulants make them much less amenable to abuse than traditional formulations.

Third, interest in ADHD in adulthood, alongside its occurrence in children and adolescents, has never been stronger. A quick perusal of book titles in the psychology and self-help sections of any major book store reveals the considerable attention now being paid by the general public to evidence of the disorder in adults.[56] Research on ADHD in adulthood comes from two primary sources. As more and more research teams are following their samples of children with ADHD into adolescence and adulthood, we are gaining a much better understanding of the long-term course of the disorder and developing a more thorough life-span perspective on ADHD. A second source of information about ADHD in adults comes from adults who present to clinics for ADHD assessments and who have never been diagnosed or sought treatment earlier in their lives. The field is wide open for careful empirical study of many aspects of the disorder in adulthood, including the impact of comorbid disorders; impairments in emotional, occupational, and social functioning; neuropsychological deficits; and the effectiveness of various pharmacological and behavioral or psychosocial treatment interventions.

Yet even as scientific understanding of ADHD advances, it is hard to imagine the social and political controversy over ADHD abating. As a diagnosis and form of treatment, ADHD and stimulant pharmacotherapy illustrate both the success that science is capable of producing—when applied to the study of mental disorders—and its limitations. Researchers have made tremendous progress over the past three decades in increasing our understanding of ADHD, but when it comes to diagnosing most mental disorders, our system is still far behind other branches of medicine. Consequently, "On an individual level, for many parents and families, the experience can be a disaster; we must say that," noted E. Jane Costello, a professor of medical psychology at Duke University Medical Center. "For these families, the search for a diagnosis is best seen as a process of trial and error that may not end with a definitive answer. "If a family can find some combination of treatments that help a child improve, she added, "then the diagnosis may not matter much at all."[57] ADHD is more straightforward and easier to diagnosis in children than, for example, bipolar disorder or autism. Yet, as previously explained, diagnosing ADHD still relies on some combination of interviews with children (who often do not exhibit symptoms in a clinician's office or are reluctant or unable to talk about themselves the way an adult would), behavioral checklists, less-than-precise rating scales (that measure the existence and severity of ADHD symptoms along the lines of "never," "occasionally," "often," and "very often"), and subjective reports from teachers and parents.

## Community Protocols and Improving Diagnosis and Treatment

Ultimately, then, diagnosing and treating mental disorders such as ADHD are still partially an art, despite the fact that the science applied to them has improved dramatically in recent decades and led to numerous advances in screening and treatment. One of the better ways for resolving this dilemma is for communities to develop protocols that integrate the communications and interactions of teachers, physicians, other school personnel (nurses, psychologists), and parents.[58] As has been successfully accomplished in two North Carolina counties, the community process through which the protocol is developed and implemented has an educational component that "increases the knowledge of school personnel about ADHD and its treatment, increasing the likelihood that referrals will be appropriate and increasing the likelihood that children will benefit from coordination of interventions among school personnel, physicians, and parents."[59]

In 2002–2003, a group of pediatric researchers from Wake Forest University School of Medicine surveyed 42 pediatricians in two rural North Carolina counties who treated most of the children with Medicaid in comprehensive pediatric clinics "known collectively as Child Health (CH). The CH pediatricians were the catalysts for the development of the community collaboration process for ADHD," noted Wake Forest pediatricians Jane Meschan Foy and Marian Earls:

> The schools were also frustrated with the haphazard referral process and the variation in treatment patterns. Teachers, psychologists, and administrators all desired better communication. School nurses were often in the untenable position of responding to questions from school personnel about ADHD medications with no information from the physician. Parents were often poorly informed and uncomfortable with medication decisions. Communication problems frequently resulted in an adversarial relationship between the parents and the school, the physician, or both.

It was in this setting that conversation among the participants became imperative.[60]

Using the American Academy of Pediatrics' (AAP's) guidelines for the assessment and treatment of children with ADHD, the CH pediatricians worked with school personnel to establish standardized screening methods at local schools for children needing assessment because of inattention and classroom behavior problems. Children who appear to need medical assessment are referred by school personnel to a contact person or team at each physician's office. After a thorough diagnostic process, as outlined by the AAP guidelines, the physicians devise individual plans for treatment and monitoring of children that involve school personnel, physicians, school nurses, and mental health professionals. The protocol concludes with forms for collecting and exchanging information at every step, "processes and key contacts for flow of communication at every step, and a plan for educating school and health care professionals about the new processes."[61]

Revisiting the communities in 2007, the Wake Forest pediatric researchers found that the protocols, continuing medical education, newsletters, and resource guides were partially successful in changing the way that pediatricians handled behavioral health problems. "Black box warnings"[62] from the U.S. Food and Drug Administration had a much bigger impact in terms of changing clinicians' prescribing practices (decreasing considerably the proportion of pediatricians who used SSRIs to treat depression in children from 52% to 26%). But in addition to the protocols and related services and informational materials, 83% of the pediatricians reported that they consulted with a mental health colleague concerning pediatric patients with mental health problems.[63]

Although it would require more effort and time, this kind of collaboration among clinicians, educators, child advocates, and parents is potentially replicable at regional and even state levels. With a community protocol, and the consensus produced in the process of developing it, undiagnosed children with ADHD are more likely to receive help (often minority children, girls, and children from low-income families), while pediatricians report being less frustrated with a lack of data for making a proper diagnosis and requests for stimulant medication from parents who have been advised by teachers to make such requests.[64] The potential of community protocols is as significant as the need for them. Without both improved communication among those in charge of children's development and significantly increased physician compliance with scientifically established diagnostic and treatment guidelines, the debates over ADHD, stimulants, and other mental disorders diagnosed in children are not likely to decrease until a clearer and more accurate set of diagnostic criteria for ADHD is developed for the DSM-V[65]—tentatively scheduled for publication in 2011—and then adhered to by most clinicians. And as difficult as this challenge will be scientifically, reforming health insurance reimbursement policies in the United States to provide clinicians with sufficient payment for performing adequately thorough diagnostic screening and chronic care management of disorders such as ADHD is an even larger challenge that presently seems politically infeasible. Thus, the controversy over disorders such as ADHD, along with their related pharmacotherapies, is only likely to continue and increase in the future.

# Notes

## 1. Introduction

1. M. Wolraich, "Attention Deficit Hyperactivity Disorder: The Most Studied and Yet the Most Controversial Diagnosis," *Mental Retardation and Developmental Disabilities Research Reviews* 5 (1999): 163–168.

2. J. Williams, K. Klinepeter, G. Palmes, et al., "Diagnosis and Treatment of Behavioral Health Disorders in Pediatric Practice," *Pediatrics* 114 (September 2004): 601–606.

3. See M. Rappley, "Attention-Deficit Hyperactivity Disorder," *New England Journal of Medicine* 352 (January 13, 2005): 165–173; S. Zuvekas, B. Vitiello, and G. Norquist, "Recent Trends in Stimulant Medication Use among U.S. Children," *American Journal of Psychiatry* 163 (May 2006): 579–585.

4. See F. Bokhari, R. Mayes, and R. Scheffler, "An Analysis of the Significant Variation in Psychostimulant Use across the U.S.," *Pharmacoepidemiology and Drug Safety* 14 (April 2005): 267–275; E. Cox, B. Motheral, R. Henderson, et al., "Geographic Variation in the Prevalence of the Stimulant Medication Use among Children 5 to 14 Years Old: Results from a Commercially Insured U.S. Sample," *Pediatrics* 111 (February 2003): 237–243; J. Zito, D. Safer, S. dosReis, et al., "Methylphenidate Patterns among Medicaid Youths," *Psychopharmacology Bulletin* 33 (1997): 143–147; J. Stevens, J. Harman, and K. Kelleher, "Race/Ethnicity and Insurance Status as Factors Associated with ADHD Treatment Patterns," *Journal of Child and Adolescent Psychopharmacology* 15 (February 2005): 88–96; J. Stevens, J. Harman, and K. Kelleher, "Ethnic and Regional Differences in Primary Care Visits for Attention-Deficit Hyperactivity Disorder," *Journal of Developmental and Behavioral Pediatrics* 25 (October 2004): 318–325; M. Radigan, P. Lannon, P. Roohan, et al., "Medication Patterns

for Attention-Deficit/Hyperactivity Disorder and Comorbid Psychiatric Conditions in a Low-Income Neighborhood," *Journal of Child and Adolescent Psychopharmacology* 15 (February 2005): 44–56.

5. See V. Bhatara, M. Feil, K. Hoagwood, et al., "National Trends in Concomitant Psychotropic Medication with Stimulants in Pediatric Visits: Practice versus Knowledge," *Journal of Attention Disorders* 7 (May 2004): 217–226; Zuvekas et al., "Recent Trends in Stimulant Medication Use among U.S. Children," 579; L. Robison, D. Sclar, and T. Skaer, "Datapoints: Trends in ADHD and Stimulant Use among Adults, 1995–2002," *Psychiatric Services* 56 (December 2005): 1497; C. Thomas, P. Conrad, R. Casler, et al., "Trends in the Use of Psychotropic Medications among Adolescents, 1994 to 2001," *Psychiatric Services* 57 (January 2006): 63–69; M. Olfson, M. Gameroff, S. Marcus, et al., "National Trends in the Treatment of Attention Deficit Hyperactivity Disorder," *American Journal of Psychiatry* 160 (June 2003): 1071–1077.

6. See M. Eberstadt, "Why Ritalin Rules," *Policy Review* 94 (April–May 1999): 24–44.

7. See R. Chiarello and J. Cole, "The Use of Psychostimulants in General Psychiatry: A Reconsideration," *Archives of General Psychiatry* 44 (March 1987): 286–295.

8. See C. Bradley, "The Behavior of Children Receiving Benzedrine," *American Journal of Psychiatry* 94 (November 1937): 577–578.

9. See R. Barkley, *Attention-Deficit Hyperactivity Disorder: A Handbook for Diagnosis and Treatment* (New York: Guilford Press, 1990), 3–38.

10. J. Swanson, M. Lerner, and L. Williams, "More Frequent Diagnosis of Attention-Deficit Hyperactivity Disorder," *New England Journal of Medicine* 333 (October 5, 1995): 944.

11. See H. Schneider and D. Eisenberg, "Who Receives a Diagnosis of Attention-Deficit/Hyperactivity Disorder in the United States Elementary School Population?" *Pediatrics* 117 (April 2006): 601–609; T. Spencer, J. Biederman, and E. Mick, "Attention-Deficit/Hyperactivity Disorder: Diagnosis, Lifespan, Comorbidities, and Neurobiology," *Ambulatory Pediatrics* 7 (January–February 2007): 73–81; Zuvekas et al., "Recent Trends in Stimulant Medication among U.S. Children," 579–585.

12. See S. Visser, C. Lesesne, and R. Perou, "National Estimates and Factors Associated with Medication Treatment for Childhood Attention-Deficit/Hyperactivity Disorder," *Pediatrics* 119 (February 2007, Suppl.): S99–S106; Centers for Disease Control and Prevention, "Mental Health in the United States: Prevalence of Diagnosis and Medication Treatment for Attention-Deficit/Hyperactivity Disorder," *MMWR: Morbidity and Mortality Weekly Report* 54 (September 2, 2005): 842–847.

13. L. Castle, R. Aubert, R. Verbrugge, et al., "Trends in Medication Treatment for ADHD," *Journal of Attention Disorders* 10 (May 2007): 335–342.

14. See R. Scotch, "Politics and Policy in the History of the Disability Rights Movement," *Milbank Quarterly* 67 (1989): 380–400; R. Sommer, "Family

Advocacy and the Mental Health System: The Recent Rise of the Alliance for the Mentally Ill," *Psychiatric Quarterly* 61 (Fall 1990): 205–221; N. Tomes, "The Patient as a Policy Factor: A Historical Case Study of the Consumer/Survivor Movement in Mental Health," *Health Affairs* 25 (May–June 2006): 720–729; A. McLean, "Empowerment and the Psychiatric Consumer/Ex-Patient Movement in the United States: Contradictions, Crisis and Change," *Social Science and Medicine* 40 (April 1995): 1053–1071; A. Hatfield, "The National Alliance for the Mentally Ill: A Decade Later," *Community Mental Health Journal* 27 (April 1991): 95–103; M. Minow and R. Weissbourd, "Social Movements for Children," *Daedalus* 122 (Winter 1993): 1–29; D. Pfeiffer, "Overview of the Disability Movement: History, Legislative Record, and Political Implications," *Policy Studies Journal* 21 (December 1993): 724–734.

15. See J. Perrin, K. Kuhlthau, T. McLaughlin, et al., "Changing Patterns of Conditions among Children Receiving Supplemental Security Income Disability Benefits," *Archives of Pediatric and Adolescent Medicine* 153 (January 1999): 80–84; R. Reid, J. Maag, and S. Vasa, "Attention Deficit Hyperactivity Disorder as a Disability Category: A Critique," *Exceptional Children* 60 (December 1993–January 1994): 198–214.

16. See Perrin et al., "Changing Patterns of Conditions among Children Receiving Supplemental Security Income Disability Benefits."

17. Reid et al., "Attention Deficit Hyperactivity Disorder as a Disability Category."

18. See S. Ettner, K. Kuhlthau, T. McLaughlin, et al., "Impact of Expanding SSI on Medicaid Expenditures of Disabled Children," *Health Care Financing Review* 21 (Spring 2000): 185–201.

19. See L. Dubay and G. Kenney, "The Effects of Medicaid Expansions on Insurance Coverage of Children," *Future of Children* 6 (Spring 1996): 152–161; K. Kronebusch, "Medicaid for Children: Federal Mandates, Welfare Reform, and Policy Backsliding," *Health Affairs* 20 (January–February 2001): 97–111.

20. See Dubay and Kenney, "The Effects of Medicaid Expansions on Insurance Coverage of Children."

21. See A. Cuellar and S. Markowitz, "Medicaid Policy Changes in Mental Health Care and Their Effect on Mental Health Outcomes," *Health Economics, Policy and Law* 2 (2007): 23–28.

22. See L. Rogler, "Making Sense of Historical Changes in the Diagnostic and Statistical Manual of Mental Disorders: Five Propositions," *Journal of Health and Social Behavior* 38 (March 1997): 9–20.

23. See J. Cook and E. Wright, "Medical Sociology and the Study of Severe Mental Illness: Reflections on Past Accomplishments and Directions for Future Research," *Journal of Health and Social Behavior* 35 (1995): 95–114; B. Ennis and T. Litwack, "Psychiatry and the Presumption of Expertise: Flipping Coins in the Courtroom," *California Law Review* 62 (1974): 693–752; R. Kendell, *The Role of Diagnosis in Psychiatry* (Oxford: Blackwell Scientific Publications, 1975).

24. See R. Mayes and A. Horwitz, "DSM-III and the Revolution in the Classification of Mental Illness," *Journal of the History of the Behavioral Sciences* 41 (Summer 2005): 249–267.

25. See G. Gabbard and J. Kay, "The Fate of Integrated Treatment: Whatever Happened to the Biopsychosocial Psychiatrist?" *American Journal of Psychiatry* 158 (December 2001): 1956–1963; G. Gabbard, "Psychotherapy in Psychiatry," *International Review of Psychiatry* 19 (February 2007): 5–12; H. Akil and S. Watson, "Science and the Future of Psychiatry," *Archives of General Psychiatry* 57 (January 2000): 86–87.

26. See R. Sturm, "How Does Risk Sharing between Employers and a Managed Behavioral Health Organization Affect Mental Health Care?" *Health Services Research* 35 (October 2000): 761–776; D. McKusick, T. Mark, E. King, et al., "Trends in Mental Health Insurance Benefits and Out-of-Pocket Spending," *Journal of Mental Health Policy and Economics* 5 (June 2002): 71–78.

27. See Mechanic, *Mental Health and Social Policy*; Goldman and Grob, "Defining 'Mental Illness' in Mental Health Policy."

28. See L. Spetie and L. Arnold, "Ethical Issues in Child Psychopharmacology Research and Practice," *Psychopharmacology* 191 (March 2007): 15–26.

29. See K. Hickey and L. Lyckholm, "Child Welfare versus Parental Autonomy: Medical Ethics, the Law, and Faith-Based Healing," *Theoretical Medicine and Bioethics* 25 (2004): 265–276; T. Kuther, "Medical Decision-Making and Minors: Issues of Consent and Assent," *Adolescence* 38 (Summer 2003): 343–358; D. Sherer, "The Capacities of Minors to Exercise Voluntariness in Medical Treatment Decisions," *Law and Human Behavior* 15 (August 1991): 431–449.

30. See J. Sparks and B. Duncan, "The Ethics and Science of Medicating Children," *Ethical Human Psychology and Psychiatry* 6 (Spring 2004): 25–39.

31. See L. Goldman, M. Genel, R. Bezman, et al., "Diagnosis and Treatment of Attention-Deficit/Hyperactivity Disorder in Children and Adolescents: Council on Scientific Affairs, American Medical Association," *Journal of the American Medical Association* 279 (April 8, 1998): 1100–1107.

32. See J. Havey, J. Olson, C. McCormick, et al., "Teachers' Perceptions of the Incidence and Management of Attention-Deficit Hyperactivity Disorder," *Applied Neuropsychology* 12 (2005): 120–127.

33. See L. Sax and K. Kautz, "Who First Suggests the Diagnosis of Attention-Deficit/Hyperactivity Disorder?" *Annals of Family Medicine* 1 (September–October 2003): 171–174.

34. See G. DuPaul and G. Stoner, *ADHD in Schools: Assessment and Intervention Strategies* (New York: Guildford Press, 2003); M. Stein, N. Marx, J. Beard, et al., "ADHD: The Diagnostic Process from Different Perspectives," *Journal of Developmental and Behavioral Pediatrics* 25 (February 2004): 53–58; J. Biederman, S. Faraone, M. Monuteaux, et al., "How In-

formative Are Parent Reports of Attention-Deficit/Hyperactivity Disorder Symptoms for Assessing Outcome in Clinical Trials of Long-Acting Treatments? A Pooled Analysis of Parents' and Teachers' Reports," *Pediatrics* 113 (June 2004): 1667–1671; J. Biederman, H. Gao, A. Rogers, et al., "Comparison of Parent and Teacher Reports of Attention-Deficit/ Hyperactivity Disorder Symptoms from Two Placebo-Controlled Studies of Atomoxetine in Children," *Biological Psychiatry* 60 (November 15, 2006): 1106–1110.

35. Havey et al., "Teachers' Perceptions of the Incidence and Management of Attention-Deficit Hyperactivity Disorder."

36. See E. Sleator and R. Ullmann, "Can the Physician Diagnose Hyperactivity in the Office?" *Pediatrics* 67 (January 1981): 13–7; T. Johnson, "Evaluating the Hyperactive Child in Your Office: Is It ADHD?" *American Family Physician* 56 (July 1997): 155–160, 168–170.

37. For more on the inherent subjectivity and clinical uncertainty in diagnosing and treating mental disorders, see T. Luhrmann, *Of Two Minds: The Growing Disorder in American Psychiatry* (New York: Vintage, 2001).

38. See M. Gordon, K. Antshel, S. Faraone, et al., "Symptoms versus Impairment: The Case for Respecting DSM-IV's Criterion D," *Journal of Attention Disorders* 9 (February 2006): 465–475.

39. See S. Timimi, "ADHD Is Best Understood as a Cultural Construct," *British Journal of Psychiatry* 184 (2004): 8–9; P. Conrad, "The Shifting Engines of Medicalization," *Journal of Health and Social Behavior* 46 (March 2005): 3–14; P. Conrad and V. Leiter, "Medicalization, Markets and Consumers," *Journal of Health and Social Behavior* 45 (2004): 158–176.

40. See S. Hinshaw and D. Cicchetti, "Stigma and Mental Disorders: Conceptions of Illness, Public Attitudes, Personal Disclosure, and Social Policy," *Development and Psychopathology* 12 (2000): 574.

41. See C. Perring, "Medicating Children: The Case of Ritalin," *Bioethics* 11 (July 1997): 228–240; M. McCubbin and D. Cohen, "Empirical, Ethical, and Political Perspectives on the Use of Methylphenidate," *Ethical Human Sciences and Services* 1 (Spring 1999): 81–101; I. Singh, "Clinical Implications of Ethical Concepts: Moral Self-Understandings in Children Taking Methylphenidate for ADHD," *Clinical Child Psychology and Psychiatry* 12 (April 2007): 167–182.

42. See Goldman et al., "Diagnosis and Treatment of Attention-Deficit/ Hyperactivity Disorder in Children and Adolescents."

43. See K. McDaniel, "Pharmacologic Treatment of Psychiatric and Neurodevelopmental Disorders in Children and Adolescents," *Clinical Pediatrics* 25 (February 1986): 65–71; J. Biederman and M. Jellinek, "Current Concepts: Psychopharmacology in Children," *New England Journal of Medicine* 310 (April 12, 1984): 968–972; D. Safer, "Broader Clinical Considerations in Child Psychopharmacology Practice," *Comprehensive Psychiatry* 24 (November–December 1983): 567–573.

44. G. Still, "The Goulstonian Lectures on Some Abnormal Psychical Conditions in Children," *Lancet* 1 (April 12, 1902): 1008–1012, (April 19, 1902): 1079–1082, (April 26, 1902): 1163–1167.

45. See R. Mayes and A. Rafalovich, "Suffer the Restless Children: The Evolution of ADHD and Pediatric Stimulant Use: 1900–1980," *History of Psychiatry* 18 (December 2007): 435–457.

46. See R. Michels and P. Marzuk, "Progress in Psychiatry," *New England Journal of Medicine* 329 (August 19, 1993): 552–560, (August 26, 1993): 628–638.

47. See M. Wilson, "DSM-III and the Transformation of American Psychiatry: A History," *American Journal of Psychiatry* 150 (March 1993): 399–410.

48. See G. Strauss, J. Yager, and G. Strauss, "The Cutting Edge in Psychiatry," *American Journal of Psychiatry* 141 (January 1984): 38–43.

49. K. Livingston, "Ritalin: Miracle Drug or Cop-Out," *Public Interest* 127 (Spring 1997): 3–18.

50. See R. Frank and S. Glied, *Better but Not Well: Mental Health Policy in the U.S. Since 1950* (Baltimore: Johns Hopkins University Press, 2006).

51. See A. Frances, H. Pincus, T. Widiger, et al., "DSM-IV: Work in Progress," *American Journal of Psychiatry* 147 (November 1990): 1439–1448.

52. See A. Horwitz, *Creating Mental Illness* (Chicago: University of Chicago Press, 2002); G. Greenberg, "Manufacturing Depression: A Journey into the Economy of Melancholy," *Harpers*, May 2007, 35–46.

53. See J. Zito and H. Koplewicz, "The Pharmaceutical Industry, Academic Medicine and the FDA," *Journal of Child and Adolescent Psychopharmacology* 17 (2007): 275–278; D. Zipkin and M. Steinman, "Interactions between Pharmaceutical Representatives and Doctors in Training," *Journal of General Internal Medicine* 20 (August 2005): 777–786; S. Paul and M. Tohen, "Conflicts of Interest and the Credibility of Psychiatric Research," *World Psychiatry* 6 (February 2007): 33–34; A. Fugh-Berman, "The Corporate Coauthor," *Journal of General Internal Medicine* 20 (June 2005): 546–548; N. Choudry, H. Stelfox, and A. Detsky, "Relationships between Authors of Clinical Practice Guidelines and the Pharmaceutical Industry," *Journal of the American Medical Association* 287 (February 6, 2002): 612–617.

54. L. Cosgrove, S. Krimsky, M. Vijayaraghavan, et al., "Financial Ties between DSM-IV Panel Members and the Pharmaceutical Industry," *Psychotherapy and Psychosomatics* 75 (2006): 154–160.

55. See E. Campbell, R. Gruen, J. Mountford, et al., "A National Survey of Physician-Industry Relationships," *New England Journal of Medicine* 356 (April 26, 2007): 1742–1750; G. Harris and J. Roberts, "Doctors' Ties to Drug Makers Are Put on Close View," *New York Times*, March 21, 2007.

56. G. Harris, B. Carey, and J. Roberts, "Psychiatrists, Children and Drug Industry's Role," *New York Times*, May 10, 2007.

57. See M. Sperber, "Short-Sheeting the Psychiatric Bed: State-Level Strategies to Curtail the Unnecessary Hospitalization of Adolescents in For-Profit

Mental Health Facilities," *American Journal of Law and Medicine* 18 (1992): 251–276; J. Lock and G. Strauss, "Psychiatric Hospitalization of Adolescents for Conduct Disorder," *Hospital and Community Psychiatry* 45 (September 1994): 925–928; L. Weithorn, "Mental Hospitalization of Troublesome Youth: An Analysis of Skyrocketing Admission Rates," *Stanford Law Review* 40 (February 1988): 773–838; S. Appelbaum, "Admitting Children to Psychiatric Hospitals: A Controversy Revived," *Hospital and Community Psychiatry* 40 (April 1989): 334–335.

58. See G. Mihalik and M. Scherer, "Fundamental Mechanisms of Managed Behavioral Health," *Journal of Health Care Finance* 24 (Spring 1998): 1–15; D. Staton, "Psychiatry's Future: Facing Reality," *Psychiatric Quarterly* 62 (Summer 1991): 165–176.

59. Tomes, "The Patient as a Policy Factor."

60. See J. Perrin, "Health Services Research for Children with Disabilities," *Milbank Quarterly* 80 (2002): 303–324.

61. See D. Safer and J. Krager, "The Increased Rate of Stimulant Treatment for Hyperactive/Inattentive Students in Secondary Schools," *Pediatrics* 94 (October 1994): 462–464.

62. See D. Callahan et al., "Special Supplement: MBD, Drug Research and the Schools," *Hastings Center Report* 6 (June 1976): 1–23; D. Safer and J. Krager, "Effect of a Media Blitz and a Threatened Lawsuit on Stimulant Treatment," *Journal of the American Medical Association* 268 (August 26, 1992): 1004–1007.

63. See L. Diller, "The Run on Ritalin: Attention Deficit Disorder and Stimulant Treatment in the 1990s," *Hastings Center Report* 26 (March–April 1996): 12–18.

64. N. Gibbs, "The Age of Ritalin," *Time*, November 30, 1998, 89–96; A. Adesman, "Does My Child Need Ritalin?" *Newsweek*, April 24, 2000, 81.

65. P. Breggin, "Treatment of Attention-Deficit/Hyperactivity Disorder," *Journal of the American Medical Association* 281 (April 28, 1999): 1490–1491; E. Marshall, "Epidemiology: Duke Study Faults Overuse of Stimulants for Children," *Science* 289 (August 4, 2000): 721.

66. See C. Milne, "Pediatric Research: Coming of Age in the New Millennium," *American Journal of Therapeutics* 6 (September 1999): 263–282; B. Vitiello, "Psychopharmacology for Young Children: Clinical Needs and Research Opportunities," *Pediatrics* 108 (October 2001): 983–989.

67. See V. Benedetto, J. Heiligenstein, M. Riddle, et al., "The Interface between Publicly Funded and Industry-Funded Research in Pediatric Psychopharmacology: Opportunities for Integration and Collaboration," *Biological Psychiatry* 56 (July 2004): 3–9.

68. See M. Stein, "Innovations in Attention-Deficit/Hyperactivity Disorder Pharmacotherapy: Long-Acting Stimulant and Nonstimulant Treatments," *American Journal of Managed Care* 10 (July 2004): S89–S98; F. Lopez, "ADHD: New Pharmacological Treatments on the Horizon," *Journal of Developmental Behavioral Pediatrics* 27 (October 2006): 410–416.

69. See J. Lear, "Health at School: A Hidden Health Care System Emerges from the Shadows," *Health Affairs* 26 (March–April 2007): 409–419.

70. See A. Campbell, "Consent, Competence, and Confidentiality Related to Psychiatric Conditions in Adolescent Medicine Practice," *Adolescent Medicine Clinics* 17 (February 2006): 25–47.

71. See L. Leslie, D. Plemmons, A. Monn, et al., "Investigating ADHD Treatment Trajectories: Listening to Families' Stories about Medication Use," *Journal of Development and Behavioral Pediatrics* 28 (June 2007): 179–188.

72. Ibid.

73. See A. Rains and L. Scahill, "New Long-Acting Stimulants in Children with ADHD," *Journal of Child and Adolescent Psychiatric Nursing* 17 (October–December 2004): 177–179.

74. See B. Carey, "What's Wrong with a Child? Psychiatrists Often Disagree," *New York Times*, November 11, 2006; T. Savage, "Ethical Issues Surrounding Attention Deficit Hyperactivity Disorder," *Pediatric Nursing* 22 (May–June 1996): 239–243; C. Malacrida, "Alternative Therapies and Attention Deficit Disorder: Discourses of Maternal Responsibility and Risk," *Gender and Society* 16 (June 2002): 366–385.

75. C. Poulin, "From Attention-Deficit/Hyperactivity Disorder to Medical Stimulant Use to the Diversion of Prescribed Stimulants to Non-Medical Stimulant Use: Connecting the Dots," *Addiction* 102 (May 2007): 740–751.

76. See N. Zamiska, "Students Turn to Drugs to Ace Admissions Exams," *Wall Street Journal*, November 8, 2004, A1.

77. See B. Carroll, T. McLaughlin, and D. Blake, "Patterns and Knowledge of Nonmedical Use of Stimulants among College Students," *Archives of Pediatric and Adolescent Medicine* 160 (May 2006): 481–485; K. Kaloyanides, S. McCabe, J. Cranford, et al., "Prevalence of Illicit Use and Abuse of Prescription Stimulants, Alcohol, and Other Drugs among College Students: Relationship with Age at Initiation of Prescription Stimulants," *Pharmacotherapy* 27 (May 2007): 666–674; S. McCabe, C. Teter, and C. Boyd, "The Use, Misuse and Diversion of Prescription Stimulants among Middle and High School Students," *Substance Use and Misuse* 39 (June 2004): 1095–1116.

78. See C. Brandon, M. Marinelli, L. Baker, et al., "Enhanced Reactivity and Vulnerability to Cocaine Following Methylphenidate Treatment in Adolescent Rats," *Neuropsychopharmacology* 25 (2001): 651–661; W. Carlezon, S. Mague, and S. Andersen, "Enduring Behavioral Effects of Early Exposure to Methylphenidate in Rats," *Biological Psychiatry* 54 (December 15, 2003): 1330–1337; M. Fischer and R. Barkley, "Childhood Stimulant Treatment and Risk for Later Substance Abuse," *Journal of Clinical Psychiatry* 63 (2003, Suppl.): 19–23.

79. See Castle et al., "Trends in Medication Treatment for ADHD."

80. See R. Friedman and A. Leon, "Expanding the Black Box: Depression, Antidepressants, and the Risk of Suicide," *New England Journal of Medicine* 356 (June 7, 2007): 2343–2346; R. Kowatch and M. Delbello, "Pediatric Bipolar Disorder: Emerging Diagnostic and Treatment Approaches," *Child*

*and Adolescent Psychiatric Clinics of North America* 15 (January 2006): 73–108; A. Dean, B. McDermott, and R. Marshall, "Psychotropic Medication Utilization in a Child and Adolescent Mental Health Service," *Journal of Child and Adolescent Psychopharmacology* 16 (June 2006): 273–285; S. Markowitz and A. Cuellar, "Antidepressants and Youth: Healing or Harmful?" *Social Science and Medicine* 64 (May 2007): 2138–2151; R. Aparasu and V. Bhatara, "Patterns and Determinants of Antipsychotic Prescribing in Children and Adolescents, 2003–2004," *Current Medical Research and Opinion* 23 (January 2007): 49–56.

81. See C. Moreno, L. Gonzalo, C. Blanco, et al., "National Trends in the Outpatient Diagnosis and Treatment of Bipolar Disorder in Youth," *Archives of General Psychiatry* 64 (September 2007): 1032–1039.

82. See S. Zuvekas, "Prescription Drugs and the Changing Patterns of Treatment for Mental Disorders, 1996–2001," *Health Affairs* 24 (January–February 2005): 195–205; R. Frank, R. Conti, and H. Goldman, "Mental Health Policy and Psychotropic Drugs," *Milbank Quarterly* 83 (2005): 271–298.

83. See A. Kleinman, "Culture and Depression," *New England Journal of Medicine* 351 (September 2, 2004): 951–953; A. Pumariega and E. Rothe, "Cultural Considerations in Child and Adolescent Psychiatric Emergencies and Crises," *Child and Adolescent Psychiatric Clinics of North America* 12 (October 2003): 723–744; L. Kirmayer and A. Young, "Culture and Context in the Evolutionary Concept of Mental Disorder," *Journal of Abnormal Psychology* 108 (August 1999): 446–452.

84. See R. Bussing, N. Schoenberg, and A. Perwien, "Knowledge and Information about ADHD: Evidence of Cultural Differences among African-American and White Parents," *Social Science and Medicine* 46 (April 1998): 919–928; J. McLeod, D. Fettes, P. Jensen, et al., "Public Knowledge, Beliefs, and Treatment Preferences Concerning Attention-Deficit Hyperactivity Disorder," *Psychiatric Services* 58 (May 2007): 626–631.

85. B. Good, "Studying Mental Illness in Context: Local, Global or Universal?" *Ethos* 25 (1997): 231.

86. See P. Breggin, *Talking Back to Ritalin* (New York: Da Capo, 2001).

87. See American Medical Association, "Report 10 of the Council on Science and Public Health: Attention Deficit Hyperactivity Disorder," June 2007, www.ama-assn.org/ama/pub/category/17738.html (accessed November 27, 2007).

88. See E. Chan, M. Hopkins, J. Perrin, et al., "Diagnostic Practices for Attention Deficit Hyperactivity Disorder: A National Survey of Primary Care Physicians," *Ambulatory Pediatrics* 5 (July–August 2005): 201–208; B. Olson, P. Rosenbaum, N. Dosa, et al., "Improving Guideline Adherence for the Diagnosis of ADHD in an Ambulatory Pediatric Setting," *Ambulatory Pediatrics* 5 (May–June 2005): 138–142; J. Rushton, K. Fant, and S. Clark, "Use of Practice Guidelines in the Primary Care of Children with Attention-Deficit/Hyperactivity Disorder," *Pediatrics* 114 (July 2004): 23–28.

89. See L. Furman, "What Is Attention-Deficit Hyperactivity Disorder (ADHD)?" *Journal of Child Neurology* 20 (December 2005): 994–1002.

90. See P. Shaw, K. Eckstrand, W. Sharp, et al., "Attention-Deficit/Hyperactivity Disorder Is Characterized by a Delay in Cortical Maturation," *Proceedings of the National Academy of Sciences* 104 (November 2007): 19649–19654.

91. See B. Lahey, W. Pelham, J. Loney, et al., "Instability of the DSM-IV Subtypes of ADHD from Preschool through Elementary School," *Archives of General Psychiatry* 62 (August 2005): 896–902.

92. See A. Rafalovich, "Exploring Clinician Uncertainty in the Diagnosis and Treatment of Attention Deficit Hyperactivity Disorder," *Sociology of Health and Illness* 27 (April 2005): 305–323; A. Kwasman, B. Tinsley, and H. Lepper, "Pediatricians' Knowledge and Attitudes Concerning Diagnosis and Treatment of Attention Deficit and Hyperactivity Disorders: A National Survey Approach," *Archives of Pediatric and Adolescent Medicine* 149 (November 1995): 1211–1216; E. Carlson, D. Jacobvitz, and L. Sroufe, "A Developmental Investigation of Inattentiveness and Hyperactivity," *Child Development* 66 (February 1995): 37–54; Chan et al., "Diagnostic Practices for Attention Deficit Hyperactivity Disorder," 23–28.

93. See L. Furman and B. Berman, "Rethinking the AAP Attention Deficit/Hyperactivity Disorder Guidelines," *Clinical Pediatrics* 43 (2004): 601–603.

94. See C. Whalen, L. Jamner, B. Henker, et al., "The ADHD Spectrum and Everyday Life: Experience Sampling of Adolescent Moods, Activities, Smoking, and Drinking," *Child Development* 73 (January–February 2002): 209–227; E. Taylor and J. Rogers, "Practitioner Review: Early Adversity and Developmental Disorders," *Journal of Child Psychology and Psychiatry* 46 (May 2005): 451–467; S. Mayes, S. Calhoun, and E. Crowell, "Learning Disabilities and ADHD: Overlapping Spectrum Disorders," *Journal of Learning Disabilities* 33 (September–October 2000): 417–424.

95. See T. Power, T. Costigan, S. Leff, et al., "Assessing ADHD across Settings: Contributions of Behavioral Assessment to Categorical Decision-Making," *Journal of Clinical Child Psychology* 30 (September 2001): 399–412.

96. See I. Singh, "A Framework for Understanding Trends in ADHD Diagnosis and Stimulant Drug Treatment: School and Schooling as a Case Study," *BioSocieties* 1 (2006): 439–452.

97. See I. Singh, "Biology in Context: Social and Cultural Perspective on ADHD," *Children and Society* 16 (2002): 360–367.

98. See S. Burt, "Sources of Covariation among Attention-Deficit/Hyperactivity Disorder, Oppositional Defiant Disorder, and Conduct Disorder: The Importance of Shared Environment," *Journal of Abnormal Psychology* 110 (November 2001): 516–525; J. Warner-Rogers, A. Taylor, E. Taylor, et al., "Inattentive Behavior in Childhood: Epidemiology and Implications for Development," *Journal of Learning Disabilities* 33 (November 2000): 520–536; S. Hinshaw, "Impulsivity, Emotion Regulation, and Developmental Psychopathology: Specificity versus Generality of Linkages," *Annals of the New York Academy of Sciences* 149 (December 2003): 149–159; Spencer et al., "Attention-Deficit/Hyperactivity Disorder: Diagnosis."

99. Sydney Z. Spiesel, clinical associate professor of pediatrics, Yale University School of Medicine, e-mail exchange with Rick Mayes, October 7, 2007.

100. See M. Wynia, D. Cummins, J. VanGeest, et al., "Physician Manipulation of Reimbursement Rules for Patients: Between a Rock and a Hard Place," *Journal of the American Medical Association* 283 (April 12, 2000): 1858–1865.

101. See J. Rushton, B. Felt, and M. Roberts, "Coding of Pediatric Behavioral and Mental Disorders," *Pediatrics* 110 (July 2002): e8; Rafalovich, "Exploring Clinician Uncertainty," 313; Carey, "What's Wrong with a Child? Psychiatrists Often Disagree."

102. See W. Gardner, K. Kelleher, K. Pajer, et al., "Primary Care Clinicians' Use of Standardized Psychiatric Diagnoses," *Child: Care, Health and Development* 30 (September 2004): 401–412.

103. See E. Campbell, "Doctors and Drug Companies—Scrutinizing Influential Relationships," *New England Journal of Medicine* 357 (November 1, 2007): 1796–1797.

104. See T. Widiger and D. Samuel, "Diagnostic Categories or Dimensions? A Question for the Diagnostic and Statistical Manual of Mental Disorders—Fifth Edition," *Journal of Abnormal Psychology* 114 (November 2005): 494–504; A. Jablensky, "Categories, Dimensions and Prototypes: Critical Issues for Psychiatric Classification," *Psychopathology* 38 (July–August 2005): 201–205.

105. See T. Beauchaine, "Taxometrics and Developmental Psychopathology," *Development and Psychopathology* 15 (Summer 2003): 501–527; S. Rosenman, "Reconsidering the Attention Deficit Paradigm," *Australasian Psychiatry* 14 (June 2006): 127–132.

106. See S. Pliszka, "Patterns of Psychiatric Comorbidity with Attention Deficit/Hyperactivity Disorder," *Child Adolescent Psychiatric Clinics of North America* 9 (2000): 525–540; T. Wilens, J. Biederman, S. Brown, et al., "Psychiatric Comorbidity and Functioning in Clinically Referred Preschool Children and School-Age Youth with ADHD," *Journal of the American Academy of Child and Adolescent Psychiatry* 41 (2002): 262–268.

107. See E. Owens, S. Hinshaw, H. Kraemer, et al., "Which Treatment for Whom for ADHD? Moderators of Treatment Response in the MTA," *Journal of Consulting and Clinical Psychology* 71 (June 2003): 540–542; S. Hinshaw, "Moderators and Mediators of Treatment Outcome for Youth with ADHD: Understanding for Whom and How Interventions Work," *Journal of Pediatric Psychology* 32 (July 2007): 664–675.

## 2. An Introduction to ADHD

1. American Psychiatric Association, *Diagnostic and Statistical Manual of Mental Disorders*, 4th ed. (Washington, DC: American Psychiatric Association, 1994).

2. B. Applegate, B. Lahey, E. Hart, et al., "Validity of the Age-of-Onset Criterion for ADHD: A Report of the DSM-IV Field Trials," *Journal of the American Academy of Child and Adolescent Psychiatry* 36 (1997): 1211–1221. Also see discussion in R. A. Barkley, *Attention-Deficit Hyperactivity Disorder: A Handbook for Diagnosis and Treatment*, 3rd ed. (New York: Guilford Press, 2006).

3. R. Barkley and C. Edelbrock, "Assessing Situational Variation in Children's Behavior Problems: The Home and School Situations Questionnaires," in *Advances in Behavioral Assessment of Children and Families*, ed. R. Prinz (Greenwich, CT: JAI Press, 1987), 157–176.

4. T. Altpeter and M. Breen, "Situational Variation in Problem Behavior at Home and School in Attention Deficit Disorder with Hyperactivity: A Factor Analytic Study," *Journal of Child Psychology and Psychiatry* 33 (1992): 741–748; G. DuPaul and R. Barkley, "Situational Variability of Attention Problems: Psychometric Properties of the Revised Home and School Situations Questionnaires," *Journal of Clinical Child Psychology* 21 (1992): 178–188.

5. A. Anastopoulos and T. Shelton, *Assessing Attention-Deficit/Hyperactivity Disorder* (New York: Kluwer Academic/Plenum Publishers, 2001).

6. D. Cantwell, "Attention Deficit Disorder: A Review of the Past 10 Years," *Journal of the American Academy of Child and Adolescent Psychiatry* 35 (1996): 978–987.

7. Anastopoulos and Shelton, *Assessing Attention-Deficit/Hyperactivity Disorder*.

8. Ibid.

9. P. Szatmari, "The Epidemiology of Attention-Deficit Hyperactivity Disorders," *Child and Adolescent Psychiatric Clinics of North America* 1 (1992): 361–372.

10. E. Nolan, K. Gadow, and J. Sprafkin, "Teacher Reports of DSM-IV ADHD, ODD, and CD Symptoms in Schoolchildren," *Journal of the American Academy of Child and Adolescent Psychiatry* 40 (2001): 241–249.

11. E. Costello, S. Mustillo, A. Erkanli, et al., "Prevalence and Development of Psychiatric Disorders in Childhood and Adolescence," *Archives of General Psychiatry* 60 (2003): 837–844.

12. Ibid.

13. For examples, see J. Breton, L. Bergeron, J. Valla, et al., "Quebec Children Mental Health Survey: Prevalence of DSM-III-R Mental Health Disorders," *Journal of Child Psychology and Psychiatry* 40 (1999): 375–384; M. Briggs-Gowan, S. Horwitz, M. Schwab-Stone, et al., "Mental Health in Pediatric Settings: Distribution of Disorders and Factors Related to Service Use," *Journal of the American Academy of Child and Adolescent Psychiatry* 39 (2000): 841–849; P. Szatmari, D. Offord, and M. Boyle, "Correlates, Associated Impairments, and Patterns of Service Utilization of Children with Attention Deficit Disorders: Findings from the Ontario Child Health Study," *Journal of Child Psychology and Psychiatry* 30 (1989): 205–217.

14. Szatmari et al., "Correlates, Associated Impairments, and Patterns of Service Utilization."
15. R. Barkley, *Attention-Deficit Hyperactivity Disorder: A Handbook for Diagnosis and Treatment*, 2nd ed. (New York: Guilford Press, 1998).
16. B. Lahey, B. Applegate, K. McBurnett, et al., "DSM-IV Field Trials for Attention Deficit/Hyperactivity Disorder in Children and Adolescents," *American Journal of Psychiatry* 151 (1994): 1673–1685.
17. Ibid.
18. J. Biederman, M. Monuteaux, E. Mick, et al., "Psychopathology in Females with Attention-Deficit/Hyperactivity Disorder: A Controlled, Five-Year Prospective Study," *Biological Psychiatry* 60 (2006): 1098–1105; S. Hinshaw, E. Owens, N. Sami, et al., "Prospective Follow-Up of Girls with Attention-Deficit/Hyperactivity Disorder into Adolescence: Evidence for Continuing Cross-Domain Impairment," *Journal of Consulting and Clinical Psychology* 74 (2006): 489–499.
19. R. Loeber, S. Green, B. Lahey, et al., "Developmental Sequences in the Age of Onset of Disruptive Child Behaviors," *Journal of Child and Family Studies* 1 (1992): 21–41.
20. Applegate et al., "Validity of the Age-of-Onset Criterion for ADHD."
21. Szatmari et al., "Correlates, Associated Impairments, and Patterns of Service Utilization."
22. E. Hart, B. Lahey, R. Loeber, et al., "Developmental Changes in Attention-Deficit Hyperactivity Disorder in Boys: A Four-Year Longitudinal Study," *Journal of Abnormal Child Psychology* 23 (1995): 729–750.
23. S. Okie, "ADHD in Adults," *New England Journal of Medicine* 354 (June 22, 2006): 2637–2641. Also see R. Barkley, K. Murphy, and M. Fischer, *ADHD in Adults: What the Science Says* (New York: Guilford Press, 2008). This text provides extensive detail on a follow-up study of adults with a history of ADHD in childhood and on a study of clinic-referred adults with ADHD. The authors report comprehensive data on the degree of impairment and disability in adulthood for individuals with ADHD and for individuals with a history of ADHD.
24. R. Gittelman, S. Mannuzza, R. Shenker, et al., "Hyperactive Boys Almost Grown Up: I. Psychiatric Status," *Archives of General Psychiatry* 42 (1985): 937–947; S. Mannuzza, R. Klein, N. Bonagura, et al., "Hyperactive Boys Almost Grown Up: V. Replication of Psychiatric Status," *Archives of General Psychiatry* 48 (1991): 77–83.
25. D. Claude and P. Firestone, "The Development of ADHD Boys: A 12-Year Follow-Up," *Canadian Journal of Behavioral Science* 27 (1995): 226–249.
26. R. Barkley, M. Fischer, L. Smallish, et al., "The Persistence of Attention-Deficit/Hyperactivity Disorder into Young Adulthood as a Function of Reporting Source and Definition of Disorder," *Journal of Abnormal Psychology* 111 (2002): 279–289. Barkley et al., *ADHD in Adults*.

27. B. Molina and W. Pelham, Jr., "Childhood Predictors of Adolescent Substance Use in a Longitudinal Study of Children with ADHD," *Journal of Abnormal Psychology* 112 (2003): 497–507.

28. J. Biederman, S. Faraone, S. Milberger, et al., "A Prospective 4-Year Follow-Up Study of Attention-Deficit Hyperactivity and Related Disorders," *Archives of General Psychiatry* 53 (1996): 437–446.

29. R. Kessler, L. Adler, R. Barkley, et al., "Patterns and Predictors of Attention-Deficit/Hyperactivity Disorder Persistence into Adulthood: Results from the National Comorbidity Survey Replication," *Biological Psychiatry* 57 (2005): 1442–1451.

30. R. Barkley, M. Fischer, C. Edelbrock, et al., "The Adolescent Outcome of Hyperactive Children Diagnosed by Research Criteria: I. An 8-Year Prospective Follow-Up Study," *Journal of the American Academy of Child and Adolescent Psychiatry* 29 (1990): 546–557; Biederman et al., "A Prospective 4-Year Follow-Up Study"; Molina and Pelham, "Childhood Predictors of Adolescent Substance Use"; Biederman et al., "Psychopathology in Females with Attention-Deficit/Hyperactivity Disorder"; Hinshaw et al., "Prospective Follow-Up of Girls with Attention-Deficit/Hyperactivity Disorder into Adolescence."

31. Barkley et al., "The Adolescent Outcome of Hyperactive Children"; Biederman et al., "A Prospective 4-Year Follow-Up Study"; M. Fischer, R. Barkley, C. Edelbrock, and L. Smallish, "The Adolescent Outcome of Hyperactive Children Diagnosed by Research Criteria: II. Academic, Attentional, and Neuropsychological Status," *Journal of Consulting and Clinical Psychology* 58 (1990): 580–588.

32. C. Bagwell, B. Molina, W. Pelham, Jr., et al., "Attention-Deficit Hyperactivity Disorder and Problems in Peer Relations: Predictions from Childhood to Adolescence," *Journal of the American Academy of Child and Adolescent Psychiatry* 40 (2001): 1285–1292; R. Barkley, M. Fischer, C. Edelbrock, and L. Smallish, "The Adolescent Outcome of Hyperactive Children Diagnosed by Research Criteria: III. Mother-Child Interactions, Family Conflicts, and Maternal Psychopathology," *Journal of Child Psychology and Psychiatry* 32 (1991): 233–255; Biederman et al., "A Prospective 4-Year Follow-Up Study."

33. Biederman et al., "A Prospective 4-Year Follow-Up Study"; M. Fischer, R. Barkley, L. Smallish, and K. Fletcher, "Young Adult Follow-Up of Hyperactive Children: Self-Reported Psychiatric Disorders, Comorbidity, and the Role of Childhood Conduct Problems and Teen CD," *Journal of Abnormal Child Psychology* 30 (2002): 463–475; Barkley et al., *ADHD in Adults.* Note that at the age 27 follow-up assessment, Barkley and colleagues distinguished between probands who had current ADHD and probands who did not. Probands with current ADHD had increased risk for any mood disorder (but not major depression alone) compared to the non-ADHD comparison group, but probands without current ADHD did not show this increased risk relative to the comparison group.

34. Claude and Firestone, "The Development of ADHD Boys"; S. Mannuzza, R. Klein, A. Bessler, et al., "Adult Outcome of Hyperactive Boys: Educa-

tional Achievement, Occupational Rank, and Psychiatric Status," *Archives of General Psychiatry* 50 (1993): 565–576; S. Mannuzza, R. Klein, A. Bessler, et al., "Adult Psychiatric Status of Hyperactive Boys Grown Up," *American Journal of Psychiatry* 155 (1998): 493–498.

35. C. Bagwell, B. Molina, T. Kashdan, et al., "Anxiety and Mood Disorders in Adolescents with Childhood Attention-Deficit/Hyperactivity Disorder," *Journal of Emotional and Behavioral Disorders* 14 (2006): 178–187; Fischer et al., "Young Adult Follow-Up of Hyperactive Children."

36. For reviews, see A. Angold, E. Costello, and A. Erkanli, "Comorbidity," *Journal of Child Psychology and Psychiatry* 40 (1999): 57–87; P. Jensen, D. Martin, and D. Cantwell, "Comorbidity in ADHD: Implications for Research, Practice, and DSM-V," *Journal of the American Academy of Child and Adolescent Psychiatry* 36 (1997): 1065–1079.

37. Angold et al., "Comorbidity."

38. Fischer et al., "Young Adult Follow-Up of Hyperactive Children"; Mannuzza et al., "Adult Outcome of Hyperactive Boys"; Mannuzza et al., "Adult Psychiatric Status of Hyperactive Boys Grown Up."

39. Jensen et al., "Comorbidity in ADHD."

40. For examples, see J. Biederman, J. Newcorn, and S. Sprich, "Comorbidity of Attention Deficit Hyperactivity Disorder with Conduct, Depressive, Anxiety, and Other Disorders," *American Journal of Psychiatry* 148 (1991): 564–577; MTA Cooperative Group, "A 14-Month Randomized Clinical Trial of Treatment Strategies for Attention Deficit Hyperactivity Disorder," *Archives of General Psychiatry* 56 (1999): 1073–1086.

41. Angold et al., "Comorbidity."

42. Ibid.

43. C. Paternite, J. Loney, H. Salisbury, et al., "Childhood Inattention-Overactivity, Aggression, and Stimulant Medication History as Predictors of Young Adult Outcomes," *Journal of Child and Adolescent Psychopharmacology* 9 (1999): 169–184.

44. Fischer et al., "Young Adult Follow-Up of Hyperactive Children."

45. Jensen et al., "Comorbidity in ADHD."

46. P. Jensen, S. Hinshaw, H. Kraemer, et al., "ADHD Comorbidity Findings from the MTA Study: Comparing Comorbid Subgroups," *Journal of the American Academy of Child and Adolescent Psychiatry* 40 (2001): 147–158.

47. S. Hinshaw, "Is ADHD an Impairing Condition in Childhood and Adolescence?" in *Attention Deficit Hyperactivity Disorder: State of the Science, Best Practices*, ed. P. Jensen and J. Cooper (Kingston, NJ: Civic Research Institute, 2002), 3–5.

48. R. Barkley, *Attention-Deficit Hyperactivity Disorder: A Handbook for Diagnosis and Treatment* (New York: Guilford Press, 1990).

49. D. Cantwell and L. Baker, "Association between Attention Deficit Hyperactivity Disorder and Learning Disorders," in *Attention Deficit Disorder Comes of Age: Toward the Twenty-First Century*, ed. S. E. Shaywitz and B. A. Shaywitz (Austin, TX: Pro-Ed, 1992), 145–164.

50. For a review, see S. Hinshaw, "Externalizing Behavior Problems and Academic Underachievement in Childhood and Adolescence: Causal Relationships and Underlying Mechanisms," *Psychological Bulletin* 111 (1992): 127–155.

51. R. Barkley, G. DuPaul, and M. McMurray, "A Comprehensive Evaluation of Attention Deficit Disorder with and without Hyperactivity," *Journal of Consulting and Clinical Psychology* 58 (1990): 775–789; S. W. Brock and P. Knapp, "Reading Comprehension Abilities of Children with Attention-Deficit/Hyperactivity Disorder," *Journal of Attention Disorders* 1 (1996): 173–186; D. Cantwell and J. Satterfield, "The Prevalence of Academic Underachievement in Hyperactive Children," *Journal of Pediatric Psychology* 3 (1978): 168–171.

52. M. Rapport, S. Scanlan, and C. Denney, "Attention-Deficit/Hyperactivity Disorder and Scholastic Achievement: A Model of Dual Developmental Pathways," *Journal of Child Psychology and Psychiatry* 40 (1999): 1169–1183.

53. W. Pelham and M. Bender, "Peer Relationships in Hyperactive Children," *Advances in Learning and Behavioral Disabilities* 1 (1982): 365–436; C. Whalen and B. Henker, "The Social Profile of Attention-Deficit Hyperactivity Disorder: Five Fundamental Facets," *Child and Adolescent Psychiatric Clinics of North America* 1 (1992): 395–410.

54. D. Erhardt and S. Hinshaw, "Initial Sociometric Impressions of Attention-Deficit Hyperactivity Disorder and Comparison Boys: Predictions from Social Behaviors and from Nonbehavioral Variables," *Journal of Consulting and Clinical Psychology* 62 (1994): 833–842; Pelham and Bender, "Peer Relationships in Hyperactive Children."

55. S. Hinshaw and S. Melnick, "Peer Relationships in Boys with Attention-Deficit Hyperactivity Disorder with and without Comorbid Aggression," *Development and Psychopathology* 7 (1995): 627–647.

56. Pelham and Bender, "Peer Relationships in Hyperactive Children."

57. A. Pope, K. Bierman, and G. Mumma, "Relations between Hyperactive and Aggressive Behavior and Peer Relations at Three Elementary Grade Levels," *Journal of Abnormal Child Psychology* 17 (1989): 253–267.

58. Hinshaw and Melnick, "Peer Relationships in Boys with Attention-Deficit Hyperactivity Disorder."

59. Ibid.

60. Pope et al., "Relations between Hyperactive and Aggressive Behavior and Peer Relations"; A. Pope and K. Bierman, "Predicting Adolescent Peer Problems and Antisocial Activities: The Relative Roles of Aggression and Dysregulation," *Developmental Psychology* 35 (1999): 335–346.

61. K. Bierman, *Peer Rejection* (New York: Guilford Press, 2004).

62. S. Hinshaw, "Preadolescent Girls with Attention-Deficit/Hyperactivity Disorder: I. Background Characteristics, Comorbidity, Cognitive and Social Functioning, and Parenting Practices," *Journal of Consulting and Clinical Psychology* 70 (2002): 1086–1098.

63. For reviews, see Bierman, *Peer Rejection*; J. Parker and S. Asher, "Peer Relations and Later Personal Adjustment: Are Low Accepted Children 'At Risk'?" *Psychological Bulletin* 102 (1987): 357–389; K. Rubin, W. Bukowski, and J. Parker, "Peer Interactions, Relationships, and Groups," in *Handbook of Child Psychology*, 6th ed., ed. N. Eisenberg, W. Damon, and R. Lerner (New York: Wiley, 1998), 571–645.

64. For further discussion, see S. Mrug, B. Hoza, and A. Gerdes, "Children with Attention-Deficit/Hyperactivity Disorder: Peer Relationships and Peer-Oriented Interventions," in *The Role of Friendship in Psychological Adjustment*, ed. D. W. Nangle and C. A. Erdley (San Francisco: Jossey-Bass, 2001), 51–77.

65. D. Blachman and S. Hinshaw, "Patterns of Friendship among Girls with and without Attention-Deficit/Hyperactivity Disorder," *Journal of Abnormal Child Psychology* 30 (2002): 625–640; Whalen and Henker, "The Social Profile of Attention-Deficit Hyperactivity Disorder." For an exception, see B. Hoza, S. Mrug, A. Gerdes, et al., "What Aspects of Peer Relationships Are Impaired in Children with Attention-Deficit/Hyperactivity Disorder?" *Journal of Consulting and Clinical Psychology* 73 (2005): 411–423.

66. J. Hubbard and A. Newcomb, "Initial Dyadic Peer Interaction of Attention Deficit-Hyperactivity Disorder and Normal Boys," *Journal of Abnormal Child Psychology* 19 (1991): 179–195.

67. Blachman and Hinshaw, "Patterns of Friendship among Girls with and without Attention-Deficit/Hyperactivity Disorder."

68. Bagwell et al., "Attention-Deficit Hyperactivity Disorder and Problems in Peer Relations."

69. S. Campbell, "Attention-Deficit/Hyperactivity Disorder: A Developmental View," in *Handbook of Developmental Psychopathology*, 2nd ed., ed. A. Sameroff, M. Lewis, and S. Miller (New York: Kluwer Academic/ Plenum Publishers, 2000), 383–401.

70. See, for example, J. Nigg, *What Causes ADHD?* (New York: Guilford Press, 2006).

71. R. Barkley, "Attention-Deficit/Hyperactivity Disorder," in *Child Psychopathology*, 2nd ed., ed. E. J. Mash and R. A. Barkley (New York: Guilford Press, 2003), 75–143.

72. C. Conners and L. Eisenberg, "The Effects of Methylphenidate on Symptomatology and Learning in Disturbed Children," *American Journal of Psychiatry* 120 (November 1963): 458–464.

73. For a review and discussion of disinhibition and other mechanisms as they relate to ADHD, see J. Nigg, "Is ADHD a Disinhibitory Disorder?" *Psychological Bulletin* 127 (2001): 571–598.

74. R. Barkley, "Behavioral Inhibition, Sustained Attention, and Executive Functions: Constructing a Unifying Theory of ADHD," *Psychological Bulletin* 121 (1997): 65–94; R. Barkley, *ADHD and the Nature of Self-Control* (New York: Guildford Press, 1997); Barkley, *Attention-Deficit Hyperactivity Disorder: A Handbook for Diagnosis and Treatment*, 3rd ed.

75. For reviews, see Nigg, "Is ADHD a Disinhibitory Disorder?"; Nigg, *What Causes ADHD?*

76. For a related model, see H. Quay, "Inhibition and Attention Deficit Hyperactivity Disorder," *Journal of Abnormal Child Psychology* 25 (1997): 7–13.

77. Barkley, "Attention-Deficit/Hyperactivity Disorder," 112.

78. For example, K. Sieg, G. Gaffney, D. Preston, et al., "SPECT Brain Imaging Abnormalities in Attention Deficit Hyperactivity Disorder," *Clinical Nuclear Medicine* 20 (1995): 55–60.

79. For examples, see A. Zametkin, L. Liebenauer, G. Fitzgerald, et al., "Brain Metabolism in Teenagers with Attention-Deficit Hyperactivity Disorder," *Archives of General Psychiatry* 50 (1993): 333–340; A. Zametkin, T. Nordahl, M. Gross, et al., "Cerebral Glucose Metabolism in Adults with Hyperactivity of Childhood Onset," *New England Journal of Medicine* 323 (1990): 1361–1366.

80. P. Berquin, J. Giedd, and L. Jacobsen, "Cerebellum in Attention-Deficit Hyperactivity Disorder: A Morphometric MRI Study," *Neurology* 50 (1998): 1087–1093; F. Castellanos, J. Giedd, P. Berquin, et al., "Quantitative Brain Magnetic Resonance Imaging in Girls with Attention-Deficit/Hyperactivity Disorder," *Archives of General Psychiatry* 58 (2001): 289–295; F. Castellanos, J. Giedd, W. Marsh, et al., "Quantitative Brain Magnetic Resonance Imaging in Attention-Deficit Hyperactivity Disorder," *Archives of General Psychiatry* 53 (1996): 607–616. F. Castellanos, W. Sharp, R. Gottesman, et al., "Anatomic Brain Abnormalities in Monozygotic Twins Discordant for Attention Deficit Hyperactivity Disorder," *American Journal of Psychiatry* 160 (2003): 1693–1695; P. Filipek, M. Semrud-Clikeman, R. Steingard, et al., "Volumetric MRI Analysis Comparing Subjects Having Attention-Deficit Hyperactivity Disorder with Normal Controls," *Neurology* 48 (1997): 589–601; D. Hill, R. Yeo, R. Campbell, et al., "Magnetic Resonance Imaging Correlates of Attention-Deficit/Hyperactivity Disorder in Children," *Neuropsychology* 17 (2003): 496–506; G. Hynd, K. Hern, E. Novey, et al., "Attention-Deficit Hyperactivity Disorder and Asymmetry of the Caudate Nucleus," *Journal of Child Neurology* 8 (1993): 339–347; G. Hynd, M. Semrud-Clikeman, A. Lorys, et al., "Brain Morphology in Developmental Dyslexia and Attention Deficit Disorder/Hyperactivity," *Archives of Neurology* 47 (1990): 919–926; Nigg, *What Causes ADHD?*; K. Plessen, R. Bansal, H. Zhu, et al., "Hippocampus and Amygdala Morphology in Attention-Deficit/Hyperactivity Disorder," *Archives of General Psychiatry* 63 (2006): 795–807; M. Semrud-Clikeman, R. Steingard, P. Filipek, et al., "Using MRI to Examine Brain-Behavior Relationships in Males with Attention Deficit Disorder with Hyperactivity," *Journal of the American Academy of Child and Adolescent Psychiatry* 39 (2000): 477–484.

81. S. Durston, "A Review of the Biological Bases of ADHD: What Have We Learned from Imaging Studies?" *Mental Retardation and Developmental Disabilities Research Reviews* 9 (2003): 184–195; R. Tannock, "Attention Deficit Hyperactivity Disorder: Advances in Cognitive, Neurobiological,

and Genetic Research," *Journal of Child Psychology and Psychiatry* 39 (1998): 65–100.

82. K. Schulz, C. Tang, J. Fan, et al., "Differential Prefrontal Cortex Activation during Inhibitory Control in Adolescents with and without Childhood Attention-Deficit/Hyperactivity Disorder," *Neuropsychology* 19 (2005): 390–402.

83. P. Shaw, K. Eckstrand, W. Sharp, et al., "Attention-Deficit/Hyperactivity Disorder Is Characterized by a Delay in Cortical Maturation," *Proceedings of the National Academy of Sciences* 104 (2007): 19649–19654.

84. Ibid.

85. Barkley, *Attention-Deficit Hyperactivity Disorder: A Handbook for Diagnosis and Treatment*, 2nd ed.

86. Barkley, *Attention-Deficit Hyperactivity Disorder: A Handbook for Diagnosis and Treatment*, 3rd ed.; J. Biederman, S. Faraone, K. Keenan, et al., "Evidence of a Familial Association between Attention Deficit Disorder and Major Affective Disorders," *Archives of General Psychiatry* 48 (1991): 633–642; J. Biederman, S. Faraone, K. Keenan, et al., "Further Evidence for Family-Genetic Risk Factors in Attention Deficit Hyperactivity Disorder: Patterns of Comorbidity in Probands and Relatives in Psychiatrically and Pediatrically Referred Samples," *Archives of General Psychiatry* 49 (2002): 728–738.

87. J. Biederman, S. Faraone, E. Mick, et al., "High Risk for Attention Deficit Hyperactivity Disorder among Children of Parents with Childhood Onset of the Disorder: A Pilot Study," *American Journal of Psychiatry* 152 (1995): 431–435.

88. J. Gilger, B. Pennington, and J. DeFries, "A Twin Study of the Etiology of Comorbidity: Attention-Deficit Hyperactivity Disorder and Dyslexia," *Journal of the American Academy of Child and Adolescent Psychiatry* 31 (1992): 343–348.

89. F. Levy, D. Hay, M. McStephen, et al., "Attention-Deficit Hyperactivity Disorder: A Category or a Continuum? Genetic Analysis of a Large-Scale Twin Study," *Journal of the American Academy of Child and Adolescent Psychiatry* 36 (1997): 737–744.

90. D. Sherman, W. Iacono, and M. McGue, "Attention-Deficit Hyperactivity Disorder Dimensions: A Twin Study of Inattention and Impulsivity-Hyperactivity," *Journal of the American Academy of Child and Adolescent Psychiatry* 54 (1997): 745–753.

91. T. Price, E. Simonoff, P. Asherson, et al., "Continuity and Change in Preschool ADHD Symptoms: Longitudinal Genetic Analysis with Contrast Effects," *Behavior Genetics* 35 (2005): 121–132.

92. For a review, see F. Levy and D. Hay, *Attention, Genes, and ADHD* (Philadelphia: Brunner-Routledge, 2001).

93. T. Bouchard, Jr., "IQ Similarity in Twins Reared Apart: Findings and Responses to Critics," in *Intelligence, Heredity, and Environment*, ed. R. J. Sternberg and E. Grigorenko (New York: Cambridge University Press,

1997), 126–160; E. Grigorenko, "Heritability and Intelligence," in *Handbook of Intelligence*, ed. R. J. Sternberg (New York: Cambridge University Press, 2000), 53–91.

94. L. Raskin, S. Shaywitz, B. Shaywitz, et al., "Neurochemical Correlates of Attention Deficit Disorder," *Pediatric Clinics of North America* 31 (1984): 387–396.

95. A. Arnsten, J. Steere, and R. Hunt, "The Contribution of alpha 2-Noradrenergic Mechanisms of Prefrontal Cortical Cognitive Function: Potential Significance for Attention-Deficit Hyperactivity Disorder," *Archives of General Psychiatry* 53 (1996): 448–455; J. Halperin, J. Newcorn, I. Kopstein, et al., "Serotonin, Aggression, and Parental Psychopathology in Children with Attention-Deficit Hyperactivity Disorder," *Journal of the American Academy of Child and Adolescent Psychiatry* 36 (1997): 1391–1398.

96. J. Quist and J. Kennedy, "Genetics of Childhood Disorders: XXIII. ADHD, Part 7: The Serotonin System," *Journal of the American Academy of Child and Adolescent Psychiatry* 40 (2001): 253–256.

97. Cantwell, "Attention Deficit Disorder: A Review of the Past 10 Years."

98. Halperin et al., "Serotonin, Aggression, and Parental Psychopathology."

99. K. Schulz, J. Newcorn, K. McKay, et al., "Relationship between Central Serotonergic Function and Aggression in Prepubertal Boys: Effect of Age and Attention-Deficit/Hyperactivity Disorder," *Psychiatry Research* 101 (2001): 1–10.

100. For example, N. Breslau, G. Brown, J. Del Dotto, et al., "Psychiatric Sequelae of Low Birth Weight at 6 Years of Age," *Journal of Abnormal Child Psychology* 24 (1996): 385–400; A. Whittaker, R. Van Rossem, J. Feldman, et al., "Psychiatric Outcomes in Low-Birth-Weight Children at Age 6 Years: Relation to Neonatal Cranial Ultrasound Abnormalities," *Archives of General Psychiatry* 54 (1997): 847–856.

101. For example, S. Milberger, J. Biederman, S. Faraone, et al., "Is Maternal Smoking during Pregnancy a Risk Factor for Attention Deficit Hyperactivity Disorder in Children?" *American Journal of Psychiatry* 153 (1996): 1138–1142.

102. For example, H. Needleman, A. Schell, D. Bellinger, et al., "The Long-Term Effects of Exposure to Low Doses of Lead in Childhood: An 11-Year Follow-Up Report," *New England Journal of Medicine* 322 (1990): 83–88.

103. For further discussion, see Barkley, *Attention-Deficit Hyperactivity Disorder: A Handbook for Diagnosis and Treatment*, 3rd ed.

104. See Nigg, *What Causes ADHD?* for a review.

105. For example, I. Silverman and D. Ragusa, "Child and Maternal Correlates of Impulse Control in 24-Month Old Children," *Genetic, Social, and General Psychology Monographs* 116 (1992): 435–473; T. Willis and I. Lovaas, "A Behavioral Approach to Treating Hyperactive Children: The Parent's Role," in *Learning Disabilities and Related Disorders*, ed. J. B. Millichap (Chicago: Year Book Medical, 1977), 119–140.

106. Levy et al., "Attention-Deficit Hyperactivity Disorder: A Category or a Continuum?"; Sherman et al., "Attention-Deficit Hyperactivity Disorder Dimensions."

107. V. Knopik, E. Sparrow, P. Madden, et al., "Contributions of Parental Alcoholism, Prenatal Substance Exposure, and Genetic Transmission to Child ADHD Risk: A Female Twin Study," *Psychological Medicine* 35 (2005): 625–635.

108. Barkley, "Attention-Deficit/Hyperactivity Disorder"; J. Nigg, S. Hinshaw, and C. Huang-Pollock, "Disorders of Attention and Impulse Regulation" in *Developmental Psychopathology,* vol. 3, *Risk, Disorder, and Adaptation,* 2nd ed., ed. D. Cicchetti and D. Cohen (New York: Wiley, 2006), 358–403. Nigg and colleagues provide a thorough discussion of transactional views of ADHD that explain how heredity is mediated by environmental factors in the development of ADHD.

109. Cantwell, "Attention Deficit Disorder: A Review of the Past 10 Years."

110. Campbell, "Attention-Deficit/Hyperactivity Disorder: A Developmental View."

111. S. Campbell, E. Pierce, G. Moore, et al., "Boys' Externalizing Problems at Elementary School Age: Pathways from Early Behavior Problems, Maternal Control, and Family Stress," *Development and Psychopathology* 8 (1996): 701–720.

112. Barkley, *Attention-Deficit Hyperactivity Disorder: A Handbook for Diagnosis and Treatment,* 2nd ed.; M. Fischer, "Parenting Stress and the Child with Attention Deficit Hyperactivity Disorder," *Journal of Clinical Child Psychology* 19 (1990): 337–346.

113. A. Sameroff, "General Systems Theories and Developmental Psychopathology," in *Developmental Psychopathology*, vol. 1, *Theory and Methods,* ed. D. Cicchetti and D. Cohen (New York: Wiley, 1995), 659–695.

114. C. Whalen, B. Henker, L. Jamner, et al., "Toward Mapping Daily Challenges of Living with ADHD: Maternal and Child Perspectives Using Electronic Devices," *Journal of Abnormal Child Psychology* 34 (2006): 15–130.

115. D. Connor, "Stimulants," in *Attention-Deficit Hyperactivity Disorder: A Handbook for Diagnosis and Treatment,* 3rd ed., by R. A. Barkley (New York: Guilford Press, 2006), 608–647; T. Spencer, J. Biederman, and T. Wilens, "Pharmacotherapy of Attention Deficit Hyperactivity Disorder," *Psychopharmacology* (2000): 77–97.

116. Connor, "Stimulants."

117. Ibid.

118. Cantwell, "Attention Deficit Disorder: A Review of the Past 10 Years."

119. D. Safer, J. Zito, and J. Gardner, "Pemoline Hepatoxicity and Postmarketing Surveillance," *Journal of the American Academy of Child and Adolescent Psychiatry* 40 (2001): 622–629.

120. Connor, "Stimulants."

121. W. Pelham, E. Gnagy, L. Burrows-Maclean, et al., "Once-a-Day Concerta Methylphenidate versus Three-Times-Daily Methylphenidate in Laboratory and Natural Settings," *Pediatrics* 107 (2001): 1417–1418; M. Wolraich, L. Greenhill, W. Pelham, et al., "Randomized, Controlled Trial of OROS Methylphenidate Once a Day in Children with Attention-Deficit/Hyperactivity Disorder," *Pediatrics* 108 (2001): 883–892.
122. Connor, "Stimulants"; T. Wigal, L. Greenhill, S. Chuang, et al., "Safety and Tolerability of Methylphenidate in Preschool Children with ADHD," *Journal of the American Academy of Child and Adolescent Psychiatry* 45 (2006): 1294–1303.
123. J. Swanson, L. Greenhill, T. Wigal, et al., "Stimulant-Related Reductions of Growth Rates in the PATS," *Journal of the American Academy of Child and Adolescent Psychiatry* 45 (2006): 1304–1313.
124. For a review, see Connor, "Stimulants"; R. Barkley, M. McMurray, C. Edelbrock, et al., "Side Effects of Methylphenidate in Children with Attention Deficit Hyperactivity Disorder: A Systemic, Placebo-Controlled Evaluation," *Pediatrics* 86 (1990): 184–192; Cantwell, "Attention Deficit Disorder: A Review of the Past 10 Years"; Swanson et al., "Stimulant-Related Reductions of Growth Rates in the PATS"; J. Swanson, G. Elliott, L. Greenhill, et al., "Effects of Stimulant Medication on Growth Rates across 3 Years in the MTA Follow-Up," *Journal of the American Academy of Child and Adolescent Psychiatry* 46 (2007): 1015–1027.
125. Connor, "Stimulants."
126. Ibid.; T. Wilens and T. Spencer, "The Stimulants Re-visited," *Child and Adolescent Psychiatric Clinics of North America* 9 (2000): 573–603.
127. Connor, "Stimulants."
128. Ibid.
129. F. Castellanos, J. Giedd, J. Elia, et al., "Controlled Stimulant Treatment of ADHD and Comorbid Tourette's Syndrome: Effects of Stimulants and Dose," *Journal of the American Academy of Child and Adolescent Psychiatry* 36 (1997): 1–8.
130. Cantwell, "Attention Deficit Disorder: A Review of the Past 10 Years."
131. For a review, see Spencer et al., "Pharmacotherapy of Attention Deficit Hyperactivity Disorder."
132. T. Spencer, "Antidepressant and Specific Norepinephrine Reuptake Inhibitor Treatments," in *Attention-Deficit Hyperactivity Disorder: A Handbook for Diagnosis and Treatment*, 3rd ed., by R. A. Barkley (New York: Guilford Press, 2006), 648–657.
133. Barkley, *Attention-Deficit Hyperactivity Disorder: A Handbook for Diagnosis and Treatment*, 2nd ed.
134. Barkley, *Attention-Deficit Hyperactivity Disorder: A Handbook for Diagnosis and Treatment*, 3rd ed.
135. K. Wells, "Parent Management Training," in *Conduct Disorders in Children and Adolescents*, ed. G. P. Sholevar (Washington, DC: American Psychiatric Association, 1995), 213–236.

136. K. Wells, W. Pelham, Jr., R. Kotkin, et al., "Psychosocial Treatment Strategies in the MTA Study: Rationale, Methods, and Critical Issues in Design and Implementation," *Journal of Abnormal Child Psychology* 28 (2000): 483–505.

137. Anastopoulos and Shelton, *Assessing Attention-Deficit/Hyperactivity Disorder*; A. Anastopoulos, T. Shelton, G. DuPaul, et al., "Parent Training for Attention-Deficit Hyperactivity Disorder: Its Impact on Parent Functioning," *Journal of Abnormal Child Psychology* 21 (1993): 581–596.

138. W. Pelham, Jr. and B. Hoza, "Intensive Treatment: A Summer Treatment Program for Children with ADHD," in *Psychosocial Treatments for Child and Adolescent Disorders: Empirically Based Strategies for Clinical Practice*, ed. E. D. Hibbs and P. S. Jensen (Washington, DC: American Psychological Association, 1996), 311–340.

139. Anastopoulos et al., "Parent Training for Attention-Deficit Hyperactivity Disorder"; Wells et al., "Psychosocial Treatment Strategies in the MTA Study."

140. For example, see Anastopoulos et al., "Parent Training for Attention-Deficit Hyperactivity Disorder."

141. Cantwell, "Attention Deficit Disorder: A Review of the Past 10 Years."

142. G. DuPaul and G. Stoner, *ADHD in the Schools: Assessment and Intervention Strategies* (New York: Guilford Press, 1994); L. Pfiffner and R. Barkley, "Treatment of ADHD in School Settings," in *Attention-Deficit Hyperactivity Disorder: A Handbook for Diagnosis and Treatment*, 2nd ed., by R. Barkley (New York: Guilford Press, 2006), 458–490.

143. Pfiffner and Barkley, "Treatment of ADHD in School Settings"; Wells et al., "Psychosocial Treatment Strategies in the MTA Study."

144. Pelham and Hoza, "Intensive Treatment."

145. W. Pelham, Jr., E. Gnagy, A. Greiner, et al., "Behavioral versus Behavioral and Pharmacological Treatment in ADHD Children Attending a Summer Treatment Program," *Journal of Abnormal Child Psychology* 28 (2000): 507–525.

146. Pelham and Hoza, "Intensive Treatment"; Wells et al., "Psychosocial Treatment Strategies in the MTA Study."

147. Pelham and Hoza, "Intensive Treatment"; Pelham et al., "Behavioral versus Behavioral and Pharmacological Treatment."

148. For examples, see W. Pelham, Jr., T. Wheeler, and A. Chronis, "Empirically Supported Psychosocial Treatments for Attention Deficit Hyperactivity Disorder," *Journal of Clinical Child Psychology* 27 (1998): 190–205; J. Swanson, K. McBurnett, T. Wigal, et al., "Effect of Stimulant Medication on Children with Attention Deficit Disorder: A 'Review of Reviews,'" *Exceptional Children* 60 (1993): 154–162.

149. For an exception, see C. Gillberg, H. Melander, A. von Knorring, et al., "Long-Term Stimulant Treatment of Children with Attention-Deficit Hyperactivity Disorder Symptoms: A Randomized, Double-Blind, Placebo-Controlled Trial," *Archives of General Psychiatry* 54 (1997): 857–864.

150. MTA Cooperative Group, "A 14-Month Randomized Clinical Trial of Treatment Strategies"; MTA Cooperative Group, "Moderators and Mediators of

Treatment Response for Children with Attention-Deficit/Hyperactivity Disorder," *Archives of General Psychiatry* 56 (1999): 1088–1096.

151. MTA Cooperative Group, "A 14-Month Randomized Clinical Trial of Treatment."

152. R. Barkley, "Commentary on the Multimodal Treatment Study of Children with ADHD," *Journal of Abnormal Child Psychology* 28 (2000): 595–599.

153. Ibid.; M. Boyle and A. Jadad, "Lessons from Large Trials: The MTA Study as a Model for Evaluating the Treatment of Childhood Psychiatric Disorder," *Canadian Journal of Psychiatry* 44 (1999): 991–998.

154. J. Swanson, H. Kraemer, S. Hinshaw, et al., "Clinical Relevance of the Primary Findings of the MTA: Success Rates Based on Severity of ADHD and ODD Symptoms at the End of Treatment," *Journal of the American Academy of Child and Adolescent Psychiatry* 40 (2001): 168–179; C.K. Conners, J. Epstein, J. March, et al., "Multimodal Treatment of ADHD in the MTA: An Alternative Outcome Analysis," *Journal of the American Academy of Child and Adolescent Psychiatry* 40 (2001): 159–167; S. Hinshaw, E. Owens, K. Wells, et al., "Family Processes and Treatment Outcome in the MTA: Negative/Ineffective Parenting Practices in Relation to Multimodal Treatment," *Journal of Abnormal Child Psychology* 28 (2000): 555–568.

155. MTA Cooperative Group, "Moderators and Mediators of Treatment."

156. MTA Cooperative Group, "A 14-Month Randomized Clinical Trial of Treatment."

157. Pelham et al., "Behavioral versus Behavioral and Pharmacological Treatment."

158. W. Pelham, Jr., "The NIMH Multimodal Treatment Study for Attention-Deficit Hyperactivity Disorder: Just Say Yes to Drugs Alone?" *Canadian Journal of Psychiatry* 44 (1999): 981–990.

159. P. Jensen, E. Arnold, J. Swanson, et al., "3-Year Follow-Up of the NIMH MTA Study," *Journal of the American Academy of Child and Adolescent Psychiatry* 46 (2007): 989–1002.

160. Ibid.

161. J. Swanson, "Secondary Evaluations of MTA 36-Month Outcomes: Propensity Score and Growth Mixture Model Analyses," *Journal of the American Academy of Child and Adolescent Psychiatry* 46 (2007): 1003–1014.

162. Jensen et al., "3-Year Follow-Up of the NIMH MTA Study."

163. Swanson et al., "Secondary Evaluations of MTA 36-Month Outcomes."

164. Ibid.

165. Ibid.

166. R. Klein, H. Abikoff, L. Hechtman, et al., "Design and Rationale of Controlled Study of Long-Term Methylphenidate and Multimodal Psychosocial Treatment in Children with ADHD," *Journal of the American Academy of Child and Adolescent Psychiatry* 43 (2004): 792–801.

167. H. Abikoff, L. Hechtman, R. Klein, et al., "Symptomatic Improvement in Children with ADHD Treated with Long-Term Methylphenidate and Multi-

modal Psychosocial Treatment," *Journal of the American Academy of Child and Adolescent Psychiatry* 43 (2004): 802–811; H. Abikoff, L. Hechtman, R. Klein, et al., "Social Functioning in Children with ADHD Treated with Long-Term Methylphenidate and Multimodal Psychosocial Treatment," *Journal of the American Academy of Child and Adolescent Psychiatry* 43 (2004): 820–829; L. Hechtman, H. Abikoff, R. G. Klein, et al., "Academic Achievement and Emotional Status of Children with ADHD Treated with Long-Term Methylphenidate and Multimodal Psychosocial Treatment," *Journal of the American Academy of Child and Adolescent Psychiatry* 43 (2004): 812–819; L. Hechtman, H. Abikoff, R. Klein, et al., "Children with ADHD Treated with Long-Term Methylphenidate and Multimodal Psychosocial Treatment: Impact on Parental Practices," *Journal of the American Academy of Child and Adolescent Psychiatry* 43 (2004): 830–838.

168. S. Kollins, L. Greenhill, J. Swanson, et al., "Rationale, Design, and Methods of the Preschool ADHD Treatment Study (PATS)," *Journal of the American Academy of Child and Adolescent Psychiatry* 45 (2006): 1275–1283.

169. L. Greenhill, S. Kollins, H. Abikoff, et al., "Efficacy and Safety of Immediate-Release Methylphenidate Treatment for Preschoolers with ADHD," *Journal of the American Academy of Child and Adolescent Psychiatry* 45 (2006): 1284–1293.

170. Wigal et al., "Safety and Tolerability of Methylphenidate in Preschool Children with ADHD."

171. Swanson et al., "Stimulant-Related Reductions of Growth Rates in the PATS."

172. Barkley, *ADHD and the Nature of Self-Control.*

173. For a review, see Barkley, *Attention-Deficit Hyperactivity Disorder: A Handbook for Diagnosis and Treatment*, 3rd ed.

## 3. A Survey of the Evolution of ADHD and Pediatric Stimulant Use, 1900–1980

1. See J. Werry, *Pediatric Psychopharmacology: The Use of Behavior Modifying Drugs in Children* (New York: Brunner/Mazel, Publishers, 1978), 113.

2. For the best and most comprehensive account of Still's analysis and the socioeconomic conditions that influenced the era in which he made them, see A. Rafalovich, "The Conceptual History of Attention Deficit Hyperactivity Disorder: Idiocy, Imbecility, Encephalitis and the Child Deviant, 1877–1929," *Deviant Behavior: An Interdisciplinary Journal* 22 (2001): 93–115.

3. G. Still, "The Goulstonian Lectures on Some Abnormal Psychical Conditions in Children," *Lancet* 1 (April 12): 1008–1012, (April 19): 1079–1082, (April 26): 1163–1167.

4. Ibid.

5. Ibid., 1166.

6. See S. Sandberg and J. Barton, "Historical Development," in *Hyperactivity Disorders of Childhood*, ed. S. Sandberg (Cambridge: Cambridge University Press, 1996), 5.

7. See I. Singh, "Biology in Context: Social and Cultural Perspectives on ADHD," *Children and Society* 16 (2002): 360–367.

8. See H. Marland and M. Gijswijt-Hofstra, *Cultures of Child Health in Britain and the Netherlands in the Twentieth Century* (New York: Rodopi Press, 2003).

9. See B. Rowntree, *Poverty: A Study of Town Life* (London: Macmillan, 1901).

10. Ibid. See also A. Newsholme, *Fifty Years in Public Health: A Personal Narrative* (London: Allen and Unwin, 1935).

11. See R. Schachar, "Hyperkinetic Syndrome: Historical Development of the Concept," in *The Overactive Child*, ed. E. Taylor, Clinics in Developmental Medicine 97 (Oxford: Blackwell, 1986), 19–40. Schachar's historical account of the evolutionary development of ADHD and stimulants is one of the best available.

12. Ibid., 20.

13. Still, "The Goulstonian Lectures on Some Abnormal Psychical Conditions in Children," 1008.

14. Rafalovich, "The Conceptual History of Attention Deficit Hyperactivity Disorder," 105–106.

15. Still, "The Goulstonian Lectures on Some Abnormal Psychical Conditions in Children," 1008.

16. See A. Lakoff, "Adaptive Will: The Evolution of Attention Deficit Disorder," *Journal of the History of the Behavioral Sciences* 36 (Spring 2000): 149–150.

17. Still, "The Goulstonian Lectures on Some Abnormal Psychical Conditions in Children," 1165.

18. C. Darwin, *On the Origin of Species by Means of Natural Selection or the Preservation of the Favoured Races in the Struggle for Life* (London: John Murray, 1859).

19. Schachar, "Hyperkinetic Syndrome," 20.

20. Still, "The Goulstonian Lectures on Some Abnormal Psychical Conditions in Children," 1165.

21. W. James, *The Principles of Psychology* (New York: Henry Holt, 1890).

22. Lakoff, "Adaptive Will," 150.

23. See E. Palmer and S. Finger, "An Early Description of ADHD (Inattentive Subtype)," *Child Psychology and Psychiatry Review* 6 (2001): 66–73; P. Neufeld and M. Foy, "Historical Reflections on the Ascendancy of ADHD in North America," *British Journal of Educational Studies* (2006): 449–470.

24. Still, "The Goulstonian Lectures on Some Abnormal Psychical Conditions in Children," 1166.

25. Ibid., 1164.

26. Schachar, "Hyperkinetic Syndrome," 22.
27. A. Tredgold, *Mental Deficiency (Amentia)*, 4th ed. (New York: William Wood, 1922), 174–201.
28. Ibid., 174.
29. Ibid., 176.
30. Ibid.
31. Ibid., 181.
32. Ibid., 181–182.
33. See M. Waldrop, F. Pederson, and R. Bell, "Minor Physical Anomalies and Behavior in Preschool Children," *Child Development* 39 (June 1968): 391–400; M. Waldrop, R. Bell, B. McLaughlin, et al., "Newborn Minor Physical Anomalies Predict Short Attention Span, Peer Aggression, and Impulsivity at Age 3," *Science* 199 (February 3, 1978): 563–565.
34. Tredgold, *Mental Deficiency*, 180, 191; see Plates II and III, in particular.
35. Waldrop et al., "Newborn Minor Physical Anomalies Predict Short Attention Span," 535–540.
36. Ibid., 535.
37. Ibid.
38. Lakoff, "Adaptive Will," 150.
39. Tredgold, *Mental Deficiency*, 178–179.
40. Sandberg and Barton, "Historical Development," 7.
41. Quoted in Schachar, "Hyperkinetic Syndrome," 22–23.
42. Tredgold, *Mental Deficiency*, 184–185.
43. Ibid., 181.
44. Ibid., 180.
45. See L. Hohman, "Post Encephalitic Behavior Disorders in Children," *Johns Hopkins Hospital Bulletin* 33 (1922): 372–375; F. Ebaugh, "Neuropsychiatric Sequelae of Acute Epidemic Encephalitis in Children," *American Journal of Diseases of Children* 25 (1923): 89–97; E. Strecker and F. Ebaugh, "Neuropsychiatric Sequelae of Cerebral Trauma in Children," *Archives of Neurology and Psychiatry* 12 (1924): 443–453.
46. See J. Barry, *The Great Influenza: The Epic Story of the Deadliest Plague in History* (New York: Viking, 2004). See also, "Influenza 1918," *The American Experience*, PBS, www.pbs.org/wgbh/amex/influenza/ (accessed July 16, 2005).
47. Rafalovich, "The Conceptual History of Attention Deficit Hyperactivity Disorder," 107.
48. P. Steen, "Epidemic Encephalitis," *American Journal of Nursing* 31 (November 1931): 1235–1239.
49. See C. Strother, "Minimal Cerebral Dysfunction: A Historical Overview," *Annals of the New York Academy of Sciences* 205 (February 28, 1973): 8–9.
50. Schachar, "Hyperkinetic Syndrome," 24; Sandberg and Barton, "Historical Development," 8.
51. Rafalovich, "The Conceptual History of Attention Deficit Hyperactivity Disorder," 111–112.

52. E. Kahn and L. Cohen, "Organic Drivenness: A Brain Stem Syndrome and an Experience with Case Reports," *New England Journal of Medicine* 210 (1934): 748–756.

53. Quoted in Sandberg and Barton, "Historical Development," 10; Schachar, "Hyperkinetic Syndrome," 25.

54. Ibid.

55. Kahn and Cohen, "Organic Drivenness."

56. M. Laufer, "In Osler's Day It was Syphilis," in *Explorations in Child Psychiatry*, ed. E. Anthony (New York: Plenum Press, 1975), 105–106.

57. Ibid.

58. Ibid., 106.

59. See W. Brown, "Images in Psychiatry: Charles Bradley, M.D., 1902–1979," *American Journal of Psychiatry* 155 (July 1998): 968.

60. Laufer, "In Osler's Day It was Syphilis," 106.

61. Ibid., 108.

62. S. Feldman, "Confessions of a Managed Behavioral Health Physician," *Developmental and Behavioral Pediatrics* 23 (February 2002): S52; Brown, "Images in Psychiatry," 968.

63. C. Elliott, *Better Than Well* (New York: Oxford University Press, 2004), 251–252.

64. C. Bradley, "Benzedrine and Dexedrine in the Treatment of Children's Behavior Disorders," *Pediatrics* 5 (January 1950): 25.

65. C. Bradley, "The Behavior of Children Receiving Benzedrine," *American Journal of Psychiatry* 94 (November 1937): 577–578.

66. Ibid., 578–580.

67. Quoted in Schachar, "Hyperkinetic Syndrome," 26.

68. E. Bromley, "Stimulating a Normal Adjustment: Misbehavior, Amphetamines, and the Electroencephalogram at the Bradley Home for Children," *Journal of the History of the Behavioral Sciences* 42 (Fall 2006): 379–398.

69. Bradley, "The Behavior of Children Receiving Benzedrine," 579.

70. M. Molitch and J. Sullivan, "The Effect of Benzedrine Sulfate on Children Taking the New Stanford Achievement Test," *American Journal of Orthopsychiatry* 7 (October 1937): 519–522.

71. Bradley, "The Behavior of Children Receiving Benzedrine," 582.

72. Ibid., 582, 584.

73. L. Grinspoon and S. Singer, "Amphetamines in the Treatment of Hyperkinetic Children," *Harvard Education Review* 43 (November 1973): 521.

74. Bradley, "Benzedrine and Dexedrine in the Treatment of Children's Behavior Disorders," 24–37.

75. Ibid., 36.

76. Sandberg and Barton, "Historical Development," 11.

77. See A. Strauss and L. Lehtinen, *Psychopathology and Education of the Brain-Injured Child* (New York: Grune and Stratton, 1947); A. Strauss and H. Werner, "Disorders of Conceptual Thinking in the Brain-Injured Child," *Journal of Nervous and Mental Disease* 96 (1942): 153–172; A. Strauss

and H. Werner, "Comparative Psychopathology of the Brain-Injured Child and the Traumatic Brain-Injured Adult," *American Journal of Psychiatry* 99 (1943): 835–838.

78. Strauss and Lehtinen, *Psychopathology and Education of the Brain-Injured Child*, 23: "In the course of development from animal to human being or from suckling newborn to grown child, the new brain develops more and more softening and inhibiting power. Sudden outbursts of laughter or of crying, extreme aggressiveness in anger, or restlessness in fear become modulated and controlled by volitional forces. Remove or diminish the inhibiting effect of the new brain by a disruption of connections or by an impairment of this balancing power and the old brain acts unchecked; excessive emotional reactions and hyperactivity are the result. This clinical picture of emotional and psychomotor disinhibition resulting from loss of control by the new brain or by the hyperexcitability of the old brain has been called by Kahn 'drivenness'. It is a disintegration of the coordinated activity of the old and new brain."

79. Ibid., 90, table 3.

80. Ibid., 90.

81. Strauss and Lehtinen, *Psychopathology and Education of the Brain-Injured Child*, 130.

82. Ibid.

83. Ibid., 131.

84. Ibid., 132–134, figures 23, 24, 25.

85. D. Ross and S. Ross, *Hyperactivity: Research, Theory, and Action* (New York: Wiley, 1976), 18.

86. W. Cruickshank, W. Bentzen, F. Ratzeburg, et al., *A Teaching Method for Brain Injured and Hyperactive Children: A Demonstration Pilot Study* (Syracuse, NY: Syracuse University Press, 1961); J. Gallagher, "Comparison of Brain-Injured and Non-Brain-Injured Mentally Retarded Children on Several Psychological Variables," *Monographs of the Society for Research in Child Development* 22 (1957): 9–76.

87. J. Weatherwax and E. Benoit, "Concrete and Abstract Thinking in Organic and Non-Organic Mentally Retarded Children," in *Readings on the Exceptional Child: Research and Theory*, ed. E. Trapp and P. Himmelstein (New York: Appleton-Century-Crofts, 1962).

88. Ross and Ross, *Hyperactivity*, 18.

89. M. Laufer, E. Denhoff, and G. Solomons, "Hyperkinetic Impulse Disorder in Children's Behavior Problems," *Psychosomatic Medicine* 19 (January–February 1957): 38–49.

90. Singh, "Biology in Context," 361.

91. Ibid., 38.

92. Ibid.

93. See M. Laufer and E. Denhoff, "Hyperkinetic Behavior Syndrome in Children," *Pediatrics* 50 (April 1957): 464.

94. Laufer et al., "Hyperkinetic Impulse Disorder in Children's Behavior Problems," 45–46.

95. Grinspoon and Singer, "Amphetamines in the Treatment of Hyperkinetic Children," 534.

96. Laufer and Denhoff, "Hyperkinetic Behavior Syndrome in Children," 467.

97. See J. Satterfield, D. Cantwell, L. Lesser, et al., "Physiological Studies of the Hyperkinetic Child," *American Journal of Psychiatry* 128 (May 1972): 1418–1424; J. Satterfield, L. Lesser, R. Saul, et al., "EEG Aspects in the Diagnosis and Treatment of Minimal Brain Dysfunction," *Annals of the New York Academy of Sciences* 205 (February 28, 1973): 274–282.

98. Laufer and Denhoff, "Hyperkinetic Behavior Syndrome in Children," 473.

99. Laufer, "In Osler's Day It was Syphilis," 113.

100. Laufer et al., "Hyperkinetic Impulse Disorder in Children's Behavior Problems," 47; Laufer and Denhoff, "Hyperkinetic Behavior Syndrome in Children," 470.

101. Ibid.

102. Laufer et al., "Hyperkinetic Impulse Disorder in Children's Behavior Problems," 45–47, 48; Laufer and Denhoff, "Hyperkinetic Behavior Syndrome in Children," 465–466.

103. Laufer et al., "Hyperkinetic Impulse Disorder in Children's Behavior Problems," 44; italics added.

104. Laufer and Denhoff, "Hyperkinetic Behavior Syndrome in Children," 474; italics added.

105. See D. Safer, "Drugs for Problem School Children," *Journal of School Health* 41 (November 1971): 491.

106. S. Fisher, ed., *Child Research in Psychopharmacology* (Springfield, IL: Charles C. Thomas Publisher, 1958), vii.

107. Ross and Ross, *Hyperactivity*, 18–19.

108. For example, see H. Freed and C. Peifer, "Treatment of Hyperkinetic Emotionally Disturbed Children with Prolonged Administration of Chlorpromazine," *American Journal of Psychiatry* 113 (July 1956): 22–26; A. Freedman, A. Effron, and L. Bender, "Pharmacotherapy in Children with Psychiatric Illness," *Journal of Nervous and Mental Disease* 122 (November 1955): 479–486.

109. Freed and Peifer, "Treatment of Hyperkinetic Emotionally Disturbed Children," 22.

110. Ibid.

111. Ibid., 25.

112. See H. Lehmann, "The Introduction of Chlorpromazine to North America," *Psychiatric Journal of the University of Ottawa* 14 (1989): 263–265; J. Swazey, *Chlorpromazine in Psychiatry: A Study of Therapeutic Innovation* (Cambridge, MA: MIT Press, 1974); H. Lehmann and G. Hanrahan, "New Inhibiting Agent for Psychomotor Excitement and Manic States," *Archives of Neurology and Psychiatry* 71 (1954): 227–237. The most serious side effect associated with use of chlorpromazine was tardive dyskinesia, in which patients suffered from severe involuntary facial grimacing and embarrassing, uncontrollable bodily movements. For more information, see www.mentalhealth.com/drug/p30-c01.html.

113. See W. Bower, "Chlorpromazine in Psychiatric Illness," *New England Journal of Medicine* 251 (October 21, 1954): 689–692; E. Shorter, *A History of Psychiatry: From the Age of the Asylum to the Age of Prozac* (New York: Wiley, 1997), 246–255.

114. See J. Ferguson, F. Linn, M. Nickels, et al., "Methylphenidate (Ritalin) Hydrochloride Parenteral Solution: Preliminary Report," *Journal of the American Medical Association* 162 (December 1, 1956): 1303–1304; Editor, "Methylphenidate Hydrochloride," *Journal of the American Medical Association* 163 (April 20, 1957): 1479–1480; P. Wax, "Analeptic Use in Clinical Toxicology: A Historical Appraisal," *Journal of Toxicology: Clinical Toxicology* 35 (March 1997): 203–209.

115. I. Singh, "Not Just Naughty: 50 Years of Stimulant Drug Advertising," in *Medicating Modern America: Prescription Drugs in History*, ed. A. Tone and A. Watkins (New York: New York University Press, 2007), 134–135.

116. Laufer and Denhoff, "Hyperkinetic Behavior Syndrome in Children," 473.

117. Ibid.

118. See R. Lipman, "NIMH-PRB Support of Research in Minimal Brain Dysfunction in Children," in *Clinical Use of Stimulant Drugs in Children*, ed. C. Conners (Amsterdam: Excerpta Medica, 1974), 203–213.

119. Fisher, *Child Research in Psychopharmacology*, vii–viii.

120. Ibid., 31–32.

121. Keith Conners, telephone interview with Mayes, July 20, 2005. When asked about the quote, however, Eisenberg claims no credit for it: "The quote about 'who is pushing them in' is not original with me, though I used it as rhetoric many times. I think I first heard it from a lovely child psychiatrist in [Washington] D.C. (Reginald Lourie), but he was probably telling a story he had heard someone else tell. So I have no reservations about acknowledging the quote but I demur at being given credit for originating it." Eisenberg, e-mail exchange with Mayes, July 25, 2005.

122. J. Swanson, K. McBurnett, D. Christian, et al., "Stimulant Medications and the Treatment of Children with ADHD," in *Advances in Clinical Child Psychology*, vol. 17, ed. T. Ollendick and R. Prinz (New York: Plenum Press, 1995), 286.

123. Fisher, *Child Research in Psychopharmacology*, xi.

124. Swanson et al., "Stimulant Medications and the Treatment of Children with ADHD," 270–271.

125. See C. Conners and L. Eisenberg, "The Effects of Methylphenidate on Symptomatology and Learning in Disturbed Children," *American Journal of Psychiatry* 120 (November 1963): 458–464.

126. Ibid., 458.

127. Ibid.

128. Conners interview with Mayes.

129. Conners and Eisenberg, "The Effects of Methylphenidate on Symptomatology and Learning in Disturbed Children," 458.

130. Ibid., 462.

131. Conners interview with Mayes.

132. Ross and Ross, *Hyperactivity*, 19.

133. See H. Birch, *Brain Damage in Children: The Biological and Social Aspects* (Baltimore, MD: Williams and Wilkins, 1964); M. Herbert, "The Concept and Testing of Brain Damage in Children: A Review," *Journal of Child Psychology and Psychiatry* 5 (1964): 197–217; I. Rapin, "Brain Damage in Children," in *Practice of Pediatrics*, ed. J. Brennemann (Hagerstown, MD: Prior, 1964); E. Denhoff, M. Laufer, and R. Holden, "The Syndromes of Cerebral Dysfunction," *Journal of the Oklahoma State Medical Association* 52 (1959): 360–366; M. Bax and R. MacKeith, "Minimal Brain Damage: A Concept Discarded," in *Minimal Cerebral Dysfunction*, ed. R. MacKeith and M. Bax, Little Club Clinics in Development Medicine 10 (London: Heinemann, 1963).

134. In Stella Chess's now famous report of 82 hyperactive children, only 14 were diagnosed as brain damaged. See S. Chess, "Diagnosis and Treatment of the Hyperactive Child," *New York State Journal of Medicine* 60 (1960): 2379–2385. For more on the lack of definitive evidence for a link between brain damage and hyperactivity, see M. Stewart, F. Pitts, A. Craig, et al., "The Hyperactive Child Syndrome," *American Journal of Orthopsychiatry* 36 (October 1966): 861–867.

135. R. Barkley, *Attention-Deficit Hyperactivity Disorder: A Handbook for Diagnosis and Treatment*, 2nd ed. (New York: Guilford Press, 1990), 10.

136. See S. Clements and J. Peters, "Minimal Brain Dysfunction in the School-Age Child," *Archives of General Psychiatry* 6 (1962): 185–197; Ross and Ross, *Hyperactivity*, 18.

137. S. Clements, "Minimal Brain Dysfunction in Children: Terminology and Identification," Task Force 1, U.S. Department of Health, Education, and Welfare, Public Health Service Publication 1415 (Washington, DC: U.S. Government Printing Office, 1966), 9–10, italics added.

138. See V. Sanua, "Leo Kanner (1894–1981): The Man and the Scientist," *Child Psychiatry and Human Development* 21 (Fall 1990): 3–23.

139. See D. Freedman, "The Search: Body, Mind and Human Purpose," *American Journal of Psychiatry* 149 (July 1992): 858–866; J. Wortis, "Adolph Meyer: Some Recollections and Impressions," *British Journal of Psychiatry* 149 (December 1986): 677–681; Shorter, *A History of Psychiatry*, 91–93, 109–112.

140. Lakoff, "Adaptive Will," 154.

141. Ibid.

142. American Psychiatric Association, *Diagnostic and Statistical Manual of Mental Disorders*, 2nd ed. (Washington, DC: American Psychiatric Association, 1968), 50.

143. Conners quoting Eisenberg in C. Conners, "The Syndrome of Minimal Brain Dysfunction: Psychological Aspects," *Pediatric Clinics of North America* 14 (November 1967): 761: "The child's parents, usually defeated, confused and angry by the time the physicians sees them, need to understand that his behavior is not malevolent and hostile but stems from a defi-

ciency in neurophysiologic control mechanisms. If they can be helped to view his symptoms as a result of a treatable illness rather than as a personal attack on them, they will be the more able to apply the consistency of discipline, the firmness without anger and the anticipatory intervention that he requires. It is sound advice to suggest to parents that they avoid shopping trips, visits to restaurants, and attendance at large parties, for children are at their worst under such circumstances . . . Similar guidance can be offered his teacher. For effective learning, class size should be small. The room should contain a minimum of distracting stimulation (i.e., materials not in use should be in cupboards out of sight). Class activities should be paced to his capacity for sustained participation, with frequent periods of guided and supervised large muscle play. Indeed, with some children, freedom to leave the class and run about the playground has proved useful when motor tension mounts beyond control. (Clearly, this option can be made available only to the relatively mature and well motivated child.)"

144. Lipman, "NIMH-PRB Support of Research in Minimal Brain Dysfunction in Children," 204.

145. Singh, "Not Just Naughty," 140.

146. Ross and Ross, *Hyperactivity*, 116.

147. Leon Eisenberg, phone interview with Mayes July 19, 2005.

148. Ibid.; Conners interview with Mayes.

149. Lipman, "NIMH-PRB Support of Research in Minimal Brain Dysfunction in Children," 204.

150. Ibid.

151. Ibid. See also Swanson et al., "Stimulant Medications and the Treatment of Children with ADHD," 286.

152. Swanson et al., "Stimulant Medications and the Treatment of Children with ADHD," 286.

153. Lipman, "NIMH-PRB Support of Research in Minimal Brain Dysfunction in Children," 208–209.

154. Ibid., 205.

155. U.S. Congress, House of Representatives, Subcommittee of the Committee on Government Operations, *Federal Involvement in the Use of Behavior Modification Drugs on Grammar School Children on the Right to Privacy Inquiry*, 91st Cong., 2nd sess., September 29, 1970, 16.

156. U.S. Bureau of the Census, Current Population Reports, Series P-25, No. 311, "Estimates of the Population of the United States by Single Years of Age, Color, and Sex, 1900 to 1959," 22–23, 42–43; Series P-25, No. 519, "Estimates of the Population of the United States, By Age, Sex, and Race: April 1, 1960 to July 1, 1973," table 2; Series P-25, No. 917, "Preliminary Estimates of the Population of the United States by Age, Sex, and Race: 1970 to 1981," Table 2.

157. R. Maynard, "Omaha Pupils Given 'Behavior Drugs,'" *Washington Post*, June 29, 1970, 1.

158. *Medical News*, August 10, 1970.

159. E. Ladd, "Pills for Classroom Peace?" *Saturday Review*, November 21, 1970, 66–68, 81–83; N. Hentoff, "The Drugged Classroom," *Evergreen Review*, December 1970, 31–33; J. Rogers, "Drug Abuse—Just What the Doctor Ordered? *Psychology Today*, September 1971, 16–24; N. Hentoff, "Drug-Pushing in the Schools," *Village Voice*, May 25, 1972, 20–21.

160. U.S. Congress, House of Representatives, Subcommittee of the Committee on Government Operations, *Federal Involvement in the Use of Behavior Modification Drugs on Grammar School Children on the Right to Privacy Inquiry*.

161. "Report on the Conference of the Use of Stimulant Drugs in the Treatment of Behaviorally Disturbed Young School Children," *Psychopharmacological Bulletin* 7 (1971): 23.

162. Office of Child Development and the Office of the Assistant Secretary for Health and Scientific Affairs, Department of Health, Education, and Welfare, *Report of the Conference on the Use of Stimulant Drugs in the Treatment of Behaviorally Disturbed Young Children*, Washington, DC, January 11–12, 1971. Reprinted in *Journal of Learning Disabilities* 4 (November 1971): 523–530.

163. U.S. Congress, House of Representatives, Subcommittee of the Committee on Government Operations, *Federal Involvement in the Use of Behavior Modification Drugs on Grammar School Children on the Right to Privacy Inquiry*, 14, 18–19.

164. J. Graham, "Amphetamine Politics on Capitol Hill," *Transaction: Social Science and Modern Society* 9 (January 1972): 14–22.

165. *Comprehensive Drug Abuse Prevention and Control Act*, Public Law 91–513, 84 Stat. 1236 (October 27, 1970).

166. Ibid.

167. Swanson et al., "Stimulant Medications and the Treatment of Children with ADHD," 288.

168. U.S. Congress, House of Representatives, Subcommittee of the Committee on Government Operations, *Federal Involvement in the Use of Behavior Modification Drugs on Grammar School Children on the Right to Privacy Inquiry*, 29: "[A]re we not really on a dangerous course when our Government . . . is encouraging growth in this area? This is the thing that troubles me, because we talk about credibility gaps and generation gaps. The U.S. Government says they [children] cannot get off these drugs [amphetamines], but on the other hand they can take them until they are 12 years old. I just wonder whether or not we are justified in proceeding in any direction until we have more certain knowledge of the total broad effect."

169. Editorial, "Speed in Sweden . . . and Pep in America," *New England Journal of Medicine* 283 (October 1, 1970): 760–762.

170. S. Smith and D. Wesson, *Uppers and Downers* (Englewood Cliffs, NJ: Prentice-Hall, 1973), 18.

171. See L. Diller, *Running on Ritalin* (New York: Bantam Books, 1998), 27; Drug and Chemical Evaluation Section, "Methylphenidate (A Background

Paper)," Washington, DC: Office of Diversion Control, Drug Enforcement Administration, Department of Justice, October 1995.

172. Conners, *Clinical Use of Stimulant Drugs in Children*, xi.

173. *National Research Act*, Public Law 93–348 (1974).

174. R. Sprague, "Principles of Clinical Trials and Social, Ethical and Legal Issues of Drug Use in Children," in *Pediatric Psychopharmacology: The Use of Behavior Modifying Drugs in Children*, ed. J. Werry (New York: Branner-Mazel, 1978), 114.

175. Ibid., 117.

176. P. Schrag and D. Divoky, *The Myth of the Hyperactive Child and Other Means of Child Control* (New York: Pantheon Books, 1975).

177. C. Conners, *Food Additives and Hyperactive Children* (New York: Plenum, 1980).

178. B. Feingold, *Why Your Child Is Hyperactive* (New York: Random House, 1975).

179. Barkley, *Attention-Deficit Hyperactivity Disorder*, 16.

180. P. Conrad, "The Discovery of Hyperkinesis: Notes on the Medicalization of Deviant Behavior," *Social Problems* 23 (1975): 12–21.

181. Ibid.

182. Ibid., 17–18.

183. Ibid., 19: "We tend to look for causes and solutions to complex social problems in the individual rather than in the social system . . . We then seek to change the "victim" rather than the society . . . Hyperkinesis serves as a good example. Both the school and the parents are concerned with the child's behavior; the child is very difficult at home and disruptive in school. No punishments or rewards seem consistently to work in modifying the behavior; and both parents and school are at their wits' end. A medical evaluation is suggested. The diagnosis of hyperkinetic behavior leads to prescribing stimulant medications. The child's behavior seems to become more socially acceptable, reducing problems in school and at home. But there is an alternative perspective. By focusing on the symptoms and defining them as hyperkinesis we ignore the possibility that behavior is not an illness but an adaptation to a social situation. It diverts our attention from the family or school and from seriously entertaining the idea that the "problem" could be in the structure of the social system. And by giving medications we are essentially supporting the existing systems and do not allow this behavior to be a factor of change in the system."

184. See Sprague, "Principles of Clinical Trials and Social, Ethical and Legal Issues of Drug Use in Children," 129–130.

185. Ibid.

186. Ibid., 109.

187. See J. Rapoport, M. Buchsbaum, T. Zahn, et al., "Dextroamphetamine: Cognitive and Behavioral Effects on Normal Prepubertal Boys," *Science* 199 (1978): 560–563; J. Rapoport, M. Buchsbaum, H. Weingartner, et al., "Dextroamphetamine: The Cognitive and Behavioral Effects in Normal

and Hyperactive Boys and Normal Men," *Archives of General Psychiatry* 37 (August 1980): 933–943.

188. Ibid.
189. See R. Mayes and A. Horwitz, "DSM-III and the Revolution in the Classification of Mental Illness," *Journal of the History of the Behavioral Sciences* 41 (Summer 2005): 249–267.
190. Conners interview with Mayes.
191. Ibid.

## 4. The Transformation of Mental Disorders in the 1980s

1. See R. Michels and P. Marzuk, "Progress in Psychiatry," *New England Journal of Medicine* 329 (August 19, 1993): 552–560, (August 26, 1993): 628–638.
2. See R. Mayes and A. Horwitz, "DSM-III and the Revolution in the Classification of Mental Illness," *Journal of the History of the Behavioral Sciences* 41 (Summer 2005): 249–267.
3. See P. Brown, "Diagnostic Conflict and Contradiction in Psychiatry," *Journal of Health and Social Behavior* 28 (March 1987): 37–50.
4. See J. Foy and M. Earls, "A Process for Developing Community Consensus Regarding the Diagnosis and Management of Attention-Deficit/Hyperactivity Disorder," *Pediatrics* 115 (January 2005): 97–104; J. Rushton, K. Fant, and S. Clark, "Use of Practice Guidelines in the Primary Care of Children with Attention-Deficit/Hyperactivity Disorder," *Pediatrics* 114 (July 2004): 23–28.
5. See T. Luhrmann, *Of Two Minds: An Anthropologist Looks at American Psychiatry* (New York: Vintage Books, 2000).
6. See W. Gardner, K. Kelleher, K. Pajer, et al., "Primary Care Clinicians' Use of Standardized Psychiatric Diagnoses," *Child: Care, Health and Development* 30 (September 2004): 401–412.
7. See W. Reich, "Psychiatry's Second Coming," *Psychiatry* 41 (August 1982): 189–196.
8. See R. Pasnau, "The Remedicalization of American Psychiatry," *Hospital and Community Psychiatry* 38 (1987): 145–151.
9. See R. Poulsen, "Some Current Factors Influencing the Prescribing and Use of Psychiatric Drugs," *Public Health Reports* 107 (January–February 1992): 47–53.
10. See N. Ware, W. Lachicotte, S. Kirschner, et al., "Clinician Experiences of Managed Mental Health Care: A Rereading of the Threat," *Medical Anthropology Quarterly* 14 (2000): 3–27.
11. K. Gadow, "Prevalence of Drug Treatment for Hyperactivity and Other Childhood Behavior Disorders," in *Psychosocial Aspects of Drug Treatment for Hyperactivity*, ed. K. Gadow and J. Loney (Boulder, CO: Westview Press, 1981); J. Swanson, M. Lerner, and L. Williams, "More Frequent Diagnosis of Attention Deficit-Hyperactivity Disorder," *New England Journal of Medicine* 333 (October 5, 1996): 994.

12. R. Bayer and R. Spitzer, "Neurosis, Psychodynamics, and DSM-III," *Archives of General Psychiatry* 42 (February 1985): 188.

13. See D. Goodwin and S. Guze, *Psychiatric Diagnosis*, 5th ed. (New York: Oxford University Press, 1996).

14. See L. Rogler, "Making Sense of Historical Changes in the Diagnostic and Statistical Manual of Mental Disorders: Five Propositions," *Journal of Health and Social Behavior* 39 (March 1997): 9–20.

15. See R. Kessler, "The Categorical versus Dimensional Assessment Controversy in the Sociology of Mental Illness," *Journal of Health and Social Behavior* 43 (June 2002): 171–188.

16. See Mayes and Horowitz, "DSM-III and the Revolution in the Classification of Mental Illness."

17. I. Galatzer-Levy and R. Galatzer-Levy, "The Revolution in Psychiatric Diagnosis: Problems at the Foundations," *Perspectives in Biology and Medicine* 50 (Spring 2007): 161–180.

18. See K. Hoagwood, "Making the Translation from Research to Its Application: The *Je Ne Sais Pas* of Evidence-Based Practices," *Clinical Psychology: Science and Practice* 9 (June 2002): 210–213.

19. See G. Strauss, J. Yager, and G. Strauss, "The Cutting Edge in Psychiatry," *American Journal of Psychiatry* 141 (January 1984): 38–43.

20. S. Kirk and H. Kutchins, *The Selling of DSM: The Rhetoric of Science in Psychiatry* (New York: Aldine Transaction, 1992), 11.

21. M. Wilson, "DSM-III and the Transformation of American Psychiatry: A History," *American Journal of Psychiatry* 150 (March 1993): 404.

22. Ibid.

23. D. Healy, *The Anti-Depressant Era* (Cambridge, MA: Harvard University Press, 1997), 233–234.

24. D. Rosenhan, "On Being Sane in Insane Places," *Science* 179 (January 19, 1973): 250–258.

25. R. Spitzer, "On Pseudoscience in Science, Logic in Remission, and Psychiatric Diagnosis: A Critique of Rosenhan's 'On Being Sane in Insane Places,'" *Journal of Abnormal Psychology* 84 (October 1975): 442–452; R. Spitzer, "More on Pseudoscience in Science and the Case for Psychiatric Diagnosis. A Critique of D.L. Rosenhan's 'On Being Sane in Insane Places' and 'The Contestual Nature of Psychiatric Diagnosis,'" *Archives of General Psychiatry* 33 (April 1976): 459–470.

26. See M. Greenblatt, "Psychiatry: The Battered Child of Medicine," *New England Journal of Medicine* 292 (January 30, 1975): 246–250.

27. See A. Spiegel, "The Dictionary of Disorder: How One Man Revolutionized Psychiatry," *New Yorker*, January 3, 2005, 56–63.

28. In addition to Spitzer, the initial assemblage consisted of Nancy Andreasen, MD, PhD, Jean Endicott, PhD, Donald F. Klein, MD, Morton Kramer, ScD, Theodore Millon, PhD, Henry Pinsker, MD, George Saslow, MD, PhD, and Robert Woodruff, MD. Most were well-recognized contributors to the research and theoretical literature.

29. Healy, *The Antidepressant Era*, 234.

30. J. Kroll, "Philosophical Foundations of French and U.S. Nosology," *American Journal of Psychiatry* 136 (1979): 1135–1138.

31. E. Shorter, *A History of Psychiatry: From the Age of the Asylum to the Age of Prozac* (New York: Wiley, 1997), 108.

32. A. Young, *The Harmony of Illusions: Inventing Post-Traumatic Stress Disorder* (Princeton, NJ: Princeton University Press, 1995), chap. 3, 89–117; E. Kraepelin, *Lectures on Clinical Psychiatry* (New York: William Wood, 1913); R. Spitzer, J. Williams, and A. Skodal, "DSM-III: The Major Achievements and an Overview," *American Journal of Psychiatry* 137 (1980): 151–164.

33. R. Spitzer, M. Sheehy, and J. Endicott, "DSM-III: Guiding Principles," in *Psychiatric Diagnosis*, ed. V. Rakoff, H. Stancer, and H. Kedward (New York: Brunner/Mazel, 1977), 4.

34. Ibid.

35. Rogler, "Making Sense of Historical Changes in the Diagnostic and Statistical Manual of Mental Disorders," 10–12.

36. Ibid.

37. Wilson, "DSM-III and the Transformation of American Psychiatry," 405: "It was the unanimous opinion of the Committee that etiology [cause] should be a classificatory principle only when it is clearly known, and that conventional speculations about etiology should be explained if they must appear . . . A diagnosis should be made if the criteria for that diagnosis are met . . . It is hoped that this will stimulate appreciation, among psychiatrists, of the distinction between the known and the assumed. In everyday practice, then, there will be fewer assignments to diagnostic categories on the basis of probable correctness, and more diagnoses which force the clinician to admit what he does not know . . . The sense of the committee is that mental disorder should be defined narrowly rather than broadly, that a definition which permits false negatives is preferable to one that encourages false positives."

38. See R. Bayer, *Homosexuality and American Psychiatry: The Politics of Diagnosis* (New York: Basic Books, 1981).

39. See R. Stoller, J. Marmor, I. Bieber, et al., "A Symposium: Should Homosexuality Be in the APA Nomenclature?" *American Journal of Psychiatry* 130 (November 1973): 1207–1216.

40. See R. Spitzer, "The Diagnostic Status of Homosexuality in DSM-III: An Insider's Perspective," *American Journal of Psychiatry* 138 (February 1981): 210–215.

41. American Psychiatric Association, *Diagnostic and Statistical Manual of Mental Disorders*, 2nd ed. (Washington, DC: American Psychiatric Association, 1968), 44: "302.0 Sexual orientation disturbance [Homosexuality]. This is for individuals whose sexual interests are directed primarily toward people of the same sex and who are either disturbed by, in conflict with, or wish to change their sexual orientation. This diagnostic category is distinguished from homosexuality, which by itself does not constitute a psychi-

atric disorder. Homosexuality *per se* is one form of sexual behavior, and with other forms of sexual behavior which are not by themselves psychiatric disorders, are not listed in this nomenclature."

42. Shorter, *A History of Psychiatry*, 303.

43. Kirk and Kutchins, *The Selling of DSM*, 30.

44. H. Berk, "Letter to the Editor," *Psychiatric News* (March 30, 1977).

45. Bayer and Spitzer, "Neurosis, Psychodynamics, and DSM-III," 189.

46. L. Madow, "The Retreat from a Psychiatry of People," *Journal of the American Academy of Psychoanalysis* 4 (1976): 131–135.

47. G. Grob, *The Mad among Us: A History of the Care of America's Mentally Ill* (New York: Free Press, 1994), 211–219.

48. American Psychiatric Association, *Diagnostic and Statistical Manual of Mental Disorders*, 3rd ed. (Washington, DC: American Psychiatric Association, 1980), 3–5; Shorter, *A History of Psychiatry*, 302.

49. See S. Hyler, J. Williams, and R. Spitzer, "Reliability in the DSM-III Field Trials," *Archives of General Psychiatry* 39 (1982): 1275–1278.

50. See A. Garmbardella, *Science and Innovation: The U.S. Pharmaceutical Industry during the 1980s* (Cambridge: Cambridge University Press, 1995).

51. L. Judd, "NIMH during the Tenure of Director Lewis L. Judd, M.D. (1987–1990): The Decade of the Brain and the Four National Research Plans," *American Journal of Psychiatry* 155 (September 1998): 25–31.

52. L. Hall, "The Biology of Mental Disorders," *Journal of the American Medical Association* 269 (February 17, 1993): 844.

53. See L. Schmied, H. Steinberg, and E. Sykes, "Psychopharmacology's Debt to Experimental Psychology," *History of Psychology* 9 (May 2006): 144–157; U. Muller, P. Fletcher, and H. Steinberg, "The Origin of Pharmacopsychology: Emil Kraepelin's Experiments in Leipzig, Dorpat and Heidelberg (1882–1892)," *Psychopharmacology* 184 (January 2006): 131–138.

54. P. Fink, "Response to the Presidential Address: Is 'Biopsychosocial' the Psychiatric Shibboleth?" *American Journal of Psychiatry* 145 (September 1988): 1065.

55. See J. Silk, S. Nath, L. Siegel, et al., "Conceptualizing Mental Disorders in Children: Where Have We Been and Where Are We Going?" *Development and Psychopathology* 12 (2000): 713–735.

56. See C. Mallett, "Behaviorally-Based Disorders: The Historical Social Construction of Youths' Most Prevalent Psychiatric Diagnoses," *History of Psychiatry* 17 (2006): 444.

57. See N. Hamm, "The Politics of Empiricism: Research Recommendations of the Joint Commission on Mental Health in Children," *American Psychologist* 29 (January 1974): 9–13; W. Taylor, "Developmental Theory: Unsolved Problem for Child Psychiatry," *American Journal of Orthopsychiatry* 41 (July 1971): 557–565; W. Goodrich, "Changes in Child Psychiatry Training Required by Developmental-Adaptive Theory," *Journal of Nervous and Mental Disease* 154 (March 1972): 213–220; C. Ramey, "Children and Public Policy: A Role for Psychologists," *American Psychologist* 29 (January

1974): 14–18; J. Dusek, "Implications of Development Theory for Child Mental Health," *American Psychologist* 29 (January 1974): 19–24; J. Segal and H. Yahraes, "Protecting Children's Mental Health," *Children Today* 7 (September–October 1978): 23–25; L. Wright, "Health Care Psychology: Prospects for the Well-Being of Children," *American Psychologist* 34 (October 1979): 1001–1006; A. Marks and M. Cohen, "Health Screening and Assessment of Adolescents," *Pediatric Annals* 7 (September 1978): 596–604; M. Laufer, "Which Adolescents Must Be Helped and by Whom?" *Journal of Adolescence* 3 (December 1980): 265–272; A. Marks, "Aspects of Biosocial Screening and Health Maintenance in Adolescents," *Pediatric Clinics of North America* 27 (February 1980): 153–161.

58. See C. Kopp and J. Krakow, "The Developmentalist and the Study of Biological Risk: A View of the Past with an Eye to the Future," *Child Development* 54 (October 1983): 1086–1108.

59. See N. Weiss, "Mother, the Invention of Necessity: Dr. Benjamin Spock's Baby and Child Care," *American Quarterly* 29 (1977): 519–546.

60. See S. Rosenbaum and P. Wise, "Crossing the Medicaid-Private Insurance Divide: The Case of EPSDT," *Health Affairs* 26 (March–April 2007): 382–393; A. Foltz, "The Development of Ambiguous Federal Policy: Early and Periodic Screening, Diagnosis and Treatment (EPSDT)," *Milbank Memorial Fund Quarterly* 53 (Winter 1975): 35–64.

61. Sec. 1905(a)(4)(B), added by sec. 302(a), Social Security Amendments of 1967, Public Law 90–248 (approved January 2, 1968) 81 Stat. 821.

62. See P. Irwin and R. Conroy-Hughes, "EPSDT Impact on Health Status," *Health Care Financing Review* 2 (Spring 1981): 25–39.

63. Silk et al., "Conceptualizing Mental Disorders in Children," 720; Joint Commission on Mental Health of Children, *Crisis in Child Mental Health: Challenge for the 1970's* (New Yorker: Harper and Row, 1970).

64. See J. Richmond, "Disadvantaged Children: What Have They Compelled Us to Learn?" *Yale Journal of Biology and Medicine* 43 (December 1970): 127–144.

65. Education of All Handicapped Children Act, Public Law 94–142 (November 29, 1975).

66. Silk et al., "Conceptualizing Mental Disorders in Children," 720.

67. See J. Carbray and C. Pitula, "Trends in Adolescent Psychiatric Hospitalization," *Journal of Child and Adolescent Psychiatric Mental Health Nursing* 4 (April–June 1991): 68–71.

68. See L. Shear, "From Competition to Complementarity: Legal Issues and Their Clinical Implications in Custody," *Child and Adolescent Psychiatric Clinics of North America* 7 (April 1998): vi–viii, 311–334.

69. See F. Blau, "Trends in the Well-Being of American Women, 1970–1995," *Journal of Economic Literature* 36 (March 1998): 112–165.

70. See J. Kendall, M. Leo, N. Perrin, et al., "Modeling ADHD Child and Family Relationships," *Western Journal of Nursing Research* 27 (2005): 500–518;

J. Morgan, D. Robinson, and J. Aldridge, "Parenting Stress and External-izing Child Behavior," *Child and Family Social Work* 7 (August 2002): 219–225.

71. See E. Kitagawa, "New Life-Styles: Marriage Patterns, Living Arrangements, and Fertility Outside of Marriage," *The Annals of the American Academy of Political and Social Science* 453 (1981): 1–27; A. Thornton and D. Freedman, "The Changing American Family," *Population Bulletin* 38 (October 1983): 1–44.

72. See B. Weiner, "An Overview of Child Custody Laws," *Hospital and Community Psychiatry* 36 (August 1985): 838–843.

73. See J. Kelly, "Children's Adjustment in Conflicted Marriage and Divorce: A Decade Review of Research," *Journal of the American Academy of Child and Adolescent Psychiatry* 39 (August 2000): 963–973.

74. See R. Doan and T. Petti, "Clinical and Demographic Characteristics of Child and Adolescent Partial Hospital Patients," *Journal of the American Academy of Child and Adolescent Psychiatry* 28 (January 1989): 66–69; J. Wallen and H. Pincus, "Care of Children with Psychiatric Disorders at Community Hospitals," *Hospital and Community Psychiatry* 39 (February 1988): 167–172; K. Pottick, D. McAlpine, and R. Andelman, "Changing Patterns of Psychiatric Inpatient Care for Children and Adolescents in General Hospitals, 1988–1995," *American Journal of Psychiatry* 157 (August 2000): 1267–1273; B. Case, M. Òlfson, S. Marcus, et al., "Trends in the Inpatient Mental Health Treatment of Children and Adolescents in U.S. Community Hospitals between 1990 and 2000," *Archives of General Psychiatry* 64 (January 2007): 89–96.

75. See J. Rushton, B. Felt, and M. Roberts, "Coding of Pediatric Behavioral and Mental Disorders," *Pediatrics* 110 (July 2002): E8.

76. See B. Fogel, "A Psychiatric Unit Becomes a Psychiatric-Medical Unit: Administrative and Clinical Implications," *General Hospital Psychiatry* 7 (January 1985): 26–35; R. Redick, M. Witkin, and R. Manderscheid, "CMHS Data Highlights On: Availability of Psychiatric Beds, United States, Selected Years, 1970–1990," *Mental Health Statistical Note* (August 1994): 1–7.

77. See S. Gaylin, "The Coming of the Corporation and the Marketing of Psychiatry," *Hospitals and Community Psychiatry* (1985): 154.

78. See R. Redick, A. Stroup, M. Witkin, et al., "Private Psychiatric Hospitals, United States: 1983–84 and 1986," *Mental Health Statistical Note* (October 1989): 1–28; E. Goplerud, "Effects of Proprietary Management in General Hospital Psychiatric Units," *Hospital Community Psychiatry* 37 (August 1986): 832–836.

79. See J. Rascati, "Commentary on Lewin and Sharfstein," *Psychiatry* 53 (May 1990): 125.

80. See M. Jellinek and B. Nurcombe, "Two Wrongs Don't Make a Right: Managed Care, Mental Health, and the Marketplace," *Journal of the American Medicine Association* 270 (October 13, 1993): 1737–1738.

81. See R. Dorwart, M. Schlesinger, H. Davidson, et al., "A National Study of Psychiatric Hospital Care," *American Journal of Psychiatry* 148 (February 1991): 204–210; C. Kiesler and C. Simpkins, "Changes in Psychiatric Inpatient Treatment of Children and Youth in General Hospitals: 1980–1985," *Hospital Community Psychiatry* 42 (June 1991): 601–604; B. Burns, "Mental Health Service Use by Adolescents in the 1970s and 1980s," *Journal of the American Academy of Child and Adolescent Psychiatry* 30 (January 1991): 144–150.

82. See L. Weithorn, "Mental Hospitalization of Troublesome Youth: An Analysis of Skyrocketing Admission Rates," *Stanford Law Review* 40 (February 1988): 817.

83. See Jellinek and Nurcombe, "Two Wrongs Don't Make a Right," 1738; R. Friedman and K. Kutash, "Challenges for Child and Adolescent Mental Health," *Health Affairs* 11 (Fall 1992): 129–130; Kiesler and Simpkins, "Changes in Psychiatric Inpatient Treatment of Children and Youth," 601.

84. Ibid.

85. See S. McDonald, "An Ethical Dilemma: Risk versus Responsibility," *Journal of Psychosocial Nursing in Mental Health Services* 32 (January 1994): 19–25.

86. See J. Lewis, "Are Adolescents Being Hospitalized Unnecessarily? The Current Use of Hospitalization in Psychiatric Treatment," *Journal of Child and Adolescent Psychiatric Mental Health Nursing* 2 (October–December 1989): 134–138.

87. J. Iglehart, "Health Policy Report: Managed Care and Mental Health," *New England Journal of Medicine* 335 (July 4, 1996): 132.

88. See C. Kiesler, C. Simpkins, and T. Morton, "The Psychiatric Inpatient Treatment of Children and Youth in General Hospitals," *American Journal of Community Psychology* 17 (December 1989): 821–830.

89. See J. Knitzer, *Unclaimed Children: The Failure of Public Responsibility to Children and Adolescents in Need of Mental Health* Services (Washington, DC: Children's Defense Fund, 1982).

90. Friedman and Kutash, "Challenges for Child and Adolescent Mental Health," 130.

91. Weithorn, "Mental Hospitalization of Troublesome Youth," 819.

92. See L. DeMilio, "Psychiatric Syndromes in Adolescent Substance Users," *American Journal of Psychiatry* 146 (September 1989): 1212–1214; G. Strauss, M. Chassin, and J. Lock, "Can Experts Agree When to Hospitalize Adolescents?" *Journal of the American Academy of Child and Adolescent Psychiatry* 34 (1994): 418–424.

93. See M. Mason and J. Gibbs, "Patterns of Adolescent Psychiatric Hospitalization: Implications for Social Policy," *American Journal of Orthopsychiatry* 62 (July 1992): 447–457.

94. See A. Relman, "The New Medical-Industrial Complex," *New England Journal of Medicine* 303 (1980): 963–970.

95. Kinkead, "Humana's Hard-Sell Hospitals," *Fortune*, November 17, 1980, 68.

96. Weithorn, "Mental Hospitalization of Troublesome Youth," 816–826.
97. Ibid., 818.
98. See R. Mayes and R. Berenson, *Medicare Prospective Payment and the Shaping of U.S. Health Care* (Baltimore, MD: Johns Hopkins University Press, 2006).
99. See C. Taube, J. Lave, A. Rupp, et al., "Psychiatry under Prospective Payment: Experience in the First Year," *American Journal of Psychiatry* 145 (February 1988): 210–213; J. English, S. Sharfstein, D. Scherl, et al., "Diagnosis-Related Groups and General Hospital Psychiatry: The APA Study," *American Journal of Psychiatry* 143 (February 1986): 131–139.
100. See C. Taube, J. Thompson, B. Burns, et al., "Prospective Payment and Psychiatric Discharges from General Hospitals with and without Psychiatric Units," *Hospital Community Psychiatry* 36 (July 1985): 754–760.
101. See Kiesler and Simpkins, "Changes in Psychiatric Inpatient Treatment of Children and Youth in General Hospitals: 1980–1985," 601–604.
102. See I. Gold, C. Heller, and B. Ritorto, "A Short-Term Psychiatric Inpatient Program for Adolescents," *Hospital Community Psychiatry* 43 (March 1992): 58–61; D. Staton, "Psychiatry's Future: Facing Reality," *Psychiatric Quality* 62 (Summer 1991): 165–176.
103. See M. Shore and A. Beigel, "Sounding Board: The Challenges Posed by Managed Behavioral Health Care," *New England Journal of Medicine* (January 11, 1986): 116–118.
104. Ibid.
105. Iglehart, "Health Policy Report," 132.
106. See D. Forbes, "The Draconian Cuts in Mental Health," *Business Month* 130 (September 1987): 41–43; A. Blostin, "Mental Health Benefits Financed by Employers," *Monthly Labor Review* 110 (July 1987): 23–27; D. Mechanic, "Emerging Trends in Mental Health Policy and Practice," *Health Affairs* 17 (November–December 1998): 91–92.
107. See R. Dorwart and M. Schlesinger, "Privatization of Psychiatric Services," *American Journal of Psychiatry* 145 (1988): 543–553.
108. See Group Health Association of America, *What Is the Profile of HMO Hospital Use? Pilot Utilization Date Supplement to the Annual HMO Industry Survey* (Washington, DC: Group Health Association of America, 1990).
109. D. Leslie, R. Rosenheck, and S. Horwitz, "Patterns of Mental Health and Utilization and Costs among Children in a Privately Insured Population," *Health Services Research* 36 (April 2001): 115–118.
110. See A. Stone, "Psychotherapy and Managed Care: The Bigger Picture," *Harvard Mental Health Letter* 11 (February 1995): 5–7.
111. See T. Mark, R. Coffey, E. King, et al., "Spending on Mental Health and Substance Abuse Treatment, 1987–1997," *Health Affairs* 19 (July–August 2000): 113–115; B. Stroul, S. Pires, M. Armstrong, et al., "The Impact of Managed Care on Mental Health Services for Children and Their Families," *Future of the Child* 8 (Summer–Fall 1998): 119–133; S. Zuvekas, "Trends in Mental Health Services Use and Spending," *Health Affairs* 20 (March–April

2001): 214–224; S. Glied and A. Cuellar, "Trends and Issues in Child and Adolescent Mental Health," *Health Affairs* 22 (September–October 2003): 39–50; D. McKusick, T. Mark, E. King, et al., "Trends in Mental Health Insurance Benefits and Out-of-Pocket Spending," *Journal of Mental Health Policy and Economics* 5 (June 2002): 71–78.

112. R. Beardsley, G. Gardocki, D. Larson, et al., "Prescribing of Psychotropic Medications by Primary Care Physicians and Psychiatrists," *Archives of General Psychiatry* 45 (1988): 1117–1119.

113. See J. Weiner, A. Lyles, D. Steinwachs, et al., "Impact of Managed Care on Prescription Use," *Health Affairs* 10 (Spring 1991): 140–154; M. Pollard, "Managed Care and a Changing Pharmaceutical Industry," *Health Affairs* 9 (Fall 1990): 55–65; M. Olfson, S. Marcus, M. Weissman, et al., "National Trends in the Use of Psychotropic Medications by Children," *Journal of the American Academy of Child and Adolescent Psychiatry* 41 (2002): 514–521.

114. Healy, *The Anti-Depressant Era*, 197.

115. Drug Price Competition and Patent Term Restoration Act, Public Law 98–417 (September 24, 1984).

116. See D. Vaczek, "The Rise of the Generic Drug Industry," *American Druggist* (April 1996): 41.

117. See J. Wechsler, "FDA: A History of Leadership, Partnership, and Transformation," *Pharmaceutical Technology* (July 2001): 14–16.

118. See M. Olson, "Political Influence and Regulatory Policy: The 1984 Drug Legislation," *Economic Inquiry* 32 (July 1994): 363–365.

119. See W. Wardell, M. May, and G. Trimble, "New Drug Development by U.S. Pharmaceutical Firms," *Clinical Pharmacology and Therapeutics* (October 1982): 407–417.

120. T. Agres, "Hatch-Waxman Act Review Incites Controversy," *Research and Development* (March 1999): 15–16.

121. See G. Mossinghoff, "Overview of the Hatch-Waxman Act and Its Impact on the Drug Development Process," *Food and Drug Law Journal* 54 (1999): 187–194.

122. Ibid.

123. See T. Lewin, "Drug Makers Fighting Back against Advance of Generics," *New York Times*, July 28, 1987, A1; Pollard, "Managed Care and a Changing Pharmaceutical Industry," 56.

124. Vaczek, "The Rise of the Generic Drug Industry," 44.

125. See H. Pincus, T. Tanielian, S. Marcus, et al., "Prescribing Trends in Psychotropic Medications: Primary Care, Psychiatry, and Other Medical Specialties," *Journal of the American Medical Association* 279 (February 18, 1998): 526–531; Zuvekas, "Trends in Mental Health Services Use and Spending," 216.

126. See B. O'Reilly, "Drugmakers under Attack," *Fortune*, July 29, 1994, 54–63.

127. Weiner et al., "Impact of Managed Care on Prescription Use," 152.

128. Pollard, "Managed Care and a Changing Pharmaceutical Industry," 62.

129. Ibid.

130. F. Curtiss, "Managed Health Care," *American Journal of Hospital Pharmacy* 46 (April 1989): 742–763.

131. See M. Gold and D. Hodges, "Health Maintenance Organizations in 1988," *Health Affairs* (Winter 1989): 127; Pollard, "Managed Care and a Changing Pharmaceutical Industry," 57.

132. See T. Raehtz, R. Milewski, and N. Massoud, "Factors Influencing Prices Offered to Pharmaceutical Purchasing Groups," *American Journal of Hospital Pharmacy* 44 (September 1987): 2073–2076; R. Yost and D. Flowers, "New Roles for Wholesalers in Hospital Drug Distribution," *Topics in Hospital Pharmacy Management* 7 (August 1987): 84–90.

133. Pollard, "Managed Care and a Changing Pharmaceutical Industry," 58.

134. See P. Kramer, *Listening to Prozac* (New York: Viking Press, 1993).

135. See S. Begley, "One Pill Makes You Larger and One Makes You Small," *Newsweek* 123 (February 7, 1994): 37–41.

136. B. McLean, "A Bitter Pill: Prozac Made Eli Lilly," *Fortune*, August 13, 2001, 118–119.

137. Ibid., 119.

138. P. Elmer-Dewitt, "Depression: The Growing Role of Drug Therapies," *Time*, July 5, 1992, 56–60.

139. See M. Smith, *A Social History of the Minor Tranquilizers: The Quest for Small Comfort in the Age of Anxiety* (New York: Haworth Press, 1991); M. Bury and J. Gabe, "Halcion Nights: A Sociological Account of a Medical Controversy," *Sociology* 30 (1996): 447–469.

140. See Healy, *The Anti-Depressant Era*, 48–64.

141. See Kramer, *Listening to Prozac*.

142. Ibid.

143. D. Rothman, "The Problem with 'Cosmetic Psychopharmacology,'" *New Republic*, February 14, 1994, 37–38.

144. See C. Lane, "How Shyness Became an Illness: A Brief History of Social Phobia," *Common Knowledge* 12 (2006): 388–409.

145. See A. Kohn, "Suffer the Restless Children," *Atlantic Monthly* 264 (November 1989): 90–98; S. Shaywitz and B. Shaywitz, "Increased Medication Use in Attention-Deficit Hyperactivity Disorder: Regressive or Appropriate?" *Journal of the American Medical Association* 260 (October 21, 1988): 2270–2273; D. Gates, "Just Saying No to Ritalin," *Newsweek*, November 23, 1987, 6.

146. See M. Olfson and G. Klerman, "Trends in the Prescription of Psychotropic Medications: The Role of Physician Specialty," *Medical Care* 31 (1993): 559–564; D. Safer and J. Krager, "A Survey of Medication Treatment for Hyperactive/Inattentive Students," *Journal of the American Medical Association* 260 (October 21, 1988): 2256–2258.

147. See D. Safer and J. Krager, "Effect of a Media Blitz and a Threatened Lawsuit on Stimulant Treatment," *Journal of the American Medical Association* 268 (August 26, 1992): 1004–1007; L. Williams, "Parents and Doctors Fear Growing Misuse of Drug Used to Treat Hyperactive Kids," *Wall Street*

*Journal*, January 15, 1988, 1; D. Moss, "Ritalin under Fire," *ABA Journal* 74 (November 1, 1988): 19.

148. See D. Rissmiller and J. Rissmiller, "Evolution of the Antipsychiatry Movement into Mental Health Consumerism," *Psychiatric Services* 57 (June 2006): 863–866.

149. See E. Ouellette, "Legal Issues in the Treatment of Children with Attention Deficit Disorder," *Journal of Child Neurology* 6 (1991, suppl.): 569–575; R. Welke, "Litigation Involving Ritalin and the Hyperactive Child," *Detroit College Law Review* (Spring 1999): 125–176.

150. W. Schmidt, "Sales of Drug Are Soaring for Treatment of Hyperactivity," *New York Times*, May 5, 1987, C3.

151. Gates, "Just Saying No to Ritalin," 6.

152. Shaywitz and Shaywitz, "Increased Medication Use in Attention-Deficit Hyperactivity Disorder," 2270–2272.

153. K. McBurnett, B. Lahey, and L. Pfiffner, "Diagnosis of Attention Deficit Disorders in DSM-IV: Scientific Basis and Implications for Education," *Exceptional Children* 60 (October–November 1993): 109.

154. Ibid., 109–110: "The syndrome of ADD without hyperactivity was not included in DSM-III-R. A separate category of undifferentiated attention deficit disorder (UADD) was placed at the end of the child disorders section. UADD had no diagnostic criteria and was described as applicable to ADD not specified by the ADHD criteria, including attention deficits unaccompanied by significant hyperactivity. The result was that UADD became an ill-defined, heterogeneous category; and research into ADD without hyperactivity was not stimulated."

155. See B. Lahey, R. Loeber, M. Stouthammer-Loeber, et al., "Comparison of DSM-III and DSM-III-R Diagnoses for Prepubertal Children: Changes in Prevalence and Validity," *Journal of the American Academy of Child and Adolescent Psychiatry* 29 (July 1990): 620–626.

156. See L. Diller, *Running on Ritalin* (New York: Bantam Books, 1999), 130–131.

157. See N. Rojas and E. Chan, "Old and New Controversies in the Alternative Treatment of Attention-Deficit Hyperactivity Disorder," *Mental Retardation and Developmental Disabilities Research Reviews* 11 (2005): 116–130.

158. See Swanson et al., "More Frequent Diagnosis of Attention Deficit-Hyperactivity Disorder," 994; Diller, *Running on Ritalin*, 146–150; U.S. General Accounting Office, *Social Security: Rapid Rise in Children on SSI Disability Rolls Follows New Regulations*, GAO/HEHS-94-225 (Washington, DC: U.S. General Accounting Office, September 1994).

159. See J. Zito, D. Safer, S. dosReis, et al., "Psychotherapeutic Medication Patterns for Youths with Attention-Deficit/Hyperactivity Disorder," *Archives of Pediatrics and Adolescent Medicine* 153 (December 1999): 1257–1265; Pincus et al., "Prescribing Trends in Psychotropic Medications," 526–531.

160. See P. Newacheck and W. Taylor, "Childhood Chronic Illness: Prevalence, Severity, and Impact," *American Journal of Public Health* 82 (1992): 364–371.

161. See K. Kelleher, G. Childs, R. Wasserman, et al., "Insurance Status and Recognition of Psychosocial Problems: A Report from PROS and ASPN," *Archives of Pediatric and Adolescent Medicine* 151 (1998): 1109–1115; K. Kelleher and M. Wolraich, "Diagnosing Psychosocial Problems," *Pediatrics* 97 (1996): 899–901; K. Kelleher and S. Scholle, "Children with Chronic Medical Conditions II: Managed Care Opportunities and Threats," *Ambulatory Child Health* 1 (1995): 139–146; K. Kelleher, S. Scholle, H. Feldman, et al., "A Fork in the Road: Decision Time for Behavioral Pediatrics," *Journal of Developmental Behavioral Pediatrics* 20 (1999): 181–186.

162. See K. Hoagwood, K. Kelleher, M. Feil, et al., "Treatment Services for Children with ADHD: A National Perspective," *Journal of the American Academy of Child and Adolescent Psychiatry* 39 (February 2000): 198–206.

163. See D. Cantwell, "Attention Deficit Disorder: A Review of the Past 10 Years," *Journal of the American Academy of Child and Adolescent Psychiatry* 35 (1996): 982–985.

164. J. Swanson, K. McBurnett, D. Christian, et al., "Stimulant Medications and the Treatment of Children with ADHD," in *Advances in Clinical Child Psychology*, vol. 17, ed. T. Ollendick and R. Prinz (New York: Plenum Press, 1995), 271.

165. K. Kelleher, T. McInerny, W. Gardner, et al., "Increasing Identification of Psychosocial Problems: 1979–1996," *Pediatrics* 105 (June 2000): 1313.

166. See C. Liu, A. Robin, S. Brenner, et al., "Social Acceptability of Methylphenidate and Behavior Modification for Treating Attention Deficit Hyperactivity Disorder," *Pediatrics* 88 (September 1991): 560–565.

167. G. Kolata, "Researchers Say Brain Abnormality May Help to Explain Hyperactivity," *New York Times*, November 15, 1990, B18.

168. Ibid.

169. A. Zametkin, T. Nordahl, M. Gross, et al., "Cerebral Glucose Metabolism in Adults with Hyperactivity of Childhood Onset," *New England Journal of Medicine* 323 (November 15, 1990): 1361–1366.

170. A. Zametkin, L. Liebenauer, G. Fitzgerald, et al., "Brain Metabolism in Teenagers with Attention-Deficit Hyperactivity Disorder," *Archives of General Psychiatry* 50 (1993): 333–340; M. Ernst, L. Liebenauer, C. King, et al., "Reduced Brain Metabolism in Hyperactive Girls," *Journal of the American Academy of Child and Adolescent Psychiatry* 33 (1994): 858–868; M. Ernst, R. Cohen, L. Liebenauer, et al., "Cerebral Glucose Metabolism in Adolescent Girls with Attention-Deficit/Hyperactivity Disorder," *Journal of the Academy of Child and Adolescent Psychiatry* 36 (1997): 1399–1406.

## 5. ADHD and the Politics of Children's Disability Policy

1. E. Kemp, "Aiding the Disabled: No Pity, Please," *New York Times*, September 3, 1981, A19.
2. P. Longmore, "Medical Decision Making and People with Disabilities: A Clash of Cultures," *Journal of Law, Medicine, and Ethics* 23 (1995): 83.
3. T. Burke, "On the Rights Track: The Americans with Disabilities Act," in *Comparative Disadvantages? American Social Regulation and the Global Economy*, ed. P. Nivola (Washington DC: Brookings Institution Press, 1997), 242–318.
4. F. Bowe, *Handicapping America: Barriers to Disabled People* (New York: Harper and Row, 1978), 224.
5. Ibid.
6. B. Ennis, *Prisoners of Psychiatry* (New York: Harcourt Brace Jovanovich, 1972), vii–viii, 82, 230.
7. J. Chamberlain, "Psychiatric Survivors: Are We Part of the Disability Rights Movement?" *Disability Rag* 16 (1995): 4.
8. H. Hahn, "Disability Policy and the Problem of Discrimination," *American Behavioral Scientist* 28 (1985): 297.
9. Ibid., 304.
10. P. Longmore, "The Second Phase: From Disability Rights to Disability Culture," *Disability Rag and Resource* (September–October 1995), www.independentliving.org/docs3/longm95.html, accessed June 23, 2003.
11. See generally J. Charlton, *Nothing About Us without Us: Disability Oppression and Empowerment* (Berkeley: University of California Press, 2000), and on the history of children's mental health, see John S. Lyons, *Redressing the Emperor: Improving Our Children's Mental Health System* (Westport, CT: Praeger, 2004).
12. Ibid.; Longmore, "The Second Phase."
13. Ibid.
14. C. Wallis, "Life in Overdrive," *Time*, July 18, 1994, 42.
15. E. Hallowell and J. Ratey, *Driven to Distraction: Recognizing and Coping with Attention Deficit Disorder from Childhood through Adulthood* (New York: Touchstone, 1995).
16. Wallis, "Life in Overdrive."
17. T. Hartmann, *The Edison Gene: ADHD and the Gift of the Hunter Child* (Rochester, VT: Inner Traditions, 2003).
18. Wallis, "Life in Overdrive."
19. J. Shapiro, *No Pity: People with Disabilities Forging a New Civil Rights Movement* (New York: Times Books, 1994), 105–141.
20. Ibid.
21. R. Katzmann, *Institutional Disability: The Saga of Transportation Policy for the Disabled* (Washington, DC: Brookings Institution Press, 1986), 111.
22. Shapiro, *No Pity*, 142–183; Chamberlain, "Psychiatric Survivors," 4.

23. J. Sealander, *The Failed Century of the Child: Governing America's Young in the Twentieth Century* (New York: Cambridge University Press, 2003), 262, 264.

24. Ibid., 264–265.

25. Ibid., 266.

26. *Pennsylvania Association for Retarded Children v. Pennsylvania*, 334 F. Supp. 1257 (E.D. Pa. 1971) and 343 F. Supp. 279 (E.D. Pa. 1972).

27. In fact, one happy advocate went so far as to claim that "*PARC* printed the bumper stickers for disability rights." Quoted in Sealander, *The Failed Century of the Child*, 272.

28. *Mills v. Board of Education for the District of Columbia*, 348 F. Supp. 866 (D.C. 1972).

29. Sealander, *The Failed Century of the Child*, 272.

30. U.S. Congress, Senate, Committee on Labor and Public Welfare, Subcommittee on the Handicapped, "Education for All Handicapped Children, 1973–1974," Hearings, 93rd Cong., 1st sess., May 7, 1973, 341.

31. States must foot the bill for a student's "related" nonmedical services necessary for his or her education. Exactly what distinguishes a "related" nonmedical service from a medical service or unrelated nonmedical service, however, has been the subject of unending lawsuits. On this and on the issue of litigiousness under special education in general and the costs of providing services to children with disabilities, see R. Melnick, *Between the Lines: Interpreting Welfare Rights* (Washington, DC: Brookings Institution Press, 1994), 161–175; Sealander, *The Failed Century of the Child*, 279–290.

32. See the accounts of this episode in J. Swanson, K. McBurnett, D. Christian, et al., "Stimulant Medications and the Treatment of Children with ADHD," in *Advances in Clinical Child Psychology*, ed. T. Ollendick and R. Prinz (New York: Plenum Press, 1995), 288–290; and L. H. Diller, *Running on Ritalin: A Physician Reflects on Children, Society, and Performance in a Pill* (New York: Bantam Books, 1998), 149–150.

33. Congress added the listing for "developmental delay" in 1997. It applies only to children ages 3 through 9, and for ages 6 through 9 is optional for states to implement.

34. *Individuals with Disabilities Education Act*, U.S. Code (2004) 20 §1401(a)(1), and *Code of Federal Regulations*, title 34, sec. 300.5 (2004). Traumatic brain injury was added to the list in 1990.

35. See *Code of Federal Regulations*, title 34, sec. 300.8(c)(9) (2004).

36. U.S. Congress, House, Committee on Education and Labor, Subcommittee on Select Education, *Hearings on the Reauthorization of the EHA Discretionary Programs*, 101st Cong., 2nd sess., 1990, 352–355.

37. U.S. Congress, House, *Education of the Handicapped Act Amendments of 1990: Report to Accompany H.R. 1013*, 101st Cong., 2nd sess., 1990, H. Rept. 101-544, 6.

38. Ibid.

39. U.S. Congress, House, Subcommittee on Select Education, *Hearings on the Reauthorization of the EHA Discretionary Programs*, 352–355.

40. Ibid.

41. R. Reid, J. Maag, and S. Vasa, "Attention Deficit Hyperactivity Disorder as a Disability Category: A Critique," *Exceptional Children* 60, (December 1992–January 1993), 198–215, http://newman.richmond.edu:3089/itx/start .do?prodId=EAIM&userGroupName=vic_uor, accessed March 25.

42. U.S. Congress, House, Subcommittee on Select Education, *Hearings on the Reauthorization of the EHA Discretionary Programs*, 60, 78, 99. See also Council for Exceptional Children, "The ADD Controversy: What Did CEC Say?" *Exceptional Children* 60 (October–November 1993): 181–182.

43. Ibid.

44. S. Aleman, *Special Education for Children with Attention Deficit Disorders: Current Issues* (Washington, DC: Congressional Research Service, 1991); L. Danielson, K. Henderson, and E. Schiller, "Education Policy—Educating Children with Attention Deficit Hyperactivity Disorder," in *Attention Deficit Hyperactivity Disorder: State of the Science, Best Practices*, ed. P. S. Jenson and J. R. Cooper (Kingston, NJ: Civic Research Institute, 2002), 26–32.

45. R. Appling and N. Jones, *The Individuals with Disabilities Education Act (IDEA): Overview of Major Provisions*, Congressional Research Service Report for Congress, January 11, 2002, 8.

46. Diller, *Running on Ritalin*, 150.

47. R. Davila, M. Williams, and J. MacDonald, *Clarification of Policy to Address the Needs of Children with Attention Deficit Disorders within General and/or Special Education* Washington, DC: Department of Education, Office of Special Education and Rehabilitation, September 16, 1991.

48. *Code of Federal Regulations*, title 34, sec. 104.3(j)(1) (2004).

49. U.S. Department of Education, *To Assure the Free Appropriate Public Education of All Children with Disabilities*, Washington, DC, 2002, II-19.

50. Ibid., II-20.

51. Ibid. Experts speculate that growth in the emotional disturbance category would be more pronounced were it not for the stigma the "emotional disturbance" listing carries, a fact that might lead administrators to seek out other labels for children with behavioral symptoms. The IDEA amendments of 1997 changed the label "serious emotional disturbance" to "emotional disturbance" in an attempt to lessen the stigma of the designation. The change carried no other substance or legal significance. *Individual with Disabilities Education Act Amendments of 1997*, Public Law 105–17, *U.S. Statutes at Large* 111 (1997): 37–157.

52. Ibid. See also II-23–II-24 for further discussion of the growth in this listing. Incidentally, the most dramatic growth of all the IDEA listings occurred in the categories for autism (1,354%) and traumatic brain injury (5,959%). But the number of children served under these categories (in 2000–2001,

78,749 for autism and 14,844 for traumatic brain injury) did not come close to rivaling the number of children classified as having an "other health impairment." In 1999, ADHD was specifically listed in the federal regulations of IDEA under the disability category of "other health impairment."

53. Ibid., II-20 to II-21. For a detailed description of how children, specifically children suspected of having ADHD, are classified under the various categories of IDEA, see S. R. Forness and K. A. Kavale, "Impact of ADHD on School Systems," in *Attention Deficit Hyperactivity Disorder: State of the Science, Best Practices*, ed. P. S. Jenson and J. R. Cooper (Kingston, NJ: Civic Research Institute, 2002), 24-3–24-7.

54. Ibid. See also J. Taylor with A. Rudolph, *White Paper: An Advance Set of Critical Issues on Special Education Funding*, Michigan Policy Network, August 1998, www.ncrel.org/policy/states/files/mispn.htm.

55. U.S. Department of Education, *To Assure the Free Appropriate Public Education*, II-22–II-24.

56. Both J. Swanson and L. Diller trace the dramatic increase in Ritalin use to that memo. Diller, *Running on Ritalin*, 146–147; J. Swanson, M. Lerner, and L. Williams, "More Frequent Diagnosis of Attention Deficit Hyperactivity Disorder," *New England Journal of Medicine* 333 (1996): 994.

57. A. Hocutt, J. McKinney, and M. Montague, "Issues in the Education of Students with Attention Deficit Disorder: Introduction to the Special Issue," *Exceptional Children* 60 (October–November 1993): 103–107; and Reid et al., "Attention Deficit Hyperactivity Disorder as a Disability Category," 198–215, http://newman.richmond.edu:3089/itx/start.do?prodId=EAIM& userGroupName=vic_uor, accessed March 25, 2005.

58. This has been the experience of the Social Security Administration with respect to SSI. J. Ritter, former executive program policy officer for the Office of Disability, Social Security Administration, interview in the Oral History Collection, August 16, 1995, transcripts in the SSA Archives, Office of the Historian, Social Security Administration, Baltimore, Maryland.

59. U.S. Department of Education, *To Assure the Free Appropriate Public Education*, II-22, II-29–II-30.

60. This story is documented more fully in J. L. Erkulwater, *Disability Rights and the American Social Safety Net* (Ithaca, NY: Cornell University Press, 2006), 132. The material on SSI in this chapter draws heavily from this book.

61. Ibid., 160.

62. U.S. Congress, House, Committee on Ways and Means, *The Social Security Amendments of 1971*, 92nd Cong., 2nd sess., 1971, H. Rept. 92-231, 603.

63. U.S. Congress, Senate, Committee on Finance, *Social Security Amendments of 1972*, 92nd Cong., 2nd sess., 1972, 385. The Finance Committee was largely mistaken. At the time, most children with disabilities were institutionalized, with the states picking up the costs of their care. While Medicaid did cover some medical expenses, in the early 1970s, Medicaid was in its infancy, and its provisions for children with disabilities were far from adequate. The financial burden for caring for a child with disabilities was alleviated somewhat

by the expansion of Medicaid in the late 1980s and the passage in 1975 of the Education for All Handicapped Children Act, which required states to provide children with disabilities with a "free and appropriate public education" and to pay for all "related services."

64. On the creation of SSI, see V. Burke and V. Burke, *Nixon's Good Deed: Welfare Reform* (New York: Columbia University Press, 1974); M.K. Bowler, *The Nixon Guaranteed Income Proposal: Substance and Process in Policy Change* (Cambridge, MA: Ballinger, 1974); M. Derthick, *Agency under Stress: The Social Security Administration and American Government* (Washington, DC: Brookings Institution Press, 1990); Erkulwater, *Disability Rights and the American Social Safety Net.*

65. U.S. Department of Health and Human Services, *Mental Health: A Report of the Surgeon General* (Washington, DC: Public Health Service, 2000), 46, 48, 123–124. See also E.N. Brandt, Jr. and A.M. Pope, eds., *Enabling America* (Washington, DC: National Academy Press, 1997), 47–51.

66. U.S. Department of Health and Human Services, *Mental Health*, 123–124, 137–138.

67. Ibid.

68. Ibid.

69. Ibid.

70. M. Ross, former career SSA official, Social Security Administration, interview in the Oral History Collection, October 26, 1995, and February 13, 1996, transcripts in the SSA Archives, Office of the Historian, Social Security Administration, Baltimore, Maryland.

71. J. Mashaw, J. Perrin, and V.P. Reno, eds., *Restructuring the SSI Disability Program for Children and Adolescents* (Washington, DC: National Academy of Social Insurance, 1996).

72. Erkulwater, *Disability Rights and the American Social Safety Net*, 132.

73. Ibid.

74. *Zebley v. Bowen*, Appeal from the United States District Court of the Eastern District of Pennsylvania, Civil Action No. 83-3314, to the United States Court of Appeals for the Third Circuit, amicus brief by the Mental Health Law Project on behalf of the American Academy of Child and Adolescent Psychiatry et al., 1988, 9–10, copy in authors' files. (The Mental Health Law Project was renamed the Bazelon Center for Mental Health in 1990.)

75. Ibid.

76. *Sullivan v. Zebley*, 493 U.S. 521 (1990).

77. For an overview of the SSA's process for evaluating childhood disability before and after *Zebley*, see Erkulwater, *Disability Rights and the American Social Safety Net*, 172–193.

78. Ibid.

79. Ibid.

80. B. Eigen, executive program policy officer in the Office of Disability, interview with Jennifer Erkulwater, Baltimore, Maryland, September 6, 2000, quoted in ibid., 185–186.

81. B. Eigen, executive program policy officer in the Office of Disability, interview with Jennifer Erkulwater, Baltimore, Maryland, September 6, 2000.

82. Mashaw, Perrin, and Reno, *Restructuring the SSI Disability Program*, 27–29.

83. U.S. General Accounting Office (GAO), *Social Security: New Functional Assessments for Children Raise Eligibility Questions*, GAO/HEHS-95-66, 1995, Figure 2, 9–10.

84. Erkulwater, *Disability Rights and the American Social Safety Net*, 172–193.

85. U.S. General Accounting Office, *Supplemental Security Income: Recent Growth in the Rolls Raises Fundamental Program Concerns*, GAO/T-HEHS-95-67, January 27, 1995, 3.

86. GAO, *Social Security: New Functional Assessments*, 9–10.

87. J. Perrin, K. Kuhlthau, T. MacLaughlin, et al., "Changing Patterns of Conditions among Children Receiving Supplemental Security Income Disability Benefits," *Archives of Pediatric and Adolescent Medicine* 153 (1999): 80–84.

88. Ibid.

89. K. Kuhlthau, J. Perrin, S. Ettner, et al., "High-Expenditure Children with Supplemental Security Income," *Pediatrics* 102 (September 1998): 610–615.

90. B. Woodward and B. Weiser, "Costs Soar for Children's Disability Program: How 26 Words Cost the Taxpayers Billions in New Entitlement Payments," *Washington Post*, February 4, 1994, A1.

91. See, among others, J. Dixon, "After 20 Years of Helping Poor, Fast-Growing SSI Dogged by Questions," Associated Press, February 23, 1994, http://newman .richmond.edu:2435/us/lnacademic/home/home.do?randomNum=0 .3782461776992677, accessed July 14, 2002; and C. M. Sennott, "Disability Grants for Children Fuel Welfare Debate," *Boston Globe*, May 12, 1994, Metro Section, 1. A full listing of media stories alleging fraud and abuse in the children's program can be found in the National Commission on Childhood Disability, *Supplemental Security Income for Children with Disabilities*, Washington, DC, 1995, copy in the SSA Archives, Office of the Historian, Social Security Administration, Baltimore, Maryland.

92. R. Weaver, *Ending Welfare as We Know It* (Washington, DC: Brookings Institution Press, 2000), 222–246.

93. L. Mueller and P. Wheeler, "The Growth in Disability Programs as Seen by SSA Field Office Managers," in *Growth in Disability Benefits*, ed. K. Rupp and D. Stapleton (Kalamazoo, MI: Upjohn Institute, 1998), 214.

94. D. Lutterbeck, "Government by Tantrum: Bill Aims to Limit Supplemental Security Income Eligibility," *Common Cause*, Summer 1995.

95. Sennott, "Disability Grants for Children Fuel Welfare Debate," 1.

96. J. Kubik, "Incentives for the Identification and Treatment of Children with Disabilities: The Supplemental Security Income Program," *Journal of Public Economics* 73 (1999): 187–215, cited in M. C. Daly and R. Burkhauser,

"Left Behind: SSI in the Era of Welfare Reform," *Focus* 22, 3 (Summer 2003): 41.

97. A. Yelowitz, "The Impact of Health Care Costs and Medicaid on SSI Participation," in *Growth in Income Entitlement Benefits for Disability: Explanations and Policy Implications*, ed. K. Rupp and D. C. Stapleton (Kalamazoo, MI: Upjohn Institute, 1998), 109–133.

98. U.S. Congress, House, Committee on Ways and Means, Subcommittee on Human Resources, *Contract with America—Welfare Reform*, 104th Cong., 1st sess., 1996, 416–417; U.S. General Accounting Office, *Social Security: Federal Disability Programs Face Major Issues*, GAO/T-HEHS-95-97, 1995, 12; J. Bound, S. Kossoudji, and G. Ricart-Moss, "The Ending of General Assistance and SSI Disability Growth in Michigan," in Rupp and Stapleton, *Growth in Disability Benefits*, 232–237; and G. Livermore, D. Stapleton, and A. Zeuschner, "Lessons from Case Studies of Recent Program Growth," in Rupp and Stapleton, *Growth in Disability Benefits*, 255–262.

99. General Accounting Office, "Supplemental Security Income: Growth and Changes" *in Recipient Population Call for Reexamining Program*, GAO/HEHS-95-137, July 7, 1995, 21.

100. Ibid., 22; J. Ritter, former executive program policy officer for the Office of Disability, Social Security Administration, interview in the Oral History Collection, August 16, 1995, transcripts in the SSA Archives, Office of the Historian, Social Security Administration, Baltimore, Maryland.

101. U.S. Congress, House, Subcommittee on Human Resources, *Contract with America*, 416–417.

102. U.S. Social Security Administration, "SSA Will Review 45,000 Cases of Children Who Had SSI Benefits Ceased, Offer Second Chance for Appeal to All," news release, December 17, 1997, www.socialsecurity.gov/pressoffice/childhood_press.html, accessed February 21, 1998. The number of children with ADHD declined slightly after the enactment of welfare reform in 1996 and then stabilized thereafter, rising slightly only in recent years. Perrin et al., "Changing Patterns of Conditions," 80–84.

103. See, for example, W. Olson, *The Excuse Factory* (New York: Free Press, 1997); R. Shalit, "Defining Disability Down: Why Johnny Can't Read, Write, or Sit Still," *New Republic*, August 25, 1997, 16; J. Greene and G. Forster, *Effects of Funding Incentives on Special Education Enrollment*, Report 32, Center for Civic Innovation, Manhattan Institute, December 2002, 1–4; P. Johnson, testimony, in U.S. Congress, House, Committee on Education and the Workforce, Subcommittee on Oversight and Investigations, *Behavioral Drugs in Schools: Questions and Concerns*, 106th Cong., 2nd sess., September 29, 2000, http://newman.richmond.edu:2054/congcomp/, accessed May 24, 2007. See also P. Johnson, "Too Much Ritalin," Independence Institute, Denver, Colorado, October 20, 1999, www.i2i.org/main/article.php?article_id=325; but also see B. Day, "Ain't Just Misbehavin'," Independence Institute, Denver, Col-

orado, November 17, 1999, www.i2i.org/main/article.php?article_id= 321.

104. P. Johnson, testimony, in U.S. Congress, House, Committee on Education and the Workforce, Subcommittee on Oversight and Investigations, *Behavioral Drugs in Schools*, http://newman.richmond.edu:2054/congcomp, accessed May 24, 2007.

105. K. Koch, "Special Education: Do Students with Disabilities Get the Help They Need?" *CQ Researcher* 10 (November 10, 2000): 911.

106. P. Schlafly, "Dumbing Down and Developing Diversity," *Phyllis Schlafly Report* 34, no. 8 (March 2001), www.eagleforum.org/psr/2001/mar01/ psrmar01.shtml.

107. Greene and Forster, *Effects of Funding Incentives*, 1–4.

108. Ibid.

109. Ibid.

110. Ibid.

111. Ibid.

112. Ibid.

113. L. Goldstein, "Special Education Growth Spurs Cap Plan in Pending IDEA," *Education Week* 22, no. 31 (April 16, 2003).

114. *Code of Federal Regulations*, title 34, sec. 104.3(j)(1) (2004).

115. Under Section 504, in order to obtain federal funds, schools cannot discriminate against children with disabilities. The law applies to virtually all public schools since almost all of them receive funding from the Elementary and Secondary Education Act. The ADA, meanwhile, applies to private schools and colleges. Appling and Jones, *The Individuals with Disabilities Education Act*, 7–10. Students with ADHD are eligible for services and accommodations under all three federal laws even though the disorder is not specifically mentioned by any of them. Which law applies, however, depends on the specific circumstances of the child, such as where the child goes to school, what kind of impairment the child has, and what kind of functional limitations the impairment imposes.

116. See, for instance, L. Sax, "Ritalin—Better Living through Chemistry?" *World and I* 15, no. 11 (November 2000); Shalit, "Defining Disability Down," 16; and, for an extension of this argument to the adult world of work, W. Olson, "Disabling America," *National Review*, May 5, 1997, 40–42. An excellent response to and analysis of the conservative attack on disability rights is F. Pelka, "Bashing the Disabled: The Right-Wing Attack on the ADA—Americans with Disabilities Act," *Humanist*, November–December 1996, 26–30.

117. Shalit, "Defining Disability Down," 16.

118. Ibid. On the limits of the ADA, see R. O' Brien, *Crippled Justice: The History of Modern Disability Policy in the Workplace* (Chicago: University of Chicago Press, 2001).

119. P. Schlafly, "Is Ritalin Raising Kids to Be Drug Addicts?" *Eagle Forum*, June 21, 2000, www.eagleforum.org/column/2000/june00/00-06-21.html.

120. J. Buchan, "ETS to Stop 'Flagging' Tests of Disabled Students after Lawsuit," *Daily Princetonian*, September 17, 2002, www.dailyprincetonian.com/archives/2002/09/17/news/5335.shtml.

121. Johnson, "Too Much Ritalin."

122. L. Rubenstein, "Unfair Portrayal of a Good Program," *Washington Post*, February 26, 1994, A24; M. Ford and R. Schulzinger, "Contention over Children's Benefits," *Washington Post*, March 2, 1994, A16.

123. Lutterbeck, "Government by Tantrum."

124. GAO, *Social Security: New Functional Assessments*, 17.

125. R. Weaver, "Controlling Entitlements," in *The New Direction in American Politics*, ed. J. Chubb and P. Peterson (Washington, DC: Brookings Institution Press, 1985), 337.

126. GAO, *Growth and Changes*, 10.

127. J. Chambers, T. Parrish, and J. Harr, "What Are We Spending on Special Education Services in the United States, 1999–2000?" Special Education Expenditure Project, Center for Special Education Finance, Office of Special Education Programs, U.S. Department of Education, 2002, 1.

128. Koch, "Special Education," 911.

129. Estimates in Forness and Kavale, "Impact of ADHD on School Systems," 24-8–24-9. Forness and Kavale use data from the Department of Education, which classifies students by impairment category, not by diagnosis. At the low end of costs are children in the learning disability and other health impairment classification who are mainstreamed into regular classrooms. The most expensive are children who are classified as emotionally disturbed and who are taught in separate classrooms. Forness and Kavale, however, caution that their estimates rely on assumptions made about the number of children with ADHD in each of the impairment categories (information the Department of Education does not provide) and the setting in which children are educated. Thus, the figures represent their best educated guess rather than statistical fact.

130. Koch, "Special Education," 911.

131. Ibid., 912–913.

132. For a more detailed description of how the SSA evaluated mental disabilities in the 1970s and early 1980s, see Erkulwater, *Disability Rights and the American Social Safety Net*, 98–105.

133. Quoted in *Mental Health Association of Minnesota v. Schweicker*, 554 F. Supp. 157, 162 (D. Minn. 1982).

134. U.S. Congress, Senate, Committee on Finance, *Social Security Disability Insurance Program*, 97th Cong., 2nd sess., 1982, 25.

135. Erkulwater, *Disability Rights and the American Social Safety Net*, 154–158, 177–181.

136. GAO, *Social Security: New Functional Assessments*, 12–14.

137. Ibid.

138. Ibid., 13.

139. Ibid., 29–30.

140. Ibid., 29.

141. A. Rafalovich, "Exploring Clinician Uncertainty in the Diagnosis and Treatment of Attention Deficit Hyperactivity Disorder," *Sociology of Health and Illness* 27 (April 2005): 305–323.

142. T. Scheff, "Decision Rules and Types of Errors, and Their Consequences in Medical Diagnosis," *Behavioral Science* 8 (1963): 97–107.

143. Appling and Jones, *The Individuals with Disabilities Education Act*, 16.

144. Ibid. See also American Academy of Child and Adolescent Psychiatry, "Practice Parameters for the Assessment and Treatment of Children, Adolescents, and Adults with Attention-Deficient/Hyperactivity Disorder," *Journal of the American Academy of Child and Adolescent Psychiatry* 36 (1997 Suppl.), 85S–121S.

145. See, for example, attempts to estimate the proportion and number of children receiving special education services who have ADHD in Forness and Kavale, "Impact of ADHD on School Systems," 24-7–24-9.

146. U.S. Congress, House, Subcommittee on Select Education, *Hearings on the Reauthorization of the EHA Discretionary Programs*, 224–225.

147. B. Eigen, executive program policy officer in the Office of Disability, Social Security Administration, interview with Jennifer Erkulwater, Baltimore, Maryland, September 6, 2000.

148. For an overview of studies on the overlap in diagnostic categories in the special education setting, see Forness and Kavale, "Impact of ADHD on School Systems," 24-3–24-7. See also E. Tirosh, J. Berger, M. Cohen-Ophir, et al., "Learning Disabilities with and without Attention Deficit-Hyperactivity Disorder: Parents' and Teachers' Perspectives," *Journal of Child Neurology* 13, no. 6 (June 1998): 270–276; P. Pastor and C. Reuben, "Attention Deficit Disorder and Learning Disability: United States, 1997–1998," *Vital and Health Statistics*, Series 10, Number 206 (Washington, DC: National Center for Health Statistics, May 2002), 1–12.

149. S. Forness, K. Kavale, I. Blum, et al., "Mega-Analysis of Meta-Analyses: What Works in Special Education and Related Services," *Teaching Exceptional Children* 29 (1997): 4–9; J. Lloyd, S. Forness, and K. Kavale, "Some Methods Are More Effective than Others," *Intervention in School and Clinic* 33 (1998): 195–200.

150. See, for example, the review of the literature in R. Miech, A. Caspi, T. Moffitt, et al., "Low Socioeconomic Status and Mental Disorders: A Longitudinal Study of Selection and Causation during Young Adulthood," *American Journal of Sociology* 104 (January 1999): 1096–1131.

151. B. Eigen, executive program policy officer in the Office of Disability, Social Security Administration, interview with Jennifer Erkulwater, Baltimore, Maryland, September 6, 2000.

152. J. Cheeseman Day with A. Jamieson, *School Enrollment: 2000* (Washington, DC: U.S. Census Bureau, August 2003), 1; U.S. Department of Education, *To Assure the Free Appropriate Public Education*, II-19.

153. U.S. Department of Education, *To Assure the Free Appropriate Public Education*, II-32–II-35.

154. J. Davison and D. Ford, "Perceptions of Attention Deficit Hyperactivity Disorder in One African American Community," *Journal of Negro Education* 70 (Autumn 2001): 264–274.

155. K.R. Weiss, "New Test-Taking Skill: Working the System," *Los Angeles Times*, January 9, 2000.

156. Ibid.

157. Ibid. On the underdiagnosis and overdiagnosis of ADHD in various age, race, gender, and income groups, see S.P. Cuffe, C.G. Moore, and R.E. McKeown, "Prevalence and Correlates of ADHD Symptoms in the National Health Interview Survey," *Journal of Attention Disorders* 9 (November 2005): 392–401.

158. Erkulwater, *Disability Rights and the American Social Safety Net*, 158–159.

159. D. Morgan, "Medicaid Costs Balloon into a Fiscal 'Time Bomb,'" *Washington Post*, January 30, 1994, A1; R. Lombardi, "The Evaluation of Children's Impairments in Determining Disability under the Supplemental Security Income Program," *Fordham Law Review* 57 (1989): 1107.

160. F. Ullman, I. Hill, and R. Almeida, "CHIP: A Look at Emerging State Programs," *New Federalism: Issues and Options for States*, Urban Institute, Series A, No. A-35, September 1999.

161. A. Cuellar and S. Markowitz, "Medicaid Policy Changes in Mental Health Care and Their Effect on Mental Health Outcomes," *Health Economics, Policy, and Law* 2 (2007): 23.

162. Ibid., 27.

163. Ibid., 29.

164. A. Martin and D. Leslie, "Trends in Psychotropic Medication Costs for Children and Adolescents, 1997–2000," *Archives of Pediatric and Adolescent Medicine* 157 (October 2003): 997–1004.

165. S.H. Zuvekas, "Prescription Drugs and the Changing Patterns of Treatment for Mental Disorders, 1996–2001," *Health Affairs* 24 (January–February 2005): 195–205.

166. Ibid; Martin and Leslie, "Trends in Psychotropic Medication Costs," 997–1004.

167. S. Crouch, "Alternative Definition of Disability for Title XVI," November 8, 1974, 12, in the Social Security Administration Archives, Office of the Historian, Social Security Administration, Baltimore, Maryland.

6. The Backlash against ADHD and Stimulants

1. T. Szasz, *The Myth of Mental Illness* (New York: Hoeber-Harper, 1961).

2. T. Scheff, *Being Mentally Ill* (Chicago: Aldine, 1966); T. Scheff, "The Societal Reaction to Deviance: Ascriptive Elements in the Psychiatric Screening of Mental Patients in a Midwestern State," in *The Mental Patient*, ed. S. Spitzer and N.K. Denzin (New York: McGraw-Hill, 1968), 276–290;

T. Scheff, "The Role of the Mentally Ill and the Dynamics of Mental Disorder: A Research Framework," *Sociometry* 26 (1963): 436–453.

3. See, for example, T. Szasz, *Law, Liberty, and Psychiatry* (New York: MacMillan, 1963); and T. Szasz, *The Manufacture of Madness* (New York: Harper and Row, 1970).

4. B. Ennis, *Prisoners of Psychiatry* (New York: Harcourt Brace Jovanovich, 1972), vii–viii, 82, 230.

5. R. DeGrandpre, *Ritalin Nation: Rapid Fire Culture and the Transformation of Human Consciousness* (New York: W. W. Norton, 1999).

6. S. Walker, *The Hyperactive Hoax: How to Stop Drugging Your Child and Find Real Medical Help* (New York: St. Martin's, 1999).

7. M. Block, *No More Ritalin: Treating ADHD without Drugs* (New York: Kensington, 1996); M. Block, *No More ADHD: 10 Steps to Help Improve Your Child's Attention and Behavior without Drugs!* (Hurst, TX: Block Center, 2001).

8. T. Armstrong, *The Myth of the ADD Child: 50 Ways to Improve Your Child's Behavior and Attention Span without Drugs, Labels, or Coercion* (New York: Plume Books, 1997); F. Baughman, *The ADHD Fraud: How Psychiatry Makes "Patients" Out of Normal Children* (Oxford: Trafford, 2006).

9. M. Freedman, "A Headache for Novartis," *Forbes*, July 23, 2001.

10. See, for example, P. Breggin, "Should the Use of Neoleptics Be Severely Limited?" in *Controversial Issues in Mental Health*, ed. S. Kirk and S. Einbinder (Boston: Allyn and Bacon, 1993), reprinted and updated in P. Breggin, "Neuroleptics, Psychiatric Drug Hazards, and Tardive Dyskinesia," www.breggin.com/neuroleptics.html.

11. P. Breggin, *Toxic Psychiatry: Why Therapy, Empathy and Love Must Replace the Drugs, Electroshock, and Biochemical Theories of the "New Psychiatry"* (New York: St. Martin's, 1991); P. Breggin with G. Breggin, *Talking Back to Prozac: What Doctors Aren't Telling You About Today's Most Controversial Drug* (New York: St. Martin's, 1995); P. Breggin with D. Cohen, *Your Drug May Be Your Problem: How and Why to Stop Taking Psychiatric Medications* (Cambridge, MA: Perseus, 2000); P. Breggin, *Talking Back to Ritalin: What Doctors Aren't Telling You about Stimulants and ADHD* (Cambridge, MA: Da Capo, 2001); P. Breggin, *The Ritalin Fact Book: What Your Doctor Won't Tell You* (Cambridge, MA: Perseus, 2002).

12. Breggin, *Talking Back to Ritalin*, 180, 171.

13. Citizens Commission on Human Rights, "Purpose," www.fightforkids.com/purpose.html.

14. P. Breggin, "Joe McCarthy Lives! He's Whispering in the Ear of Eli Lily and Company, the Manufacturer of Prozac," 1994, www.breggin.com/Joemccarthylives.html.

15. G. Gugliotta, "Mixing Business, Advocacy," *Washington Post*, June 18, 2000, A15.

16. Ablechild, "About Us," www.ablechild.org/about%20us.htm.

17. National Alliance against Mandated Mental Health Screening and Psychiatric Drugging of Children, "Death from Ritalin: The Truth Behind ADHD," www.ritalindeath.com.

18. National Alliance against Mandated Mental Health Screening and Psychiatric Drugging of Children, "What Drugmakers Don't Want You to Know: Children's Deaths Caused from ADD and ADHD Drugs," http://ritalindeath .com/ADHD-Drug-Deaths.htm.

19. P. Schlafly, "Can Courts Order Kids to Take Drugs?" *Phyllis Schlafly Report*, September 13, 2000, www.eagleforum.org/column/2000/sept00/00 -09-13.shtml.

20. P. Johnson, "Too Much Ritalin," October 20, 1999, Independence Institute, Denver, Colorado, www.i2i.org/main/article.php?article_id=325; and P. Johnson, testimony, in U.S. House of Representatives, Committee on Education and the Workforce, Subcommittee on Oversight and Investigations, *Behavioral Drugs in Schools: Questions and Concerns*, 106th Cong., 2nd sess., September 29, 2000.

21. See, for example, L. H. Diller, *Running on Ritalin: A Physician Reflects on Children, Society, and Performance in a Pill* (New York: Bantam Books, 1998). For the social science perspective on ADHD, see D. Kindlon and M. Thompson, *Raising Cain: Protecting the Emotional Lives of Boys* (New York: Ballantine Books, 1999); W. Pollack, *Real Boys: Rescuing Our Sons from the Myths of Boyhood* (New York: Random House, 1998). Though these researchers accept the medical reality of ADHD, they are nonetheless troubled by the large number of children diagnosed with the disorder and correspondingly placed on stimulants. They direct their attention to the cultural and social antecedents that contribute to a child being diagnosed with ADHD.

22. Diller captures this tendency well in his discussion of the various patients he has treated over the years, but see especially Diller, *Running on Ritalin*, 214–253.

23. Ibid., 345n33.

24. See, for example, M. Nahata, "More Conflicts of Interest: Review Articles Sponsored by the Pharmaceutical Industry," *Journal of the American Medical Association* 272, no. 16 (October 26, 1994): 1253–1254; K. Wahlback and C. Adams, "Beyond Conflicts of Interest: Sponsored Drug Trials Show More Favorable Outcomes," *British Medical Journal* 318, no. 7181 (February 13, 1999): 465.

25. R. Perils, C. Perils, Y. Wu, et al., "Industry Sponsorship and Financial Conflict of Interest in the Reporting of Clinical Trials in Psychiatry," *American Journal of Psychiatry* 162, no. 10 (October 2005): 1957–1960.

26. Ibid., 365.

27. Both Horton and Angell are quoted in R. Smith, "Medical Journals Are an Extension of the Marketing Arm of Pharmaceutical Companies," *PloS Medicine* 2, no. 5 (May 2005): 364–366.

28. C. Phillips, "Medicine Goes to School: Teachers as Sickness Brokers for ADHD," *PloS Medicine* 3 (April 2006): 434.

29. J. Hunter, *Culture Wars: The Struggle to Define America* (New York: Basic Books, 1992).

30. P. Schlafly, "Is Ritalin Raising Kids to be Drug Addicts?" June 21, 2000, www.eagleforum.org/column/2000/june00/00-06-21.html; M. Eberstadt, "Why Ritalin Rules," *Policy Review* 94 (April–May 1999).

31. J. Garreau, " 'Smart Pills' Are on the Rise, but Is Taking Them Wise?" *Washington Post*, June 11, 2005, D1.

32. K. Thomas, "Stealing, Dealing, and Ritalin: Adults and Students are Involved in Abuse of Drug," *USA Today*, November 27, 2000, 1D.

33. P. Zielbauer, "New Campus High: Illicit Prescription Drugs," *New York Times*, March 24, 2000, A1.

34. K. Thomas, "Ritalin Maker's Ties to Advocates Probed," *USA Today*, November 16, 1995, 14D.

35. W. Leary, "Blunder Limits Supply of Crucial Drug," *New York Times*, November 14, 1993.

36. Diller, *Running on Ritalin*, 34, 38–40.

37. Public Broadcasting Stations, "The Merrow Report—ADD, Ritalin, CHADD (CH.A.D.D.), and Ciba-Geigy: Transcript of a Special Report," October 20, 1995, www.add-adhd.org/textonly/ritalin_CHADD_A.D.D.html; W. Goodman, "Questioning Treatment for Attention Disorder," *New York Times*, October 20, 1995, B18; Thomas, "Ritalin Maker's Ties to Advocates Probed," 4D.

38. Diller, *Running on Ritalin*, 40.

39. U.S. Department of Justice, Drug Enforcement Administration, Drug and Chemical Evaluation Section, Office of Diversion Control, "Methylphenidate: A Background Paper," October 1995, www.ablechild.org/dea%20report%2010-1-95.htm.

40. Diller, *Running on Ritalin*, 40.

41. J. Zito, D. Safer, S. dosReis, et al., "Trends in the Prescribing of Psychotropic Medications to Preschoolers," *Journal of the American Medical Association* 283 (2000): 1025–1030.

42. M. Nahata, "Inadequate Pharmacotherapeutic Data for Drugs Used in Children: What Can Be Done?" *Pediatric Drugs* 1 (1999): 245–249; J. T. Wilson, "An Update on the Therapeutic Orphan," *Pediatrics* 104 (1999): 585–590.

43. R. Pear, "White House Seeks to Curb Pills Used to Calm the Young; Risks Would Be Outlined," *New York Times*, March 20, 2000, A1.

44. E. Goode, "Fury, Not Facts, in the Battle over Childhood Behavior," *New York Times*, April 9, 2000, WK1.

45. J. Zito, D. Safer, S. dosReis, et al., "Psychotropic Practice Patterns for Youth: A 10-Year Perspective," *Archives of Pediatric and Adolescent Medicine* 157 (2003): 17–25. See also Goode, "Fury, Not Facts."

46. E. Goode, "Study Finds Jump in Children Taking Psychiatric Drugs," *New York Times*, January 14, 2003, A21.

47. J. Coyle, "Psychotropic Drug Use in Very Young Children," *Journal of the American Medical Association* 283 (2000): 1059–1060. See also S. Okie, "Behavioral Drug Use in Toddlers up Sharply; Research Lacking Effects, Safety," *Washington Post*, February 23, 2000, A1.

48. Goode, "Study Finds Jump in Children Taking Psychiatric Drugs," A21. For example, T. Robinson and B. Kolb, "Persistent Structural Modifications in the Nucleus Accumbens and Prefrontal Cortex Neurons Produced by Previous Experience with Amphetamine," *Journal of Neuroscience* 17 (1997): 8491–8497. See, in addition, works cited in Breggin, *Talking Back to Ritalin*, 70–74.

49. Breggin, *Talking Back to Ritalin*, 79, 80.

50. S. Stolberg, "Preschool Meds," *New York Times*, November 17, 2002, E58.

51. Ibid.

52. Ibid.

53. R. Pear, "Effort on Mood Drugs for Young Is Backed; Doctors, Teachers, and Business Endorse White House Plan," *New York Times*, March 21, 2000, A18.

54. U.S. Department of Health and Human Services, "First Lady Hillary Rodham Clinton Launches New Public-Private Effort to Improve the Diagnosis and Treatment of Children with Behavioral and Mental Conditions," press release, March 20, 2000, www.hhs.gov/news/press/2000pres/20000320.html.

55. Ibid.

56. Ibid. See also Pear, "White House Seeks to Curb Pills," A1.

57. U.S. Department of Health and Human Services, "First Lady Hillary Rodham Clinton Launches New Public-Private Effort."

58. Pear, "Effort on Mood Drugs for Young Is Backed," A18.

59. R. Merill, "Modernizing the FDA: An Incremental Revolution," *Health Affairs* 18 (1999): 96–111.

60. Ibid.; P. Rheinstein, "Overview of the US Food and Drug Administration's Reform Legislation," *Clinical Therapeutics* 20 (1998): C4–C11.

61. "FDA Draft Sets 50,000 Pediatric Prescription Mentions/Year Threshold for Research List," *FDC Reports* 60 (1998): 11–12; C. Lehmann, "Extension Likely for a Law Encouraging Medication Studies in Children," *Psychiatric News* 36 (July 20, 2001): 4.

62. Lehmann, "Extension Likely for a Law," 4.

63. Ibid.

64. Ibid.

65. B. Strauch, "Use of Antidepression Medicine for Young Patients Has Soared; To Bolster Market, Makers Seek F.D.A. Sanction," *New York Times*, August 10, 1997, 1.

66. Lehmann, "Extension Likely for a Law," 4.

67. Ibid.

68. K. Rodgers, "ADHD Med Reformulated: An Old Drug Reenters Market," *Drug Topics* 140, no. 6 (March 18, 1996): 31–32.

69. K. Thomas, "Back to School for ADHD Drugs," *USA Today*, August 28, 2001, 1D.

70. Ibid. See also A. Martin and D. Leslie, "Trends in Psychotropic Medication Costs for Children and Adolescents, 1997–2000," *Archives of Pediatric and Adolescent Medicine* 157 (2003): 997–1004; A. McCarthy, M. Kelly, S. Johnson, et al., "Changes in Medications Administered in Schools," *Journal of School Nursing* 22 (April 2006): 102–107.

71. Thomas, "Back to School for ADHD Drugs," 1D.

72. Ibid.; Frontline, "Medicating Kids: Backlash: The Business of ADHD," Public Broadcasting Service, 2001, www.pbs.org/wgbh/pages/frontline/shows/medicating/experts/business.html.

73. Thomas, "Back to School for ADHD Drugs," 1D.

74. These campaigns described in Ibid.

75. Frontline, "Medicating Kids: Backlash: The Business of ADHD."

76. C. Phillips, "Medicine Goes to School," 433–435. The examples in this paragraph are taken from this article.

77. Ibid., 434.

78. Ibid., 434–435.

79. Thomas, "Back to School for ADHD Drugs," 1D.

80. M. Angell, *The Truth about the Drug Companies* (New York: Random House, 2004); S. Fried, *Bitter Pills* (New York: Bantam Books, 1998); G. Harris, "At FDA, Strong Drug Ties and Less Monitoring," *New York Times*, December 6, 2004, A1; M. Kaufman and B. Masters, "FDA Is Flexing Less Muscle," *Washington Post*, November 18, 2004, A1; M. Ferris, "Drug Safety: Does the FDA Adequately Protect the Public?" *CQ Researcher* 15 (March 11, 2005): 221–244.

81. Frontline, "Medicating Kids: Backlash: ADHD Lawsuits," Public Broadcasting Service, 2001, www.pbs.org/wgbh/pages/frontline/shows/medicating/backlash/lawsuits.html.

82. Ibid.

83. Ibid.

84. Ibid.

85. R. Scruggs in foreword to Breggin, *Talking Back to Ritalin* (2001 edition), xiii.

86. Frontline, "Medicating Kids: Backlash: ADHD Lawsuits"; T. Locy, "Fight over Ritalin Is Heading to Court," *USA Today*, September 15, 2000, 3A.

87. Locy, "Fight over Ritalin Is Heading to Court," 3A.

88. R. Scruggs in foreword to Breggin, *Talking Back to Ritalin*, xiii.

89. Locy, "Fight over Ritalin Is Heading to Court," 3A.

90. "Another Group of Plaintiffs Drops Ritalin Lawsuit," *Psychiatric News* 36, no. 8 (September 21, 2001): 1.

91. D. Young, "FDA Ponders Cardiovascular Risks of ADHD Drugs," *American Journal of Health-Systems Pharmacy* 63 (March 15, 2006): 492–494;

"Debate over Warnings for ADHD Stimulants," *Child Health Alert* 24 (April 2006): 1.

92. R. Sherer, "FDA Panel: No Black Box Warning for ADHD Drugs," *Psychiatric Times* 23 (May 1, 2006): 1–2, http://psychiatrictimes.com/Children-and-Adolescents/ADD-in-Children//showArticle.jhtml?articleId=187202607; American Psychiatric Association, "APA Urges FDA to Rely on Science, Not Anecdote Alone, for Regulating ADHD Drugs," press release, March 22, 2006, www.psych.org/news_room/press_releases/06-17fdaadhdhearing.pdf; and L. Greenhill, "American Academy of Child and Adolescent Psychiatry: Testimony to the FDA Pediatric Advisory Committee Meeting," March 22, 2006, www.aacap.org/galleries/Psychiatric Medication/Greenhill_Testimony_0306.pdf.

93. See, for example, the Web sites for plaintiffs' attorneys firms: Weitz and Luxenberg (www.weitzlux.com/adhd/adderall/ritalin/strokeheartattackdeath_156854.html); Schmidt and Clark (www.schmidtandclark.com/Ritalin/); and Oshman and Mirisola (www.oshmanlaw.com/pharmaceutical_litigation/Ritalin.html).

94. American Psychiatric Association, *Diagnostic and Statistical Manual of Mental Disorders*, 4th ed. (Washington, DC: American Psychiatric Association, 1994).

95. In a limited study of physicians in Washington, D.C., researchers found that almost half the time parents took children to clinics for an ADHD diagnosis, the reason had been a teacher's suggestion rather than a parent's suspicion. See L. Sax and K. Kautz, "Who First Suggests the Diagnosis of Attention-Deficit/Hyperactivity Disorder?" *Annals of Family Medicine* 1 (September–October 2003): 171–174. However, there are cross-national variations in teachers' receptivity to ADHD. See C. Malacrida, "Medicalization, Ambivalence, and Social Control: Mothers' Descriptions of Educators and ADD/ADHD," *Health* 8 (2004): 61–80.

96. *Valerie J. and Michael J. v. Derry Cooperative School District*, 771 F. Supp. 483 (1991), affirmed 825 F. Supp. 434 (1993).

97. *Valerie J.*, 771 F. Supp. at 489 (1991).

98. "Court Criticizes School's Ordering Drugs for Boy," *New York Times*, August 8, 1991, C9; A. Komoroski, "Stimulant Drug Therapy for Hyperactive Children: Adjudicating Disputes between Parents and Educators," *Boston Public Interest Law Journal* 11 (Fall 2001): 100–101.

99. N. Porter, "Who Decides What's Best for Your Child?" *Pennsylvania Lawyer* 23 (January–February 2001): 16–17. In fact, the Jesson case was the only lawsuit of the late 1980s and early 1990s to end favorably for plaintiffs.

100. C. Lenz, "Prescribing a Legislative Response: Educators, Physicians, and Psychotropic Medication for Children," *Journal of Contemporary Health Law and Policy* 22 (Fall 2005): 81.

101. J. Caher, "Ritalin Case Puts Parents, Courts on a Collision Course," *New York Law Journal*, August 17, 2000, 1.

102. Ibid.

103. U.S. Congress, House, Committee on Government Reform, *Attention Deficit/Hyperactivity Disorder—Are We Over-Medicating Our Children?* 107th Cong., 2nd sess., September 26, 2002, 26–27.

104. U.S. Congress, House, Committee on Government Reform, *Attention Deficit/Hyperactivity Disorder*, 26–27; Komoroski, "Stimulant Drug Therapy for Hyperactive Children," 102.

105. Schlafly, "Is Ritalin Raising Kids to Be Drug Addicts?"; P. Schlafly, "Who Decides What Drugs Are Forced on Children?" *Phyllis Schlafly Report* 34, no. 7 (February 2001), www.eagleforum.org/psr/2001/feb01/psrfeb01.shtml.

106. S. Gilles, "Liberal Parentalism and Children's Educational Rights," *Capital University Law Review* 26 (1997): 9–10, quoted in Komoroski, "Stimulant Drug Therapy for Hyperactive Children," 119.

107. D. Montero, "I Was Told to Dope My Kid: RX Cocktail Making Her Son Psychotic," *New York Post*, August 7, 2002, 6; D. Montero, "Mom's Private RX: Transfers Son over PS 28 Ritalin Push," *New York Post*, August 8, 2002, 9; D. Montero, "Schools Pill-Oriented: Parents Forced to Drug Kids: Activist," *New York Post*, August 9, 2002, 11; D. Montero, "Parents Tell of School Pill Pushers' Extortion," *New York Post*, August 11, 2002, 8; D. Montero, "Give Pill Parents a Hot Line, Not a Cold Shoulder," *New York Post*, August 12, 2002, 6.

108. Lenz, "Prescribing a Legislative Response," 99.

109. M. Janofsky, "Colorado Fuels U.S. Debate over the Use of Behavioral Drugs," *New York Times*, November 25, 1999, A1. Resolution quoted in Lenz, "Prescribing a Legislative Response," 93–94.

110. Janofsky, "Colorado Fuels U.S. Debate over the Use of Behavioral Drugs," A1.

111. Ibid.

112. Ibid.

113. Lenz, "Prescribing a Legislative Response," 94–95.

114. Ibid.

115. K. Zernike and M. Petersen, "Schools' Backing of Behavior Drugs Comes under Fire; Legislatures Set Limits," *New York Times*, August 19, 2001, 1; and the Citizens Commission for Human Rights, "Bills and Resolutions," www.fightforkids.com/bills_resolutions.htm.

116. For an overview of congressional action, see Lenz, "Prescribing a Legislative Response," 98–99.

117. E. Berntsen, "The Child Medication Safety Act: Special Treatment for the Parents of Children with ADHD?" *Washington University Law Quarterly* 83 (2005): 1585n130. On the politics of the bill, see 1585–1593.

118. C. Lehmann, "Bill Would Regulate ADHD Discussions in School," *Psychiatric News* 38 (May 16, 2003): 10.

119. Ibid.

120. J. Vascellaro, "Kennedy Ties up Drug Bill," *Boston Globe*, July 2, 2004, 2.

121. U.S. Congress, House, *Improving Education Results for Children with Disability Act of 2003*, Report No. 108-77, 108th Cong., 1st sess., 2003, 99.

122. Ibid.

123. P. Schlafly, "No Child Left Unmedicated," *Phyllis Schlafly Report*, 38, no. 8 (March 2005), www.eagleforum.org/psr/2005/mar05/psrmar05.html.

124. President's New Freedom Commission on Mental Health, *Achieving the Promise: Transforming Mental Health Care in America, Final Report*, DHHS Pub. No. SMA-03-3832, Rockville, MD, July 2003, 57–65.

125. Schlafly, "No Child Left Unmedicated."

126. Tracked on U.S. Library of Congress, THOMAS, H.R. 181: Parental Consent Act of 2005, and H.R. 1790: Child Medication Safety Act of 2005.

127. P. Johnson, "Too Much Ritalin," October 20, 1999, Independence Institute, Denver, Colorado, www.i2i.org/main/article.php?article_id=325.

128. Eberstadt, "Why Ritalin Rules."

129. Porter, "Who Decides What's Best for Your Child," 16.

130. C. Sommers, *The War against Boys: How Misguided Feminism Is Harming Our Young Men* (New York: Simon and Schuster, 2001), 95; Diller, *Running on Ritalin*, 90–91; Sax, "Ritalin—Better Living through Chemistry?" Note, however, that although Sommers believes that schools are asking too much of young children to sit still for long periods of time, she does not believe that ADHD is merely an outgrowth of a mismatch between the school environment and a child's temperament. She believes that ADHD is a legitimate medical disorder. See M. Fumento, "Trick Question—A Liberal 'Hoax' Turns out to Be True," *New Republic*, February 3, 2003, 19.

131. P. Schlafly, "Dumbing Down and Developing Diversity," *Phyllis Schlafly Report* 34, no. 8 (March 2001), www.eagleforum.org/psr/2001/mar01/psrmar01.shtml.

132. National Commission on Excellence in Education, *A Nation At Risk* (Washington, DC: Department of Education, 1983).

133. B. Mantel, "No Child Left Behind: Is the Law Improving Student Performance?" *CQ Researcher* 15, no. 20 (May 27, 2005): 469–492.

134. L. Sax, "Ritalin: Better Living through Chemistry," *World and I* 15, no, 11 (November 2000): 286.

135. Ibid.

136. Ibid.; Johnson, "Too Much Ritalin"; Schlafly, "Dumbing Down and Developing Diversity."

137. Sommers, *The War against Boys*, 95; Diller, *Running on Ritalin*, 90–91; Sax, "Ritalin—Better Living through Chemistry?"

138. S. Dillon, "Schools Cut Back Subjects to Push Reading and Math," *New York Times*, March 26, 2006, A1; C. Hemphill, "In Kindergarten Playtime, A New Meaning for 'Play,'" *New York Times*, July 26, 2006, A1.

139. Johnson, "Too Much Ritalin."

140. The most cogent statement of this viewpoint is Eberstadt, "Why Ritalin Rules." But on the topic of the medicalization of everyday problems, in general, see, for instance, J. Nolan, *The Therapeutic State* (New York: New York University Press, 1998); F. Fukuyama, *Our Posthuman Future: Con-*

*sequences of the Biotechnology Revolution* (New York: Picador, 2003); Sommers, *The War against Boys;* C. Sommers and S. Satel, *One Nation under Therapy: How the Helping Culture Is Eroding Self-Reliance* (New York: St. Martin's Press, 2005). However, Sommers and Satel, even while criticizing the rise of the therapeutic ethos, do not cite ADHD as an example of this. Fukuyama, on the other hand, devotes an entire chapter to ADHD and Ritalin, though he admits that ADHD might be a legitimate brain disorder, albeit one that is overdiagnosed.

141. See, for instance, Fukuyama, *Our Posthuman Future.*
142. T. Sowell, "Drugging Children," Townhall.com, August 23, 2001, www .townhall.com/columnists/ThomasSowell/2001/08/23/drugging-children.
143. Fukuyama, *Our Posthuman Future,* 52.
144. Fumento, "Trick Question," 18–21.
145. M. Kimmel, "A War against Boys?" *Dissent* 53, (Fall 2006): 65–70.
146. See, for example, M. Pipher, *Reviving Ophelia: Saving the Selves of Adolescent Girls* (New York: Ballantine, 1995). These events are described in C. Goldberg, "After Girls Get the Attention, Focus Shifts to Boys' Woes," *New York Times,* April 23, 1998, A1; T. Lewin, "How Boys Lost Out to Girl Power," *New York Times,* December 13, 1998, WK3.
147. See Kindlon and Thompson, *Raising Cain;* Pollack, *Real Boys;* and M. Gurian, *The Wonder of Boys* (New York: Tarcher, 1996).
148. See, for instance, N. Angier, "The Debilitating Malady Called Boyhood," *New York Times,* July 24, 1998, E1; Goldberg, "After Girls Get the Attention, Focus Shifts to Boys' Woes," A1; and Lewin, "How Boys Lost Out to Girl Power," WK3.
149. Angier, "The Debilitating Malady Called Boyhood," E1.
150. G. Gilder, "The Idea of the (Feminized) University: Coeds Are One Thing . . . ," *National Review,* December 31, 2005, www.discovery.org/ scripts/viewDB/index.php?command=view&id=3187.
151. Goldberg, "After Girls Get the Attention, Focus Shifts to Boys' Woes," A1.
152. Ibid.; Johnson, "Too Much Ritalin."
153. See, for instance, Sommers, *The War against Boys;* and Goldberg, "After Girls Get the Attention, Focus Shifts to Boys' Woes," A1. For a feminist response to the suggestion that boys are falling behind because of feminism, see S. Mead, *The Evidence Suggests Otherwise: The Truth about Boys and Girls,* report by the Education Sector, Washington, DC, June 2006.
154. For an insightful critique of the conservative exaltation of maleness, see Kimmel, "A War against Boys?" 65–70.
155. Mead, *The Evidence Suggests Otherwise,* 4–9.
156. D. I. MacLeod, *Building Character in the American Boy: The Boys Scouts, YMCA, and Their Forerunners* (Madison: University of Wisconsin Press, 1983).
157. Sommers, *The War against Boys.*
158. Fumento, "Trick Question," 19.

159. Ibid.
160. Sommers and Satel, *One Nation under Therapy*.
161. Fumento, "Trick Question," 20, 21.
162. Koch, "Special Education," 913–914.
163. Ibid.
164. V. Clayton, "Seeking Straight A's, Parents Push for Pills," MSNBC, September 7, 2006, www.msnbc.msn.com/id/14590058/.
165. C. Malacrida, *Cold Comfort: Mothers, Professionals, and Attention Deficit Disorder* (Toronto: Toronto University Press, 2003), 186–189.
166. Ibid.
167. For the exception that proves the rule, see, for example, the story of Sam and his parents, Tom and Susan, and the parents of Jennifer Conrad in Diller, *Running on Ritalin*, 65–70, 147–148. On the other hand, stories of parents reluctant to turn to Ritalin run throughout the book.
168. See Malacrida, *Cold Comfort*. Two sociologists found that even in underserved urban African American communities that can be expected to have high rates of ADHD, both parents and educators resisted attributing children's attention and behavior problems to ADHD. See J. C. Davison and D. Y. Ford, "Perceptions of Attention Deficit Hyperactivity Disorder in One African American Community," *Journal of Negro Education* 70 (Autumn 2001): 264–274.
169. Malacrida, *Cold Comfort*, 179.
170. Ibid., 181–242.
171. Ibid.; Diller, *Running on Ritalin*. Malacrida's and Diller's books contain many poignant stories of parents and children negotiating the emotionally laden decisions about whether to accept or resist the ADHD label and whether to engage in stimulant therapy.

## 7. Current Questions about Stimulant Treatment for ADHD

1. C. Dellaverson, "Students Self-Medicate," *Collegian*, February 9, 2006, 1.
2. Ibid., 9.
3. A. Harmon, "Young, Assured and Playing Pharmacist to Friends," *New York Times*, November 16, 2005, A-1.
4. Ibid.
5. L. Johnston, P. O'Malley, J. Bachman, et al., *Monitoring the Future National Survey Results on Drug Use, 1975–2004*, vol. 1, *Secondary School Students*, NIH Publication No. 05-5727 (Bethesda, MD: National Institute on Drug Abuse, 2005); L. Johnston, P. O'Malley, J. Bachman, et al., *Monitoring the Future National Survey Results on Drug Use, 1975–2004*, vol. 2, *College Students and Adults Ages 19–45*, NIH Publication No. 05-5728 (Bethesda, MD: National Institute on Drug Abuse, 2005).
6. 2003 National Survey on Drug Use and Health. U.S. Department of Health and Human Services, Substance Abuse and Mental Health Services Administration, Office of Applied Studies, http://oas.samhsa.gov/nhsda/

2k3nsduh/2k3Results.htm (accessed March 10, 2006); 2002 National Survey on Drug Use and Health. U.S. Department of Health and Human Services, Substance Abuse and Mental Health Services Administration, Office of Applied Studies, http://oas.samhsa.gov/nhsda2k2.htm (accessed March 10, 2006).

7. A. Arria and E. Wish, "Nonmedical Use of Prescription Stimulants among Students," *Psychiatric Annals* 35 (2005): 228–235.

8. L. Kroutil, D. Van Brunt, M. Herman-Stahl, et al., "Nonmedical Use of Prescription Stimulants in the United States," *Drug and Alcohol Dependence* 84 (2006): 135–143.

9. M. Herman-Stahl, C. Krebs, L. Kroutil, et al., "Risk and Protective Factors for Methamphetamine Use and Nonmedical Use of Prescription Stimulants among Young Adults Aged 18 to 25," *Addictive Behaviors* 32 (2007): 1003–1015.

10. Ibid.

11. Q. Babcock and T. Byrne, "Student Perceptions of Methylphenidate Abuse at a Public Liberal Arts College," *Journal of American College Health* 49 (2000): 143–145.

12. K. Low and A. Gendaszek. "Illicit Use of Psychostimulants among College Students: A Preliminary Study," *Psychology, Health and Medicine* 7 (2002): 283–287.

13. K. Hall, M. Irwin, K. Bowman, et al., "Illicit Use of Prescribed Stimulant Medication among College Students," *Journal of American College Health* 53 (2005): 167–174.

14. C. Teter, S. McCabe, C. Boyd, et al., "Illicit Methylphenidate Use in an Undergraduate Student Sample: Prevalence and Risk Factors," *Pharmacotherapy* 23 (2003): 609–617.

15. Ibid.

16. T. Wilens, M. Gignac, A. Swezey, et al., "Characteristics of Adolescents and Young Adults with ADHD Who Divert or Misuse Their Prescribed Medications," *Journal of the American Academy of Child and Adolescent Psychiatry* 45 (2006): 408–414.

17. Ibid.

18. C. Teter, S. McCabe, J. Cranford, et al., "Prevalence and Motives for Illicit Use of Prescription Stimulants in an Undergraduate Student Sample," *Journal of American College Health* 53 (2005): 253–262.

19. Ibid.

20. S. McCabe, J. Knight, C. Teter, et al., "Non-Medical Use of Prescription Stimulants among US College Students: Prevalence and Correlates from a National Survey," *Addiction* 99 (2005): 96–106.

21. Babcock and Byrne, "Student Perceptions of Methylphenidate Abuse"; Low and Gendaszek, "Illicit Use of Psychostimulants among College Students."

22. S. Kollins, E. MacDonald, and C. Rush, "Assessing the Abuse Potential of Methylphenidate in Nonhuman and Human Subjects: A Review," *Pharmacology, Biochemistry, and Behavior* 68 (2001): 611–627.

23. Babcock and Byrne, "Student Perceptions of Methylphenidate Abuse."

24. R. Kadison, "Getting an Edge—Use of Stimulants and Antidepressants in College," *New England Journal of Medicine* 353 (2005): 1089–1091.

25. S. McCabe, C. Teter, and C. Boyd, "The Use, Misuse and Diversion of Prescription Stimulants among Middle and High School Students," *Substance Use and Misuse* 39 (2004): 1095–1116.

26. S. McCabe, C. Teter, and C. Boyd, "Medical Use, Illicit Use and Diversion of Prescription Stimulant Medication," *Journal of Psychoactive Drugs* 31 (2006): 43–56; Teter et al., "Prevalence and Motives for Illicit Use of Prescription Stimulants."

27. Arria and Wish, "Nonmedical Use of Prescription Stimulants among Students."

28. Low and Gendaszek, "Illicit Use of Psychostimulants among College Students."

29. Teter et al., "Illicit Methylphenidate Use"; Teter et al., "Prevalence and Motives for Illicit Use of Prescription Stimulants."

30. Teter et al., "Prevalence and Motives for Illicit Use of Prescription Stimulants."

31. See Kollins et al., "Assessing the Abuse Potential of Methylphenidate in Nonhuman and Human Subjects," for a review of the abuse potential of methylphenidate.

32. N. Volkow, Y. Ding, J. Fowler, et al., "Is Methylphenidate Like Cocaine? Studies on Their Pharmacokinetics and Distribution in the Human Brain," *Archives of General Psychiatry* 52 (1995): 456–463; N. Volkow, G. Wang, S. Gatley, et al., "Temporal Relationships between the Pharmacokinetics of Methylphenidate in the Human Brain and Its Behavioral and Cardiovascular Effects," *Psychopharmacology* 123 (1996): 26–33.

33. Kollins et al., "Assessing the Abuse Potential of Methylphenidate in Nonhuman and Human Subjects."

34. Volkow et al., "Is Methylphenidate Like Cocaine?"

35. J. Biederman, T. Wilens, E. Mick, et al., "Is ADHD a Risk Factor for Psychoactive Substance Use Disorders? Findings from a Four-Year Prospective Follow-up Study," *Journal of the American Academy of Child and Adolescent Psychiatry* 36 (1997): 21–29.

36. R. Gittelman, S. Mannuzza, and R. Shenker, "Hyperactive Boys Almost Grown Up: I. Psychiatric Status," *Archives of General Psychiatry* 42 (1985): 937–947.

37. Biederman et al., "Is ADHD a Risk Factor for Psychoactive Substance Use Disorders?"

38. J. Burke, R. Loeber, and B. Lahey, "Which Aspects of ADHD Are Associated with Tobacco Use in Early Adolescence?" *Journal of Child Psychology and Psychiatry* 42 (2001): 493–502.

39. B. Molina and W. Pelham, Jr., "Childhood Predictors of Adolescent Substance Use in a Longitudinal Study of Children with ADHD," *Journal of Abnormal Psychology* 112 (2003): 497–507.

40. Ibid.

41. B. Molina, K. Flory, S. Hinshaw, et al., "Delinquent Behavior and Emerging Substance Use in the MTA at 36 Months: Prevalence, Course, and Treatment Effects," *Journal of the American Academy of Child and Adolescent Psychiatry* 46 (2007): 1028–1040.

42. Ibid., 1036.

43. J. Loney, J. Kramer, and H. Salisbury, "Medicated vs. Unmedicated ADHD Children—Involvement with Legal and Illegal Drugs," in *Attention Deficit Hyperactivity Disorder: State of the Science; Best Practices,* ed. P. S. Jensen and J. R. Cooper (Kingston, NJ: Civic Research Institute, 2002), 17-1–17-16.

44. R. Barkley, M. Fischer, L. Smallish, et al., "Does the Treatment of Attention-Deficit/Hyperactivity Disorder with Stimulants Contribute to Drug Use/Abuse? A 13-Year Prospective Study," *Pediatrics* 111 (2003): 97–109.

45. N. Lambert, "Stimulant Treatment as a Risk Factor for Nicotine Use and Substance Abuse," in *Attention Deficit Hyperactivity Disorder: State of the Science; Best Practices,* ed. P. S. Jensen and J. R. Cooper (Kingston, NJ: Civic Research Institute, 2002), 18-1–18-24.

46. S. Schenk and B. Partridge, "Sensitization and Tolerance in Psychostimulant Self-Administration," *Pharmacology, Biochemistry and Behavior* 57 (1997): 543–550; see also Lambert, "Stimulant Treatment as a Risk Factor for Nicotine Use and Substance Abuse," for a brief review.

47. S. Schenk and B. Partridge, "Cocaine-Seeking Produced by Experimenter-Administered Drug Injections: Dose-Effect Relationships in Rats," *Psychopharmacology* 147 (1999): 285–290.

48. R. Klein, "Alcohol, Stimulants, Nicotine, and Other Drugs in ADHD," in *Attention Deficit Hyperactivity Disorder: State of the Science; Best Practices,* ed. P. S. Jensen and J. R. Cooper (Kingston, NJ: Civic Research Institute, 2002), 16-1–16-17; Lambert, "Stimulant Treatment as a Risk Factor for Nicotine Use and Substance Abuse."

49. Barkley et al., "Does the Treatment of Attention-Deficit/Hyperactivity Disorder with Stimulants Contribute to Drug Use/Abuse?"

50. Ibid.

51. Ibid.

52. Ibid.

53. Lambert, "Stimulant Treatment as a Risk Factor for Nicotine Use and Substance Abuse."

54. See discussion in Barkley et al., "Does the Treatment of Attention-Deficit/Hyperactivity Disorder with Stimulants Contribute to Drug Use/Abuse?"

55. L. Goldman, M. Genel, R. Bezman, et al., "Diagnosis and Treatment of Attention-Deficit/Hyperactivity Disorder in Children and Adolescents," *Journal of the American Medical Association* 279 (1998): 1100–1107.

56. J. Biederman, T. Wilens, E. Mick, et al., "Pharmacotherapy of Attention-Deficit/Hyperactivity Disorder Reduces Risk for Substance Use Disorder," *Pediatrics* 104 (1999): 20–24.

57. For a recent example, see S. Katusic, W. Barbaresi, R. Colligan, et al., "Psychostimulant Treatment and Risk for Substance Abuse among Young Adults with a History of Attention-Deficit/Hyperactivity Disorder: A Population-Based, Birth Cohort Study," *Journal of Child and Adolescent Psychopharmacology* 15 (2005): 764–776.

58. T. Wilens, S. Faraone, J. Biederman, et al., "Attention-Deficit/Hyperactivity Disorder Beget Later Substance Abuse? A Meta-Analytic Review of the Literature," *Pediatrics* 111 (2003): 179–185; S. Faraone and T. Wilens, "Does Stimulant Treatment Lead to Substance Use Disorders?" *Journal of Clinical Psychiatry* 64 (suppl. 11; 2003): 9–13.

59. Klein, "Alcohol, Stimulants, Nicotine, and Other Drugs in ADHD."

60. Loney et al., "Medicated vs. Unmedicated ADHD Children."

61. Molina et al., "Delinquent Behavior and Emerging Substance Use in the MTA at 36 Months."

62. Ibid.

63. Lambert, "Stimulant Treatment as a Risk Factor for Nicotine Use and Substance Abuse."

64. Ibid.

65. T. Dishion, G. Patterson, M. Stoolmiller, et al., "Family, School, and Behavioral Antecedents to Early Adolescent Involvement with Antisocial Peers," *Developmental Psychology* 27 (1991): 172–180.

66. T. Dishion and L. Owen, "A Longitudinal Analysis of Friendships and Substance Use: Bidirectional Influence from Adolescence to Adulthood," *Developmental Psychology* 38 (2002): 480–491.

67. R. Millstein, T. Wilens, J. Biederman, et al., "Presenting ADHD Symptoms and Subtypes in Clinically Referred Adults with ADHD," *Journal of Attention Disorders* 2 (1997): 159–166; R. Barkley, K. Murphy, and M. Fischer, *ADHD in Adults: What the Science Says* (New York: Guilford Press, 2008). Barkley and colleagues present the most thorough and comprehensive contemporary report and analysis of ADHD in adults. They present data from a study of children with ADHD followed into adulthood and from a study of clinic-referred adults with ADHD.

68. S. Okie, "ADHD in Adults," *New England Journal of Medicine* 354 (June 22, 2006): 2637–2641.

69. Barkley et al., *ADHD in Adults*; R. Barkley, *Attention-Deficit Hyperactivity Disorder: A Handbook for Diagnosis and Treatment*, 3rd ed. (New York: Guilford Press, 2006).

70. R. Resnick, "Attention Deficit Hyperactivity Disorder in Teens and Adults: They Don't All Outgrow It," *Journal of Clinical Psychology* 61 (2005): 529–533.

71. Ibid.

72. P. Wender, *Attention-Deficit Hyperactivity in Adults* (New York: Oxford University Press, 1995); P. Wender, *ADHD: Attention-Deficit Hyperactivity Disorder in Children and Adults* (New York: Oxford University Press, 2000).

73. R. Kessler, L. Adler, R. Barkley, et al., "The Prevalence and Correlates of Adult ADHD in the United States: Results from the National Comorbidity Survey Replication," *American Journal of Psychiatry* 163 (2006): 716–723.

74. For a thorough discussion, see Barkley et al., *ADHD in Adults*.

75. M. Weiss, L. Hechtman, G. Weiss, *ADHD in Adulthood: A Guide to Current Theory, Diagnosis, and Treatment* (Baltimore: Johns Hopkins University Press, 1999).

76. Resnick, "Attention Deficit Hyperactivity Disorder in Teens and Adults." See also diagnostic criteria for ADHD in American Psychiatric Association, *Diagnostic and Statistical Manual of Mental Disorders,* 4th ed. (Washington, DC: American Psychiatric Association, 1994), 83–85.

77. K. Murphy and S. LeVert, *Out of the Fog: Treatment Options and Coping Strategies for Adult Attention Deficit Disorder* (New York: Hyperion, 1995); Weiss et al., *ADHD in Adulthood*.

78. Weiss et al., *ADHD in Adulthood*.

79. Ibid., 7.

80. Murphy and LeVert, *Out of the Fog*.

81. Ibid.; Weiss et al., *ADHD in Adulthood*.

82. Millstein et al., "Presenting ADHD Symptoms and Subtypes in Clinically Referred Adults with ADHD."

83. For discussion of this issue, see R. Barkley, *Attention-Deficit Hyperactivity Disorder: A Handbook for Diagnosis and Treatment*, 3rd ed.; Weiss et al., *ADHD in Adulthood*.

84. Barkley, *Attention-Deficit Hyperactivity Disorder: A Handbook for Diagnosis and Treatment*, 3rd ed., 88.

85. See E. Hallowell and J. Ratey, *Driven to Distraction* (New York: Pantheon Books, 1994); Wender, *Attention-Deficit Hyperactivity in Adults*; Wender, *ADHD: Attention-Deficit Hyperactivity Disorder in Children and Adults*; R. Barkley and K. Murphy, *Attention-Deficit Hyperactivity Disorder: A Clinical Workbook*, 3rd ed. (New York: Guilford Press, 2006).

86. For examples, see Barkley and Murphy, *Attention-Deficit Hyperactivity Disorder: A Clinical Workbook*. See also C. Conners, D. Erhardt, and E. Sparrow, *Conners Adult ADHD Rating Scales* (North Tonawanda, NY: Multi-Health Systems, 2000).

87. B. McCann and P. Roy-Byrne, "Screening and Diagnostic Utility of Self-Report Attention Deficit Hyperactivity Disorder Scales in Adults," *Comprehensive Psychiatry* 45 (2004): 175–183.

88. T. Spencer, J. Biederman, T. Wilens, et al., "Pharmacotherapy of Attention-Deficit Hyperactivity Disorder across the Life Cycle," *Journal of the American Academy of Child and Adolescent Psychiatry* 35 (1996): 409–432.

89. J. Mattes, L. Boswell, and H. Oliver, "Methylphenidate Effects on Symptoms of Attention Deficit Disorder in Adults," *Archives of General Psychiatry* 41 (1985): 1059–1063; P. Wender, F. Reimherr, D. Wood, et al., "A Controlled Study of Methylphenidate in the Treatment of Attention Deficit

Disorder, Residual Type, in Adults," *American Journal of Psychiatry* 142 (1995): 547–552; D. Wood, F. Reimherr, P. Wender, et al., "Diagnosis and Treatment of Minimal Brain Dysfunction in Adults," *Archives of General Psychiatry* 33 (1976): 1453–1460.

90. For brief reviews, see T. Spencer, T. Wilens, J. Biederman, et al., "A Double-Blind, Crossover Comparison of Methylphenidate and Placebo in Adults with Childhood-Onset Attention-Deficit Hyperactivity Disorder," *Archives of General Psychiatry* 52 (1995): 434–443; Weiss et al., *ADHD in Adulthood*.

91. Spencer et al., "A Double-Blind, Crossover Comparison of Methylphenidate and Placebo."

92. Ibid.

93. S. Faraone, T. Spencer, M. Aleardi, et al., "Meta-Analysis of the Efficacy of Methylphenidate for Treating Adult Attention-Deficit/Hyperactivity Disorder," *Journal of Clinical Psychopharmacology* 24 (2004): 24–29.

94. T. Spencer, J. Biederman, T. Wilens, et al., "Efficacy of a Mixed Amphetamine Salts Compound in Adults with Attention-Deficit/Hyperactivity Disorder," *Archives of General Psychiatry* 58 (2001): 775–782.

95. J. Prince, T. Wilens, T. Spencer, et al., "Pharmacotherapy of ADHD in Adults," in *Attention-Deficit Hyperactivity Disorder: A Handbook for Diagnosis and Treatment*, 3rd ed., by R. A. Barkley (New York: Guilford Press, 2006), 704–736.

96. T. Wilens, T. Spencer, and J. Biederman, "Pharmacotherapy of Adult ADHD," in *Attention-Deficit Hyperactivity Disorder: A Handbook for Diagnosis and Treatment*, 2nd ed., by R. Barkley (New York: Guilford Press, 1998), 592–606.

97. Barkley, *Attention-Deficit Hyperactivity Disorder: A Handbook for Diagnosis and Treatment*, 3rd ed.

98. W. Dodson, "Pharmacotherapy of Adult ADHD," *Journal of Clinical Psychology* 61 (2005): 589–606; P. Wender and F. Reimherr, "Buproprion Treatment of Attention Deficit Hyperactivity Disorder in Adults," *American Journal of Psychiatry* 147 (1990): 1018–1020; T. Wilens, J. Biederman, J. Prince, et al., "Six-Week, Double-Blind, Placebo-Controlled Study of Desipramine for Adult Attention Deficit Hyperactivity Disorder," *American Journal of Psychiatry* 153 (1996): 1147–1153.

99. Wilens et al., "Pharmacotherapy of Adult ADHD."

100. S. Safren, M. Otto, S. Sprich, et al., "Cognitive-Behavioral Therapy for ADHD in Medication-Treated Adults with Continued Symptoms," *Behaviour Research and Therapy* 43 (2005): 831–842.

101. Weiss et al., *ADHD in Adulthood*, 132.

102. Goldman et al., "Diagnosis and Treatment of Attention-Deficit/Hyperactivity Disorder in Children and Adolescents"; M. Olfson, M. Gameroff, S. Marcus, et al., "National Trends in the Treatment of Attention Deficit Hyperactivity Disorder," *American Journal of Psychiatry* 160 (2003): 1071–1077; D. Safer, J. Zito, and E. Fine, "Increased

Methylphenidate Usage for Attention Deficit Disorder in the 1990s," *Pediatrics* 98 (1996): 1084–1088.

103. J. Biederman, T. Wilens, E. Mick, et al., "Psychoactive Substance Use Disorder in Adults with Attention Deficit Hyperactivity Disorder: Effects of ADHD and Psychiatric Comorbidity," *American Journal of Psychiatry* 152 (1995): 1652–1658; Biederman et al., "Is ADHD a Risk Factor for Psychoactive Substance Use Disorders?"; Goldman et al., "Diagnosis and Treatment of Attention-Deficit/Hyperactivity Disorder in Children and Adolescents."

## 8. Conclusion

1. See J. Kuntsi, G. McLoughlin, and P. Asherson, "Attention Deficit Hyperactivity Disorder," *Neuromolecular Medicine* 8 (2006): 461–484.

2. See L. Ben Amor, N. Grizenko, G. Schwartz, et al., "Perinatal Complications in Children with Attention-Deficit Hyperactivity Disorder and Their Unaffected Siblings," *Journal of Psychiatry and Neuroscience* 30 (March 2005): 120–126.

3. R. Brown, R. Amler, W. Freeman, et al., "Treatment of Attention-Deficit/ Hyperactivity Disorder: Overview of the Evidence," *Pediatrics* 115 (June 2005): e749–e757.

4. National Institutes of Health, "Diagnosis and Treatment of Attention Deficit Hyperactivity Disorder," *NIH Consensus Statement* 16, no. 2 (November 16–18, 1990): 1–37, http://consensus.nih.gov/1998/1998Attention DeficitHyperactivityDisorder110html.htm (accessed July 10, 2006).

5. "International Consensus Statement on ADHD," *Clinical Child and Family Psychology Review* 5 (2002): 89–111.

6. R. Barkley, *Attention-Deficit Hyperactivity Disorder: A Handbook for Diagnosis and Treatment*, 3rd ed. (New York: Guilford Press, 2006), 38–39.

7. "International Consensus Statement on ADHD," 89.

8. J. Goldstein, "Is ADHD a Growth Industry?" *Journal of Attention Disorders* 9 (February 2006): 461–464.

9. See R. Shader and J. Oesterheld, "Facts and Public Policy: Should I Keep My Child on ADHD Drugs?" *Journal of Clinical Psychopharmacology* 26 (June 2006): 223–224.

10. See S. Mintz, *Huck's Raft: A History of American Childhood* (Cambridge, MA: Belknap Press, 2004).

11. Jerry Rushton, Director of the Pediatrics Residency Program, Indiana University School of Medicine, e-mail exchange with Mayes, November 6, 2007.

12. See H. Niederhofer, B. Hackenberg, and K. Lazendorfer, "Family Conflict Tendency and ADHD," *Psychological Reports* 94 (April 2004): 577–580.

13. E. Goode, "Fury, Not Facts, in the Battle over Childhood Behavior," *New York Times*, April 9, 2000, WK1.

14. See L. Castle, R. Aubert, R. Verbrugge, et al., "Trends in Medication Treatment for ADHD," *Journal of Attention Disorders* 10 (May 2007): 335–342;

T. Froehlich, B. Lanphear, J. Epstein, et al., "Prevalence, Recognition, and Treatment of Attention-Deficit/Hyperactivity Disorder in a National Sample of U.S. Children," *Archives of Pediatrics and Adolescent Medicine* 161 (September 2007): 857–864.

15. L. Diller, *Running on Ritalin: A Physician Reflects on Children, Society, and Performance in a Pill* (New York: Bantam Books, 1998), 194.

16. See D. Stone, *The Disabled State* (Philadelphia: Temple University Press, 1979); J. Erkulwater, *Disability Rights and the American Social Safety Net* (Ithaca, NY: Cornell University Press, 2006).

17. Diller, *Running on Ritalin*, 194.

18. See J. Gross, "Checklist for Camp: Bug Spray, Sunscreen, Pills," *New York Times*, July 16, 2006, 1; F. Bokhari, R. Mayes, and R. Scheffler, "An Analysis of the Significant Variation in Stimulant Use across the U.S.," *Pharmacoepidemiology and Drug Safety* 14 (April 2005): 267–275; E. Cox, B. Motheral, R. Henderson, et al., "Geographic Variation in the Prevalence of Stimulant Medication Use among Children 5 to 14 Years Old: Results from a Commercially Insured US Sample," *Pediatrics* 111 (February 2003): 237–243; A. Angold, A. Erkanli, H. Egger, et al., "Stimulant Treatment for Children: A Community Perspective," *Journal of the American Academy of Child and Adolescent Psychiatry* 39 (August 2000): 975–984; P. Jensen, L. Kettle, M. Roper, et al., "Are Stimulants Overprescribed? Treatment of ADHD in Four U.S. Communities," *Journal of the American Academy of Child and Adolescent Psychiatry* 38 (July 1999): 797–804.

19. Ibid.

20. L. Goldman, M. Genel, R. Bezman, et al., "Diagnosis and Treatment of Attention-Deficit/Hyperactivity Disorder in Children and Adolescents: Council on Scientific Affairs, American Medical Association," *Journal of the American Medical Association* 279 (April 8, 1998): 1100–1107.

21. See A. Kwasman, B. Tinsley, and H. Lepper, "Pediatricians' Knowledge and Attitudes Concerning Diagnosis and Treatment of Attention Deficit and Hyperactivity Disorders: A National Survey Approach," *Archives of Pediatrics and Adolescent Medicine* 149 (November 1995): 1211–1216; J. Williams, K. Klinepeter, G. Palmes, et al., "Diagnosis and Treatment of Behavioral Health Disorders in Pediatric Practice," *Pediatrics* 114 (September 2004): 601–606; J. Rushton, K. Fant, and S. Clark, "Use of Practice Guidelines in the Primary Care of Children with Attention-Deficit/Hyperactivity Disorder," *Pediatrics* 114 (July 2004): 23–28.

22. See L. Culpepper, "Primary Care Treatment of Attention-Deficit/ Hyperactivity Disorder," *Journal of Clinical Psychiatry* 67 (Suppl. 2006): 51–58; J. Zito, D. Safer, S. dosReis, et al., "Psychotherapeutic Medication Patterns for Youths with Attention-Deficit/Hyperactivity Disorder," *Archives of Pediatrics and Adolescent Medicine* 153 (1999): 1257–1263.

23. See A. Pellegrini and M. Horvat, "A Developmental Contextualist Critique of Attention Deficit Hyperactivity Disorder," *Educational Researcher* 24 (January–February 1995): 13–19; P. Jensen, D. Mrazek, P. Knapp, et al., "Evolution and Revolution in Child Psychiatry: ADHD as a Disorder of

Adaptation," *Journal of the American Academy of Child and Adolescent Psychiatry* 36 (December 1997): 1672–1681.

24. There are 5 criteria that must be satisfied for the disorder to exist: (1) a sufficient number of *symptoms* of inattention, hyperactivity, and/or impulsivity; (2) *onset and course* (symptoms must have been present before the age of 7); (3) *pervasiveness* (impairment from the symptoms must exist in 2 or more settings, such as school and home); (4) *impairment* (clear evidence of impairment in social, academic, or occupational functioning); and (5) *differential diagnosis* (the symptoms are not due to another mental disorder).

25. See A. Rowland, D. Umbach, K. Catoe, et al., "Studying the Epidemiology of Attention-Deficit Hyperactivity Disorder: Screening Method and Pilot Results," *Canadian Journal of Psychiatry* 46 (December 2001): 931–940; Centers for Disease Control and Prevention, "Mental Health in the United States: Prevalence of Diagnosis and Medication Treatment for Attention-Deficit/Hyperactivity Disorder," *MMWR: Morbidity and Mortality Weekly Report* 54 (September 2, 2005): 842; P. Jensen, "Epidemiological Research on ADHD: What We Know and What We Need to Learn" (paper presented at the conference ADHD: A Public Health Perspective, Centers for Disease Control and Prevention, Atlanta, GA, September 23–24, 1999), www.cdc.gov/ncbddd/adhd/confepi.htm (accessed November 5, 2007).

26. See Jensen et al., "Are Stimulants Overprescribed?"

27. See Angold et al., "Stimulant Treatment for Children."

28. See J. Rapoport, M. Buchsbaum, T. Zahn, et al., "Dextroamphetamine: Cognitive and Behavioral Effects on Normal Prepubertal Boys," *Science* 199 (1978): 560–563; J. Rapoport, M. Buchsbaum, H. Weingartner, et al., "Dextroamphetamine: The Cognitive and Behavioral Effects in Normal and Hyperactive Boys and Normal Men," *Archives of General Psychiatry* 37 (August 1980): 933–943.

29. See T. Zahn, J. Rapoport, and C. Thompson, "Autonomic and Behavioral Effects of Dextroamphetamine and Placebo in Normal and Hyperactive Prepubertal Boys," *Journal of Abnormal Child Psychology* 8 (June 1980): 145–160; Rapoport et al., "Dextroamphetamine: Its Cognitive and Behavioral Effects in Normal and Hyperactive Boys and Normal Men."

30. See A. Tone and E. Watkins, eds., *Medicating Modern America: Prescription Drugs in History* (New York: New York University Press, 2007).

31. See D. Safer, "Are Stimulants Overprescribed for Youths with ADHD?" *Annals of Clinical Psychiatry* 12 (March 2000): 55–62.

32. See A. Adesman, "The Diagnosis and Management of Attention-Deficit/Hyperactivity Disorder in Pediatric Patients," *Primary Care Companion to the Journal of Clinical Psychiatry* 3 (2001): 66–77.

33. L. Furman, "What Is Attention-Deficit/Hyperactivity Disorder (ADHD)?" *Journal of Child Neurology* 20 (December 2005): 995.

34. S. Faraone, J. Sergeant, C. Gillberg, et al., "The Worldwide Prevalence of ADHD: Is It an American Condition?" *World Psychiatry* 2 (June 2003): 104–113.

35. See M. Skounti, A. Philalithis, and E. Galanakis, "Variations in Prevalence of Attention Deficit Hyperactivity Disorder Worldwide," *European Journal of Pediatrics* 166 (February 2007): 117–123.

36. International Narcotics Control Board, *Psychotropic Drugs: Statistics for 2005: Assessment of Annual Medical and Scientific Requirement* (New York: United Nations, 2006), 269.

37. See J. Buitelaar and A. Rothenberger, "Foreword—ADHD in the Scientific and Political Context," *European Child and Adolescent Psychiatry* 13 (Suppl. 2004): 11–16; H. Hick, J. Kaye, and C. Black, "Incidence and Prevalence of Drug-Treated Attention Deficit Disorder among Boys in the U.K.," *British Journal of General Practitioners* 54 (May 2004): 345–347.

38. P. Jensen, quoted in "Medicating Kids," *Frontline*, Public Broadcasting Service, www.pbs.org/wgbh/pages/frontline/shows/medicating/experts/explosion.html (accessed November 5, 2007).

39. See L. Rohde, C. Szobot, G. Polanczyk, et al., "Attention-Deficit/ Hyperactivity Disorder in a Diverse Culture: Do Research and Clinical Findings Support the Notion of a Cultural Construct for the Disorder?" *Biological Psychiatry* 57 (June 2005): 1436–1441; Faraone et al., "The Worldwide Prevalence of ADHD: Is It an American Condition?"; G. Polanczyk, M. de Lima, B. Horta, et al., "The Worldwide Prevalence of ADHD: A Systematic Review and Metaregression Analysis," *American Journal of Psychiatry* 164 (June 2007): 942–948.

40. O. Amaral, "Psychiatric Disorders as Social Constructs: ADHD as a Case in Point," *American Journal of Psychiatry* 164 (October 2007): 1612.

41. See R. Miller, *Children, Ethics and Modern Medicine* (Bloomington: Indiana University Press, 2003).

42. See D. Gill, "Anything You Can Do, I Can Do Bigger? The Ethics and Equity of Human Growth Hormone for Small Normal Children," *Archives of Disease in Childhood* 91 (March 2006): 270–272.

43. See Tone and Watkins, *Medicating Modern America*.

44. M. Konner, "One Pill Makes You Larger," *American Prospect*, November 30, 2002.

45. Garreau, " 'Smart Pills' Are on the Rise," D1.

46. M. Olfson, S. Marcus, M. Weissman, et al., "National Trends in the Use of Psychotropic Medications by Children," *Journal of the American Academy of Child and Adolescent Psychiatry* 41 (2002): 514–521.

47. B. Vitiello, S. Zuvekas, and G. Norquist, "National Estimates of Antidepressant Medication Use among U.S. Children," *Journal of the American Academy of Child and Adolescent Psychiatry* 45 (2006): 271–279.

48. See M. Olfson, C. Blanco, L. Liu, et al., "National Trends in the Outpatient Treatment of Children and Adolescents with Antipsychotic Drugs," *Archives of General Psychiatry* 63 (2006): 679–685; C. Moreno, G. Laje, C. Blanco, et al., "National Trends in the Outpatient Diagnosis and Treatment of Bipolar Disorder in Youth," *Archives of General Psychiatry* 64 (September 2007): 1032–1039.

49. Olfson et al., "National Trends in the Outpatient Treatment of Children and Adolescents with Antipsychotic Drugs"; Olfson et al., "National Trends in the Use of Psychotropic Medications by Children."

50. S. Okie, "ADHD in Adults," *New England Journal of Medicine* 354 (2006): 2637–2641.

51. For example, see G. Emslie, A. Rush, W. Weiberg, et al., "A Double-Blind, Randomized, Placebo-Controlled Trial of Fluoxetine in Children and Adolescents with Depression," *Archives of General Psychiatry* 54 (1997): 1031–1037.

52. See, for example, R. A. Barkley, K. M. Smith, M. Fischer, et al., "An Examination of the Behavioral and Neuropsychological Correlates of Three ADHD Candidate Gene Polymorphisms (DRD4 7+, DBH TaqI A2, and DAT1 40 bp VNTR) in Hyperactive and Normal Children Followed to Adulthood," *American Journal of Medical Genetics Part B* 141 (2006): 487–498. See also S. Faraone, A. Doyle, E. Mick, et al., "Meta-Analysis of the Association between the 7-Repeat Allele of the Dopamine D4 Receptor Gene and Attention Deficit Hyperactivity Disorder," *American Journal of Psychiatry* 158 (2001): 1052–1057.

53. J. Nigg, *What Causes ADHD? Understanding What Goes Wrong and Why* (New York: Guilford Press, 2006).

54. See P. Jensen, L. Arnold, J. Swanson, et al., "3-Year Follow Up of the NIMH MTA Study," *Journal of the American Academy of Child and Adolescent Psychiatry* 46 (August 2007): 989–1002.

55. MTA Cooperative Group, "Moderators and Mediators of Treatment Response for Children with Attention-Deficit/Hyperactivity Disorder," *Archives of General Psychiatry* 56 (1999): 1088–1096.

56. R. Barkley, K. Murphy, and M. Fischer, *ADHD in Adults: What the Science Says* (New York: Guilford Press, 2007).

57. B. Carey, "What's Wrong with a Child? Psychiatrists Often Disagree," *New York Times*, November 11, 2006, A1.

58. See J. Foy and M. Earls, "A Process for Developing Community Consensus Regarding the Diagnosis and Management of Attention-Deficit/Hyperactivity Disorder," *Pediatrics* 115 (January 2005): 97–104.

59. Ibid., 97.

60. Foy and Earls, "A Process for Developing Community Consensus Regarding the Diagnosis and Management of Attention-Deficit/Hyperactivity Disorder," 99.

61. Ibid., 98.

62. See Williams K. Klinepeter, G. Palmes, et al., "Behavioral Health Practices in the Midst of Black Box Warnings and Mental Health Reform," *Clinical Pediatrics* 46 (2007): 424.

63. Ibid., 98.

64. Ibid., 99.

65. See R. Barkley, "What May Be in Store for ADHD in DSM-V," *ADHD Report* 15 (2007): 1–6.

# Selected Bibliography

Abikoff, H., L. Hechtman, R. Klein, R. Gallagher, K. Fleiss, J. Etcovitch, et al. 2004. "Social Functioning in Children with ADHD Treated with Long-Term Methylphenidate and Multimodal Psychosocial Treatment." *Journal of the American Academy of Child and Adolescent Psychiatry* 43: 820–829.

Abikoff, H., L. Hechtman, R. Klein, G. Weiss, K. Fleiss, J. Etcovitch, et al. 2004. "Symptomatic Improvement in Children with ADHD Treated with Long-Term Methylphenidate and Multimodal Psychosocial Treatment." *Journal of the American Academy of Child and Adolescent Psychiatry* 43: 802–811.

Adesman, A. 2000. "Does My Child Need Ritalin?" *Newsweek*, April 24, 81.

———. 2001. "The Diagnosis and Management of Attention-Deficit/ Hyperactivity Disorder in Pediatric Patients." *Primary Care Companion to the Journal of Clinical Psychiatry* 3: 66–77.

Agres, T. 1999. "Hatch-Waxman Act Review Incites Controversy." *Research and Development* (March): 15–16.

Akil, H., and S. Watson. 2000. "Science and the Future of Psychiatry." *Archives of General Psychiatry* 57 (January): 86–87.

Aleman, S. 1991. *Special Education for Children with Attention Deficit Disorders: Current Issues*. Washington, DC: Congressional Research Service.

Altpeter, T., and M. Breen. 1992. "Situational Variation in Problem Behavior at Home and School in Attention Deficit Disorder with Hyperactivity: A Factor Analytic Study." *Journal of Child Psychology and Psychiatry* 33: 741–748.

Amaral, O. 2007. "Psychiatric Disorders as Social Constructs: ADHD as a Case in Point." *American Journal of Psychiatry* 164 (October): 1612.

American Medical Association. 2007. "Report 10 of the Council on Science and Public Health: Attention Deficit Hyperactivity Disorder." June. http:// www.ama-assn.org/ama/pub/category/17738.html. Accessed November 27, 2007.

American Psychiatric Association. 1952, 1968, 1980, 1987, 1994. *Diagnostic and Statistical Manual of Mental Disorders.* 1st, 2nd, 3rd, 3rd rev., 4th eds. Washington, DC: American Psychiatric Association.

Anastopoulos, A., and T. Shelton. 2001. *Assessing Attention-Deficit/ Hyperactivity Disorder.* New York: Kluwer Academic/Plenum Publishers.

Anastopoulos, A., T. Shelton, G. DuPaul, and D. Guevremont. 1993. "Parent Training for Attention-Deficit Hyperactivity Disorder: Its Impact on Parent Functioning." *Journal of Abnormal Child Psychology* 21: 581–596.

Angell, M. 2004. *The Truth about the Drug Companies.* New York: Random House.

Angold, A., E. Costello, and A. Erkanli. 1999. "Comorbidity." *Journal of Child Psychology and Psychiatry* 40: 57–87.

Aparasu, R., and V. Bhatara. 2007. "Patterns and Determinants of Antipsychotic Prescribing in Children and Adolescents, 2003–2004." *Current Medical Research and Opinion* 23 (January): 49–56.

Appelbaum, S. 1989. "Admitting Children to Psychiatric Hospitals: A Controversy Revived." *Hospital and Community Psychiatry* 40 (April): 334–335.

Applegate, B., B. Lahey, E. Hart, I. Waldman, J. Biederman, G. Hynd, et al. 1997. "Validity of the Age-of-Onset Criterion for ADHD: A Report of the DSM-IV Field Trials." *Journal of the American Academy of Child and Adolescent Psychiatry* 36: 1211–1221.

Appling, R., and N. Jones. 2002. *The Individuals with Disabilities Education Act (IDEA): Overview of Major Provisions.* Congressional Research Service Report for Congress, January 11.

Armstrong, T. 1997. *The Myth of the ADD Child: 50 Ways to Improve Your Child's Behavior and Attention Span without Drugs, Labels, or Coercion.* New York: Plume Books.

Arnsten, A., J. Steere, and R. Hunt. 1996. "The Contribution of alpha sub-2-Noradrenergic Mechanisms to Prefrontal Cortical Cognitive Function: Potential Significance for Attention-Deficit Hyperactivity Disorder." *Archives of General Psychiatry* 53: 448–455.

Arria, A., and E. Wish. 2005. "Nonmedical Use of Prescription Stimulants among Students." *Psychiatric Annals* 35: 228–235.

Babcock, Q., and T. Byrne. 2000. "Student Perceptions of Methylphenidate Abuse at a Public Liberal Arts College." *Journal of American College Health* 49: 143–145.

Bagwell, C., B. Molina, T. Kashdan, W. Pelham, Jr., and B. Hoza. 2006. "Anxiety and Mood Disorders in Adolescents with Childhood Attention-Deficit/ Hyperactivity Disorder." *Journal of Emotional and Behavioral Disorders* 14: 178–187.

Bagwell, C., B. Molina, W. Pelham, Jr., and B. Hoza. 2001. "Attention-Deficit Hyperactivity Disorder and Problems in Peer Relations: Predictions from Childhood to Adolescence." *Journal of the American Academy of Child and Adolescent Psychiatry* 40: 1285–1292.

Barkley, R. 1990. *Attention-Deficit Hyperactivity Disorder: A Handbook for Diagnosis and Treatment.* New York: Guilford Press.

———. 1997. *ADHD and the Nature of Self-Control.* New York: Guildford Press.

———. 1997. "Behavioral Inhibition, Sustained Attention, and Executive Functions: Constructing a Unifying Theory of ADHD." *Psychological Bulletin* 121: 65–94.

———. 1998. *Attention-Deficit Hyperactivity Disorder: A Handbook for Diagnosis and Treatment.* 2nd ed. New York: Guilford Press.

———. 2000. "Commentary on the Multimodal Treatment Study of Children with ADHD." *Journal of Abnormal Child Psychology* 28: 595–599.

———. 2003. "Attention-Deficit/Hyperactivity Disorder." In *Child Psychopathology.* 2nd ed., ed. E. J. Mash and R. A. Barkley, 75–143. New York: Guilford Press.

———. 2006. *Attention-Deficit Hyperactivity Disorder: A Handbook for Diagnosis and Treatment.* 3rd ed. New York: Guilford Press.

———. 2007. "What May Be in Store for ADHD in DSM-V." *ADHD Report* 15:1–6.

Barkley, R., G. DuPaul, and M. McMurray. 1990. "A Comprehensive Evaluation of Attention Deficit Disorder with and without Hyperactivity." *Journal of Consulting and Clinical Psychology* 58: 775–789.

Barkley, R., and C. Edelbrock. 1987. "Assessing Situational Variation in Children's Behavior Problems: The Home and School Situations Questionnaires." In *Advances in Behavioral Assessment of Children and Families,* ed. R. Prinz, 157–176. Greenwich, CT: JAI Press.

Barkley, R., M. Fischer, C. Edelbrock, and L. Smallish. 1990. "The Adolescent Outcome of Hyperactive Children Diagnosed by Research Criteria: I. An 8-Year Prospective Follow-Up Study." *Journal of the American Academy of Child and Adolescent Psychiatry* 29: 546–557.

———. 1991. "The Adolescent Outcome of Hyperactive Children Diagnosed by Research Criteria: III. Mother-Child Interactions, Family Conflicts, and Maternal Psychopathology." *Journal of Child Psychology and Psychiatry* 32: 233–255.

Barkley, R., M. Fischer, L. Smallish, and K. Fletcher. 2002. "The Persistence of Attention-Deficit/Hyperactivity Disorder into Young Adulthood as a Function of Reporting Source and Definition of Disorder." *Journal of Abnormal Psychology* 111: 279–289.

———. 2003. "Does the Treatment of Attention-Deficit/Hyperactivity Disorder with Stimulants Contribute to Drug Use/Abuse? A 13-Year Prospective Study." *Pediatrics* 111: 97–109.

Barkley, R., M. McMurray, C. Edelbrock, and K. Robbins. 1990. "Side Effects of Methylphenidate in Children with Attention Deficit Hyperactivity Disorder: A Systemic, Placebo-Controlled Evaluation." *Pediatrics* 86: 184–192.

Barkley, R., K. Murphy, and M. Fischer. 2008. *ADHD in Adults: What the Science Says.* New York: Guilford Press.

Barkley, R., K. Smith, M. Fischer, and B. Navia. 2006. "An Examination of the Behavioral and Neuropsychological Correlates of Three ADHD Candidate Gene Polymorphisms (DRD4 7+, DBH TaqI A2, and DAT1 40 bp VNTR) in Hyperactive and Normal Children Followed to Adulthood." *American Journal of Medical Genetics Part B* 141: 487–498.

Barry, J. 2004. *The Great Influenza: The Epic Story of the Deadliest Plague in History*. New York: Viking.

Baughman, F. 2006. *The ADHD Fraud: How Psychiatry Makes "Patients" Out of Normal Children*. Oxford: Trafford.

Bax, M., and R. MacKeith. 1963. "Minimal Brain Damage: A Concept Discarded." In *Minimal Cerebral Dysfunction*, ed. R. MacKeith and M. Bax. Little Club Clinics in Development Medicine. London: Heinemann.

Bayer, R. 1981. *Homosexuality and American Psychiatry: The Politics of Diagnosis*. New York: Basic Books.

Bayer, R., and R. Spitzer. 1985. "Neurosis, Psychodynamics, and DSM-III." *Archives of General Psychiatry* 42 (February): 187–196.

Beardsley, R., G. Gardocki, D. Larson, and J. Hidalso. 1988. "Prescribing of Psychotropic Medications by Primary Care Physicians and Psychiatrists." *Archives of General Psychiatry* 45: 1117–1119.

Beauchaine, T. 2003. "Taxometrics and Developmental Psychopathology." *Development and Psychopathology* 15 (Summer): 501–527.

Begley, S. 1994. "One Pill Makes You Larger and One Makes You Small." *Newsweek*, February 7, 37–41.

Ben Amor, L., N. Grizenko, G. Schwartz, P. Lageix, C. Baron, M. Ter-Stepanian, et al. 2005. "Perinatal Complications in Children with Attention-Deficit Hyperactivity Disorder and Their Unaffected Siblings." *Journal of Psychiatry and Neuroscience* 30 (March): 120–126.

Benedetto, V., J. Heiligenstein, M. Riddle, L. Greenhill, and J. Fegert. 2004. "The Interface between Publicly Funded and Industry-Funded Research in Pediatric Psychopharmacology: Opportunities for Integration and Collaboration." *Biological Psychiatry* 56 (July): 3–9.

Berquin, P., J. Giedd, and L. Jacobsen. 1998. "Cerebellum in Attention-Deficit Hyperactivity Disorder: A Morphometric MRI Study." *Neurology* 50: 1087–1093.

Bhatara, V., M. Feil, K. Hoagwood, B. Vitiello, and B. Zima. 2004. "National Trends in Concomitant Psychotropic Medication with Stimulants in Pediatric Visits: Practice versus Knowledge." *Journal of Attention Disorders* 7 (May): 217–226.

Biederman, J., S. Faraone, K. Keenan, J. Benjamin, B. Krifcher, C. Moore, et al. 2002. "Further Evidence for Family-Genetic Risk Factors in Attention Deficit Hyperactivity Disorder: Patterns of Comorbidity in Probands and Relatives in Psychiatrically and Pediatrically Referred Samples." *Archives of General Psychiatry* 49: 728–738.

Biederman, J., S. Faraone, K. Keenan, and M. Tsuang. 1991. "Evidence of a Familial Association between Attention Deficit Disorder and Major Affective Disorders." *Archives of General Psychiatry* 48: 633–642.

Biederman, S. Faraone, E. Mick, T. Spencer, T. Wilens, K. Kiely, et al. 1995. "High Risk for Attention Deficit Hyperactivity Disorder among Children of Parents with Childhood Onset of the Disorder: A Pilot Study." *American Journal of Psychiatry* 152: 431–435.

Biederman, J., S. Faraone, S. Milberger, J. Guite, E. Mick, L. Chen, et al. 1996. "A Prospective 4-Year Follow-Up Study of Attention-Deficit Hyperactivity and Related Disorders." *Archives of General Psychiatry* 53: 437–446.

Biederman, J., S. Faraone, M. Monuteaux, and J. Grossbard. 2004. "How Informative Are Parent Reports of Attention-Deficit/Hyperactivity Disorder Symptoms for Assessing Outcome in Clinical Trials of Long-Acting Treatments? A Pooled Analysis of Parents' and Teachers' Reports." *Pediatrics* 113 (June): 1667–1671.

Biederman, J., H. Gao, A. Rogers, and T. Spencer. 2006. "Comparison of Parent and Teacher Reports of Attention-Deficit/Hyperactivity Disorder Symptoms from Two Placebo-Controlled Studies of Atomoxetine in Children." *Biological Psychiatry* 60 (November 15): 1106–1110.

Biederman, J., and M. Jellinek. 1984. "Current Concepts: Psychopharmacology in Children." *New England Journal of Medicine* 310 (April 12): 968–972.

Biederman, J., J. Newcorn, and S. Sprich. 1991. "Comorbidity of Attention Deficit Hyperactivity Disorder with Conduct, Depressive, Anxiety, and Other Disorders." *American Journal of Psychiatry* 148: 564–577.

Biederman, J., T. Wilens, E. Mick, S. Faraone, W. Weber, S. Curtis, et al. 1997. "Is ADHD a Risk Factor for Psychoactive Substance Use Disorders? Findings from a Four-Year Prospective Follow-up Study." *Journal of the American Academy of Child and Adolescent Psychiatry* 36: 21–29.

Birch, H. 1964. *Brain Damage in Children: The Biological and Social Aspects.* Baltimore: Williams and Wilkins.

Blachman, D., and S. Hinshaw. 2002. "Patterns of Friendship among Girls with and without Attention-Deficit/Hyperactivity Disorder." *Journal of Abnormal Child Psychology* 30: 625–640.

Blau, F. 1998. "Trends in the Well-Being of American Women, 1970–1995." *Journal of Economic Literature* 36 (March): 112–165.

Block, M. 1996. *No More Ritalin: Treating ADHD without Drugs.* New York: Kensington.

———. 2001. *No More ADHD: 10 Steps to Help Improve Your Child's Attention and Behavior without Drugs!* Hurst, TX: Block Center.

Blostin, A. 1987. "Mental Health Benefits Financed by Employers." *Monthly Labor Review* 110 (July): 23–27.

Bokhari, F., R. Mayes, and R. Scheffler. 2005. "An Analysis of the Significant Variation in Psychostimulant Use across the U.S." *Pharmacoepidemiology and Drug Safety* 14 (April): 267–275.

Bouchard, T. 1997. "IQ Similarity in Twins Reared Apart: Findings and Responses to Critics." In *Intelligence, Heredity, and Environment*, ed. R. J. Sternberg and E. Grigorenko, 126–160. New York: Cambridge University Press.

Bowe, F. 1978. *Handicapping America: Barriers to Disabled People.* New York: Harper and Row.

Bower, W. 1954. "Chlorpromazine in Psychiatric Illness." *New England Journal of Medicine* 251 (October 21): 689–692.

Bowler, M. 1974. *The Nixon Guaranteed Income Proposal: Substance and Process in Policy Change.* New York: Ballinger.

Boyle, M., and A. Jadad. 1999. "Lessons from Large Trials: The MTA Study as a Model for Evaluating the Treatment of Childhood Psychiatric Disorder." *Canadian Journal of Psychiatry* 44: 991–998.

Bradley, C. 1937. "The Behavior of Children Receiving Benzedrine." *American Journal of Psychiatry* 94 (November): 577–578.

———. 1950. "Benzedrine and Dexedrine in the Treatment of Children's Behavior Disorders." *Pediatrics* 5 (January): 25.

Brandon, C., M. Marinelli, L. Baker, and F. White. 2001. "Enhanced Reactivity and Vulnerability to Cocaine Following Methylphenidate Treatment in Adolescent Rats." *Neuropsychopharmacology* 25: 651–661.

Breggin, P. 1991. *Toxic Psychiatry: Why Therapy, Empathy and Love Must Replace the Drugs, Electroshock, and Biochemical Theories of the "New Psychiatry."* New York: St. Martin's Press.

———. 1993. "Should the Use of Neoleptics Be Severely Limited?" In *Controversial Issues in Mental Health*, ed. S. Kirk and S. Einbinder. Boston: Allyn and Bacon.

———. 1999. "Treatment of Attention-Deficit/Hyperactivity Disorder." *Journal of the American Medical Association* 281 (April 28): 1490–1491.

———. 2001. *Talking Back to Ritalin: What Doctors Aren't Telling You about Stimulants and ADHD.* New York: Da Capo.

———. 2002. *The Ritalin Fact Book: What Your Doctor Won't Tell You.* Cambridge, MA: Perseus.

Breggin, P., and G. Breggin. 1995. *Talking Back to Prozac: What Doctors Aren't Telling You about Today's Most Controversial Drug.* New York: St. Martin's Press.

Breggin, P., and D. Cohen. 2000. *Your Drug May Be Your Problem: How and Why to Stop Taking Psychiatric Medications.* Cambridge, MA: Perseus.

Breslau, N., G. Brown, J. Del Dotto, S. Kumar, S. Exhuthachan, P. Andreski, et al. 1996. "Psychiatric Sequelae of Low Birth Weight at 6 Years of Age." *Journal of Abnormal Child Psychology* 24: 385–400.

Breton, J., L. Bergeron, J. Valla, C. Berthiaume, N. Gaudet, J. Lambert, et al. 1999. "Quebec Children Mental Health Survey: Prevalence of DSM-III-R Mental Health Disorders." *Journal of Child Psychology and Psychiatry* 40: 375–384.

Briggs-Gowan, M., S. Horwitz, M. Schwab-Stone, J. Leventhal, and P. Leaf. 2000. "Mental Health in Pediatric Settings: Distribution of Disorders and Factors Related to Service Use." *Journal of the American Academy of Child and Adolescent Psychiatry* 39: 841–849.

Brock, S. W., and P. Knapp. 1996. "Reading Comprehension Abilities of Children with Attention-Deficit/Hyperactivity Disorder." *Journal of Attention Disorders* 1:173–186.

Bromley, E. 2006. "Stimulating a Normal Adjustment: Misbehavior, Amphetamines, and the Electroencephalogram at the Bradley Home for Children." *Journal of the History of the Behavioral Sciences* 42 (Fall): 379–398.

Brown, P. 1987. "Diagnostic Conflict and Contradiction in Psychiatry." *Journal of Health and Social Behavior* 28 (March): 37–50.

Brown, R., R. Amler, W. Freeman, J. Perrin, M. Stein, H. Feldman, et al. 2005. "Treatment of Attention-Deficit/Hyperactivity Disorder: Overview of the Evidence." *Pediatrics* 115 (June): e749–e757.

Brown, W. 1998. "Images in Psychiatry: Charles Bradley, M.D., 1902–1979." *American Journal of Psychiatry* 155 (July): 968.

Buitelaar, J., and A. Rothenberger. 2004. "Foreword—ADHD in the Scientific and Political Context." *European Child and Adolescent Psychiatry* 13 (Suppl.): 11–16.

Burke, J., R. Loeber, and B. Lahey. 2001. "Which Aspects of ADHD Are Associated with Tobacco Use in Early Adolescence?" *Journal of Child Psychology and Psychiatry* 42: 493–502.

Burke, T. 1997. "On the Rights Track: The Americans with Disabilities Act." In *Comparative Disadvantages? American Social Regulation and the Global Economy*, ed. P. Nivola. Washington DC: Brookings Institution Press, 242–318.

Burns, B. 1991. "Mental Health Service Use by Adolescents in the 1970s and 1980s." *Journal of the American Academy of Child and Adolescent Psychiatry* 30 (January): 144–150.

Burt, S. 2001. "Sources of Covariation among Attention-Deficit/Hyperactivity Disorder, Oppositional Defiant Disorder, and Conduct Disorder: The Importance of Shared Environment." *Journal of Abnormal Psychology* 110 (November): 516–525.

Bury, M., and J. Gabe. 1996. "Halcion Nights: A Sociological Account of a Medical Controversy." *Sociology* 30: 447–469.

Bussing, R., N. Schoenberg, and A. Perwien. 1998. "Knowledge and Information about ADHD: Evidence of Cultural Differences among African-American and White Parents." *Social Science and Medicine* 46 (April): 919–928.

Caher, J. 2000. "Ritalin Case Puts Parents, Courts on a Collision Course." *New York Law Journal* (August 17): 1.

Callahan, D., L. Dach, H. Edgar, W. Gaylin, G. Klerman, R. Macklin, et al. 1976. "Special Supplement: MBD, Drug Research and the Schools." *Hastings Center Report* 6 (June): 1–23.

Campbell, A. 2006. "Consent, Competence, and Confidentiality Related to Psychiatric Conditions in Adolescent Medicine Practice." *Adolescent Medicine Clinics* 17 (February): 25–47.

Campbell, E. 2007. "Doctors and Drug Companies—Scrutinizing Influential Relationships." *New England Journal of Medicine* 357 (November 1): 1796–1797.

Campbell, E., R. Gruen, J. Mountford, L. Miller, P. Cleary, and D. Blumenthal. 2007. "A National Survey of Physician-Industry Relationships." *New England Journal of Medicine* 356 (April 26): 1742–1750.

Campbell, S. 2000. "Attention-Deficit/Hyperactivity Disorder: A Developmental View." In *Handbook of Developmental Psychopathology.* 2nd ed., ed. A. Sameroff, M. Lewis, and S. Miller, 383–401. New York: Kluwer Academic/Plenum Publishers.

Campbell, S., E. Pierce, G. Moore, S. Marakovitz, and K. Newby. 1996. "Boys' Externalizing Problems at Elementary School Age: Pathways from Early Behavior Problems, Maternal Control, and Family Stress." *Development and Psychopathology* 8: 701–720.

Cantwell, D. 1996. "Attention Deficit Disorder: A Review of the Past 10 Years." *Journal of the American Academy of Child and Adolescent Psychiatry* 35: 978–987.

Cantwell, D., and L. Baker. 1992. "Association between Attention Deficit Hyperactivity Disorder and Learning Disorders." In *Attention Deficit Disorder Comes of Age: Toward the Twenty-First Century*, ed. S. E. Shaywitz and B. A. Shaywitz, 145–164. Austin, TX: Pro-Ed.

Cantwell, D., and J. Satterfield. 1978. "The Prevalence of Academic Underachievement in Hyperactive Children." *Journal of Pediatric Psychology* 3: 168–171.

Carbray, J., and C. Pitula. 1991. "Trends in Adolescent Psychiatric Hospitalization." *Journal of Child and Adolescent Psychiatric Mental Health Nursing* 4 (April–June): 68–71.

Carey, B. 2006. "What's Wrong with a Child? Psychiatrists Often Disagree." *New York Times*, November 11.

Carlezon, W., S. Mague, and S. Andersen. 2003. "Enduring Behavioral Effects of Early Exposure to Methylphenidate in Rats." *Biological Psychiatry* 54 (December 15): 1330–1337.

Carlson, E., D. Jacobvitz, and L. Sroufe. 1995. "A Developmental Investigation of Inattentiveness and Hyperactivity." *Child Development* 66 (February): 37–54.

Carroll, B., T. McLaughlin, and D. Blake. 2006. "Patterns and Knowledge of Nonmedical Use of Stimulants among College Students." *Archives of Pediatric and Adolescent Medicine* 160 (May): 481–485.

Case, B., M. Olfson, S. Marcus, and C. Siegel. 2007. "Trends in the Inpatient Mental Health Treatment of Children and Adolescents in U.S. Community Hospitals between 1990 and 2000." *Archives of General Psychiatry* 64 (January): 89–96.

Castellanos, F., J. Giedd, P. Berquin, J. Walter, W. Sharp, T. Tran, et al. 2001. "Quantitative Brain Magnetic Resonance Imaging in Girls with Attention-Deficit/Hyperactivity Disorder." *Archives of General Psychiatry* 58: 289–295.

Castellanos, F., J. Giedd, J. Elia, W. Marsh, G. Ritchie, S. Hamburger, et al. 1997. "Controlled Stimulant Treatment of ADHD and Comorbid Tourette's Syndrome: Effects of Stimulants and Dose." *Journal of the American Academy of Child and Adolescent Psychiatry* 36: 1–8.

Castellanos, F., J. Giedd, W. Marsh, S. Hamburger, A. Vaituzis, D. Dickstein, et al. 1996. "Quantitative Brain Magnetic Resonance Imaging in Attention-Deficit Hyperactivity Disorder." *Archives of General Psychiatry* 53: 607–616.

Castellanos, F., W. Sharp, R. Gottesman, D. Greenstein, J. Giedd, and J. Rapoport. 2003. "Anatomic Brain Abnormalities in Monozygotic Twins Discordant for Attention Deficit Hyperactivity Disorder." *American Journal of Psychiatry* 160: 1693–1695.

Castle, L., R. Aubert, R. Verbrugge, M. Khalid, and R. Epstein. 2007. "Trends in Medication Treatment for ADHD." *Journal of Attention Disorders* 10 (May): 335–342.

Centers for Disease Control and Prevention. 2005. "Mental Health in the United States: Prevalence of Diagnosis and Medication Treatment for Attention-Deficit/Hyperactivity Disorder." *MMWR: Morbidity and Mortality Weekly Report* 54 (September 2): 842–847.

Chan, E., M. Hopkins, J. Perrin, C. Herrerias, and C. Homer. 2005. "Diagnostic Practices for Attention Deficit Hyperactivity Disorder: A National Survey of Primary Care Physicians." *Ambulatory Pediatrics* 5 (July–August): 201–208.

Charlton, J. 2000. *Nothing About Us without Us: Disability Oppression and Empowerment*. Berkeley: University of California Press.

Chess, S. 1960. "Diagnosis and Treatment of the Hyperactive Child." *New York State Journal of Medicine* 60: 2379–2385.

Chiarello, R., and J. Cole. 1987. "The Use of Psychostimulants in General Psychiatry: A Reconsideration." *Archives of General Psychiatry* 44 (March): 286–295.

Choudry, N., H. Stelfox, and A. Detsky. 2002. "Relationships between Authors of Clinical Practice Guidelines and the Pharmaceutical Industry." *Journal of the American Medical Association* 287 (February 6): 612–617.

Claude, D., and P. Firestone. 1995. "The Development of ADHD Boys: A 12-Year Follow-Up." *Canadian Journal of Behavioral Science* 27: 226–249.

Clements, S. 1966. "Minimal Brain Dysfunction in Children: Terminology and Identification." Task Force 1, U.S. Department of Health, Education, and Welfare. Public Health Service Publication 1415. Washington, DC: U.S. Government Printing Office.

Clements, S., and J. Peters. 1962. "Minimal Brain Dysfunction in the School-Age Child." *Archives of General Psychiatry* 6: 185–197.

Connor, D. 2006. "Stimulants." In *Attention-Deficit Hyperactivity Disorder: A Handbook for Diagnosis and Treatment*. 3rd ed., by R. Barkley, 608–647. New York: Guilford Press.

Conners, C. 1980. *Food Additives and Hyperactive Children*. New York: Plenum.

Conners, C., and L. Eisenberg. 1963. "The Effects of Methylphenidate on Symptomatology and Learning in Disturbed Children." *American Journal of Psychiatry* 120 (November): 458–464.

Conrad, P. 1975. "The Discovery of Hyperkinesis: Notes on the Medicalization of Deviant Behavior." *Social Problems* 23: 12–21.

——. 2005. "The Shifting Engines of Medicalization." *Journal of Health and Social Behavior* 46 (March): 3–14.

Conrad, P., and V. Leiter. 2004. "Medicalization, Markets and Consumers." *Journal of Health and Social Behavior* 45: 158–176.

Cook, J., and E. Wright. 1995. "Medical Sociology and the Study of Severe Mental Illness: Reflections on Past Accomplishments and Directions for Future Research." *Journal of Health and Social Behavior* (special issue) 95–114.

Cosgrove, L., S. Krimsky, M. Vijayaraghavan, and L. Schneider. 2006. "Financial Ties between DSM-IV Panel Members and the Pharmaceutical Industry." *Psychotherapy and Psychosomatics* 75: 154–160.

Costello, E., S. Mustillo, A. Erkanli, G. Keeler, and A. Angold. 2003. "Prevalence and Development of Psychiatric Disorders in Childhood and Adolescence." *Archives of General Psychiatry* 60: 837–844.

Cox, E., B. Motheral, R. Henderson, and D. Mager. 2003. "Geographic Variation in the Prevalence of the Stimulant Medication Use among Children 5 to 14 Years Old: Results from a Commercially Insured U.S. Sample." *Pediatrics* 111 (February): 237–243.

Coyle, J. 2000. "Psychotropic Drug Use in Very Young Children." *Journal of the American Medical Association* 283: 1059–1060.

Cruickshank, W., W. Bentzen, F. Ratzeburg, and M. Tannhauser. 1961. *A Teaching Method for Brain Injured and Hyperactive Children: A Demonstration Pilot Study*. Syracuse, NY: Syracuse University Press.

Cuellar, A., and S. Markowitz. 2007. "Medicaid Policy Changes in Mental Health Care and Their Effect on Mental Health Outcomes." *Health Economics, Policy and Law* 2: 23–28.

Cuffe, S., C. Moore, and R. McKeown. 2005. "Prevalence and Correlates of ADHD Symptoms in the National Health Interview Survey." *Journal of Attention Disorders* 9 (November): 392–401.

Culpepper, L. 2006. "Primary Care Treatment of Attention-Deficit/Hyperactivity Disorder." *Journal of Clinical Psychiatry* 67 (Suppl.): 51–58.

Curtiss, F. 1989. "Managed Health Care." *American Journal of Hospital Pharmacy* 46 (April): 742–763.

Danielson, L., K. Henderson, and E. Schiller. 2002. "Education Policy—Educating Children with Attention Deficit Hyperactivity Disorder." In *Attention Deficit Hyperactivity Disorder: State of the Science, Best Practices*, ed. P. S. Jenson and J. R. Cooper, 26–32. Kingston, NJ: Civic Research Institute.

Darwin, C. 1859. *On the Origin of Species by Means of Natural Selection or the Preservation of the Favoured Races in the Struggle for Life*. London: John Murray.

Davila, R., M. Williams, and J. MacDonald. 1991. *Clarification of Policy to Address the Needs of Children with Attention Deficit Disorders within General and/or Special Education*. Washington, DC: Department of Education, Office of Special Education and Rehabilitation, September 16.

Davison, J. C., and D. Y. Ford. 2001. "Perceptions of Attention Deficit Hyperactivity Disorder in One African American Community." *Journal of Negro Education* 70 (Autumn): 264–274.

Dean, A., B. McDermott, and R. Marshall. 2006. "Psychotropic Medication Utilization in a Child and Adolescent Mental Health Service." *Journal of Child and Adolescent Psychopharmacology* 16 (June): 273–285.

DeGrandpre, R. 1999. *Ritalin Nation: Rapid Fire Culture and the Transformation of Human Consciousness.* New York: W. W. Norton.

DeMilio, L. 1989. "Psychiatric Syndromes in Adolescent Substance Users." *American Journal of Psychiatry* 146 (September): 1212–1214.

Denhoff, E., M. Laufer, and R. Holden. 1959. "The Syndromes of Cerebral Dysfunction." *Journal of the Oklahoma State Medical Association* 52: 360–366.

Derthick, M. 1990. *Agency under Stress: The Social Security Administration and American Government.* Washington, DC: Brookings Institution Press.

Diller, L. 1996. "The Run on Ritalin: Attention Deficit Disorder and Stimulant Treatment in the 1990s." *Hastings Center Report* 26 (March–April): 12–18.

———. 1998. *Running on Ritalin: A Physician Reflects on Children, Society, and Performance in a Pill.* New York: Bantam Books.

Dishion, T., and L. Owen. 2002. "A Longitudinal Analysis of Friendships and Substance Use: Bidirectional Influence from Adolescence to Adulthood." *Developmental Psychology* 38: 480–491.

Dishion, T., G. Patterson, M. Stoolmiller, and M. Skinner. 1991. "Family, School, and Behavioral Antecedents to Early Adolescent Involvement with Antisocial Peers." *Developmental Psychology* 27: 172–180.

Doan, R., and T. Petti. 1989. "Clinical and Demographic Characteristics of Child and Adolescent Partial Hospital Patients." *Journal of the American Academy of Child and Adolescent Psychiatry* 28 (January): 66–69.

Dodson, W. 2005. "Pharmacotherapy of Adult ADHD." *Journal of Clinical Psychology* 61: 589–606.

Dorwart, R., and M. Schlesinger. 1988. "Privatization of Psychiatric Services." *American Journal of Psychiatry* 145: 543–553.

Dorwart, R., M. Schlesinger, H. Davidson, S. Epstein, and C. Hoover. 1991. "A National Study of Psychiatric Hospital Care." *American Journal of Psychiatry* 148 (February): 204–210.

Dubay, L., and G. Kenney. 1996. "The Effects of Medicaid Expansions on Insurance Coverage of Children." *Future of Children* 6 (Spring): 152–161.

DuPaul, G., and R. Barkley. 1992. "Situational Variability of Attention Problems: Psychometric Properties of the Revised Home and School Situations Questionnaires." *Journal of Clinical Child Psychology* 21: 178–188.

DuPaul, G., and G. Stoner. 1994. *ADHD in the Schools: Assessment and Intervention Strategies.* New York: Guilford Press.

———. 2003. *ADHD in Schools: Assessment and Intervention Strategies.* New York: Guilford Press.

Durston, S. 2003. "A Review of the Biological Bases of ADHD: What Have We Learned from Imaging Studies?" *Mental Retardation and Developmental Disabilities Research Reviews* 9: 184–195.

Dusek, J. 1974. "Implications of Development Theory for Child Mental Health." *American Psychologist* 29 (January): 19–24.

Ebaugh, F. 1923. "Neuropsychiatric Sequelae of Acute Epidemic Encephalitis in Children." *American Journal of Diseases of Children* 25: 89–97.

Eberstadt, M. 1999. "Why Ritalin Rules." *Policy Review* 94 (April–May): 24–44.

Elliott, C. 2004. *Better Than Well*. New York: Oxford University Press.

Elmer-Dewitt, P. 1992. "Depression: The Growing Role of Drug Therapies." *Time*, July 5, 56–60.

Emslie, G., A. Rush, W. Weinberg, R. Kowatch, C. Hughes, T. Carmody, et al. 1997. "A Double-Blind, Randomized, Placebo-Controlled Trial of Fluoxetine in Children and Adolescents with Depression." *Archives of General Psychiatry* 54: 1031–1037.

English, J., S. Sharfstein, D. Scherl, B. Astrachan, and I. Muszynski. 1986. "Diagnosis-Related Groups and General Hospital Psychiatry: The APA Study." *American Journal of Psychiatry* 143 (February): 131–139.

Ennis, B. 1972. *Prisoners of Psychiatry*. New York: Harcourt Brace Jovanovich.

Ennis, B., and T. Litwack. 1974. "Psychiatry and the Presumption of Expertise: Flipping Coins in the Courtroom." *California Law Review* 62: 693–752.

Erhardt, D., and S. Hinshaw. 1994. "Initial Sociometric Impressions of Attention-Deficit Hyperactivity Disorder and Comparison Boys: Predictions from Social Behaviors and from Nonbehavioral Variables." *Journal of Consulting and Clinical Psychology* 62: 833–842.

Erkulwater, J. 2006. *Disability Rights and the American Social Safety Net*. Ithaca, NY: Cornell University Press.

Ernst, M., R. Cohen, et al. 1997. "Cerebral Glucose Metabolism in Adolescent Girls with Attention-Deficit/Hyperactivity Disorder." *Journal of the Academy of Child and Adolescent Psychiatry* 36: 1399–1406.

Ernst, M., L. Liebenauer, et al. 1994. "Reduced Brain Metabolism in Hyperactive Girls." *Journal of the American Academy of Child and Adolescent Psychiatry* 33: 858–868.

Ettner, S., K. Kuhlthau, T. McLaughlin, J. Perrin, and S. Gortmaker. 2000. "Impact of Expanding SSI on Medicaid Expenditures of Disabled Children." *Health Care Financing Review* 21 (Spring): 185–201.

Faraone, S., A. Doyle, E. Mick, and J. Biederman. 2001. "Meta-Analysis of the Association between the 7-Repeat Allele of the Dopamine D4 Receptor Gene and Attention Deficit Hyperactivity Disorder." *American Journal of Psychiatry* 158: 1052–1057.

Faraone, S., J. Sergeant, C. Gillberg, and J. Biederman. 2003. "The Worldwide Prevalence of ADHD: Is It an American Condition?" *World Psychiatry* 2 (June): 104–113.

Faraone, S., T. Spencer, M. Aleardi, C. Pagano, and J. Biederman. 2004. "Meta-Analysis of the Efficacy of Methylphenidate for Treating Adult Attention-

Deficit/Hyperactivity Disorder." *Journal of Clinical Psychopharmacology* 24: 24–29.

Faraone, S., and T. Wilens. 2003. "Does Stimulant Treatment Lead to Substance Use Disorders?" *Journal of Clinical Psychiatry* 64 (Suppl. 11): 9–13.

Feingold, B. 1975. *Why Your Child Is Hyperactive.* New York: Random House.

Feldman, S. 2002. "Confessions of a Managed Behavioral Health Physician." *Developmental and Behavioral Pediatrics* 23 (February): S52.

Ferguson, J., F. Linn, M. Nickels, and J. Sheets. 1956. "Methylphenidate (Ritalin) Hydrochloride Parenteral Solution: Preliminary Report." *Journal of the American Medical Association* 162 (December 1): 1303–1304.

Ferris, M. 2005. "Drug Safety: Does the FDA Adequately Protect the Public?" *CQ Researcher* 15 (March 11): 221–244.

Filipek, P., M. Semrud-Clikeman, R. Steingard, P. Renshaw, D. Kennedy, and J. Biederman. 1997. "Volumetric MRI Analysis Comparing Subjects Having Attention-Deficit Hyperactivity Disorder with Normal Controls." *Neurology* 48: 589–601.

Fink, P. 1988. "Response to the Presidential Address: Is 'Biopsychosocial' the Psychiatric Shibboleth?" *American Journal of Psychiatry* 145 (September): 1065.

Fischer, M. 1990. "Parenting Stress and the Child with Attention Deficit Hyperactivity Disorder." *Journal of Clinical Child Psychology* 19: 337–346.

Fischer, M., and R. Barkley. 2003. "Childhood Stimulant Treatment and Risk for Later Substance Abuse." *Journal of Clinical Psychiatry* 63 (Suppl.): 19–23.

Fischer, M., R. Barkley, C. Edelbrock, and L. Smallish. 1990. "The Adolescent Outcome of Hyperactive Children Diagnosed by Research Criteria: II. Academic, Attentional, and Neuropsychological Status." *Journal of Consulting and Clinical Psychology* 58: 580–588.

Fischer, M., R. Barkley, L. Smallish, and K. Fletcher. 2002. "Young Adult Follow-Up of Hyperactive Children: Self-Reported Psychiatric Disorders, Comorbidity, and the Role of Childhood Conduct Problems and Teen CD." *Journal of Abnormal Child Psychology* 30: 463–475.

Fisher, S., ed. 1958. *Child Research in Psychopharmacology.* Springfield, IL: Charles C. Thomas Publisher.

Fogel, B. 1985. "A Psychiatric Unit Becomes a Psychiatric-Medical Unit: Administrative and Clinical Implications." *General Hospital Psychiatry* 7 (January): 26–35.

Foltz, A. 1975. "The Development of Ambiguous Federal Policy: Early and Periodic Screening, Diagnosis and Treatment (EPSDT)." *Milbank Memorial Fund Quarterly* 53 (Winter): 35–64.

Forbes, D. 1987. "The Draconian Cuts in Mental Health." *Business Month* 130 (September): 41–43.

Forness, S., and K. Kavale. 2002. "Impact of ADHD on School Systems." In *Attention Deficit Hyperactivity Disorder: State of the Science, Best Practices,* ed. P. S. Jenson and J. R. Cooper. Kingston, NJ: Civic Research Institute.

Forness, S., K. Kavale, I. Blum, and J. Lloyd. 1997. "Mega-Analysis of Meta-Analyses: What Works in Special Education and Related Services." *Teaching Exceptional Children* 29: 4–9.

Foy, J., and M. Earls. 2005. "A Process for Developing Community Consensus Regarding the Diagnosis and Management of Attention-Deficit/Hyperactivity Disorder." *Pediatrics* 115 (January): 97–104.

Frances, A., H. Pincus, T. Widiger, W. Davis, and M. First. 1990. "DSM-IV: Work in Progress." *American Journal of Psychiatry* 147 (November): 1439–1448.

Frank, R., R. Conti, and H. Goldman. 2005. "Mental Health Policy and Psychotropic Drugs." *Milbank Quarterly* 83: 271–298.

Frank, R., and S. Glied. 2006. *Better but Not Well: Mental Health Policy in the U.S. since 1950.* Baltimore: Johns Hopkins University Press.

Freed, H., and C. Peifer. 1956. "Treatment of Hyperkinetic Emotionally Disturbed Children with Prolonged Administration of Chlorpromazine." *American Journal of Psychiatry* 113 (July): 22–26.

Freedman, A., A. Effron, and L. Bender. 1955. "Pharmacotherapy in Children with Psychiatric Illness." *Journal of Nervous and Mental Disease* 122 (November): 479–486.

Freedman, D. 1992. "The Search: Body, Mind and Human Purpose." *American Journal of Psychiatry* 149 (July): 858–866.

Fried, S. 1998. *Bitter Pills.* New York: Bantam Books.

Friedman, R., and K. Kutash. 1992. "Challenges for Child and Adolescent Mental Health." *Health Affairs* 11 (Fall): 129–130.

Friedman, R., and A. Leon. 2007. "Expanding the Black Box: Depression, Antidepressants, and the Risk of Suicide." *New England Journal of Medicine* 356 (June 7): 2343–2346.

Froehlich, T., B. Lanphear, J. Epstein, W. Barbaresi, S. Katusic, and R. Kahn. 2007. "Prevalence, Recognition, and Treatment of Attention-Deficit/Hyperactivity Disorder in a National Sample of U.S. Children." *Archives of Pediatrics and Adolescent Medicine* 161 (September): 857–864.

Fugh-Berman, A. 2005. "The Corporate Coauthor." *Journal of General Internal Medicine* 20 (June): 546–548.

Fukuyama, F. 2003. *Our Posthuman Future: Consequences of the Biotechnology Revolution.* New York: Picador.

Furman, L. 2005. "What Is Attention-Deficit Hyperactivity Disorder (ADHD)?" *Journal of Child Neurology* 20 (December): 994–1002.

Furman, L., and B. Berman. 2004. "Rethinking the AAP Attention Deficit/Hyperactivity Disorder Guidelines." *Clinical Pediatrics* 43: 601–603.

Gabbard, G. 2007. "Psychotherapy in Psychiatry." *International Review of Psychiatry* 19 (February): 5–12.

Gabbard, G., and J. Kay. 2001. "The Fate of Integrated Treatment: Whatever Happened to the Biopsychosocial Psychiatrist?" *American Journal of Psychiatry* 158 (December): 1956–1963.

Gadow, K. 1981. "Prevalence of Drug Treatment for Hyperactivity and Other Childhood Behavior Disorders." In *Psychosocial Aspects of Drug Treatment for Hyperactivity*, ed. K. Gadow and J. Loney. Boulder, CO: Westview Press.

Galatzer-Levy, I., and R. Galatzer-Levy. 2007. "The Revolution in Psychiatric Diagnosis: Problems at the Foundations." *Perspectives in Biology and Medicine* 50 (Spring): 161–180.

Gallagher, J. 1957. "Comparison of Brain-Injured and Non-Brain-Injured Mentally Retarded Children on Several Psychological Variables." *Monographs of the Society for Research in Child Development* 22.

Gardner, W., K. Kelleher, K. Pajer, and J. Campo. 2004. "Primary Care Clinicians' Use of Standardized Psychiatric Diagnoses." *Child: Care, Health and Development* 30 (September): 401–412.

Garmbardella, A. 1995. *Science and Innovation: The U.S. Pharmaceutical Industry during the 1980s*. Cambridge: Cambridge University Press.

Gates, D. 1987. "Just Saying No to Ritalin." *Newsweek*, November 23, 6.

Gaylin, S. 1985. "The Coming of the Corporation and the Marketing of Psychiatry." *Hospitals and Community Psychiatry*: 154–159.

Gibbs, N. 1998. "The Age of Ritalin." *Time*, November 30, 89–96.

Gilger, J., B. Pennington, and J. DeFries. 1992. "A Twin Study of the Etiology of Comorbidity: Attention-Deficit Hyperactivity Disorder and Dyslexia." *Journal of the American Academy of Child and Adolescent Psychiatry* 31: 343–348.

Gill, D. 2006. "Anything You Can Do, I Can Do Bigger? The Ethics and Equity of Human Growth Hormone for Small Normal Children." *Archives of Disease in Childhood* 91 (March): 270–272.

Gillberg, C., H. Melander, A. von Knorring, L. Janols, G. Thernlund, B. Hagglof, et al. 1997. "Long-Term Stimulant Treatment of Children with Attention-Deficit Hyperactivity Disorder Symptoms: A Randomized, Double-Blind, Placebo-Controlled Trial." *Archives of General Psychiatry* 54: 857–864.

Gittelman, R., S. Mannuzza, R. Shenker, and N. Bonagura. 1985. "Hyperactive Boys Almost Grown Up: I. Psychiatric Status." *Archives of General Psychiatry* 42: 937–947.

Glied, S., and A. Cuellar. 2003. "Trends and Issues in Child and Adolescent Mental Health." *Health Affairs* 22 (September–October): 39–50.

Gold, I., C. Heller, and B. Ritorto. 1992. "A Short-Term Psychiatric Inpatient Program for Adolescents." *Hospital Community Psychiatry* 43 (March): 58–61.

Gold, M., and D. Hodges. 1989. "Health Maintenance Organizations in 1988." *Health Affairs* (Winter): 127.

Goldman, H., and G. Grob. 2006. "Defining 'Mental Illness' in Mental Health Policy." *Health Affairs* 25 (May–June): 737–749.

Goldman, L., M. Genel, R. Bezman, and P. Slanetz. 1998. "Diagnosis and Treatment of Attention-Deficit/Hyperactivity Disorder in Children and Adolescents: Council on Scientific Affairs, American Medical Association." *Journal of the American Medical Association* 279 (April 8): 1100–1107.

Goldstein, J. 2006. "Is ADHD a Growth Industry?" *Journal of Attention Disorders* 9 (February): 461–464.

Good, B. 1997. "Studying Mental Illness in Context: Local, Global or Universal?" *Ethos* 25: 230–248.

Goodrich, W. 1972. "Changes in Child Psychiatry Training Required by Developmental-Adaptive Theory." *Journal of Nervous and Mental Disease* 154 (March): 213–220.

Goodwin, D., and S. Guze. 1996. *Psychiatric Diagnosis.* 5th ed. New York: Oxford University Press.

Goplerud, E. 1986. "Effects of Proprietary Management in General Hospital Psychiatric Units." *Hospital Community Psychiatry* 37 (August): 832–836.

Gordon, M., K. Antshel, S. Faraone, R. Barkley, L. Lewandowski, J. Hudziak, et al. 2006. "Symptoms versus Impairment: The Case for Respecting DSM-IV's Criterion D." *Journal of Attention Disorders* 9 (February): 465–475.

Graham, J. 1972. "Amphetamine Politics on Capitol Hill." *Transaction: Social Science and Modern Society* 9 (January): 14–22.

Greenberg, G. 2007. "Manufacturing Depression: A Journey into the Economy of Melancholy." *Harpers,* May, 35–46.

Greenblatt, M. 1975. "Psychiatry: The Battered Child of Medicine." *New England Journal of Medicine* 292 (January 30): 246–250.

Greenhill, L., S. Kollins, H. Abikoff, J. McCracken, M. Riddle, J. Swanson, et al. 2006. "Efficacy and Safety of Immediate-Release Methylphenidate Treatment for Preschoolers with ADHD." *Journal of the American Academy of Child and Adolescent Psychiatry* 45: 1284–1293.

Grigorenko, E. 2000. "Heritability and Intelligence." In *Handbook of Intelligence,* ed. R. J. Sternberg, 53–91. New York: Cambridge University Press.

Grinspoon, L., and S. Singer. 1973. "Amphetamines in the Treatment of Hyperkinetic Children." *Harvard Education Review* 43 (November): 521.

Grob, G. 1994. *The Mad among Us: A History of the Care of America's Mentally Ill.* New York: Free Press.

Gurian, M. 1996. *The Wonder of Boys.* New York: Tarcher.

Hahn, H. 1985. "Disability Policy and the Problem of Discrimination." *American Behavioral Scientist* 28: 293–318.

Hall, K., M. Irwin, K. Bowman, W. Frankenberger, and D. Jewett. 2005. "Illicit Use of Prescribed Stimulant Medication among College Students." *Journal of American College Health* 53: 167–174.

Hall, L. 1993. "The Biology of Mental Disorders." *Journal of the American Medical Association* 269 (February 17): 844.

Hallowell, E., and J. Ratey. 1994. *Driven to Distraction: Recognizing and Coping with Attention Deficit Disorder from Childhood Through Adulthood.* New York: Touchstone.

Halperin, J., J. Newcorn, I. Kopstein, K. McKay, S. Schwartz, L. Siever, et al. 1997. "Serotonin, Aggression, and Parental Psychopathology in Children with Attention-Deficit Hyperactivity Disorder." *Journal of the American Academy of Child and Adolescent Psychiatry* 36: 1391–1398.

Hamm, N. 1974. "The Politics of Empiricism: Research Recommendations of the Joint Commission on Mental Health in Children." *American Psychologist* 29 (January): 9–13.

Harmon, A. 2005. "Young, Assured and Playing Pharmacist to Friends." *New York Times*, November 16.

Harris, G., B. Carey, J. Roberts. 2007. "Psychiatrists, Children and Drug Industry's Role." *New York Times*, May 10.

Harris, G., and J. Roberts. 2007. "Doctors' Ties to Drug Makers Are Put on Close View." *New York Times*, March 21.

Hart, E., B. Lahey, R. Loeber, B. Applegate, and P. Frick. 1995. "Developmental Changes in Attention-Deficit Hyperactivity Disorder in Boys: A Four-Year Longitudinal Study." *Journal of Abnormal Child Psychology* 23: 729–750.

Hartmann, T. 2003. *The Edison Gene: ADHD and the Gift of the Hunter Child.* Rochester, VT: Inner Traditions.

Hatfield, A. 1991. "The National Alliance for the Mentally Ill: A Decade Later." *Community Mental Health Journal* 27 (April): 95–103.

Havey, J., J. Olson, C. McCormick, and G. Cates. 2005. "Teachers' Perceptions of the Incidence and Management of Attention-Deficit Hyperactivity Disorder." *Applied Neuropsychology* 12: 120–127.

Healy, D. 1997. *The Anti-Depressant Era.* Cambridge, MA: Harvard University Press.

Hechtman, L., H. Abikoff, R. Klein, B. Greenfield, J. Etcovitch, L. Cousins, et al. 2004. "Children with ADHD Treated with Long-Term Methylphenidate and Multimodal Psychosocial Treatment: Impact on Parental Practices." *Journal of the American Academy of Child and Adolescent Psychiatry* 43: 830–838.

Hechtman, L., H. Abikoff, R. G. Klein, G. Weiss, C. Respitz, J. Kouri, et al. 2004. "Academic Achievement and Emotional Status of Children with ADHD Treated with Long-Term Methylphenidate and Multimodal Psychosocial Treatment." *Journal of the American Academy of Child and Adolescent Psychiatry* 43: 812–819.

Hentoff, N. 1970. "The Drugged Classroom." *Evergreen Review*, December, 31–33.

———. 1972. "Drug-Pushing in the Schools." *Village Voice*, May 25, 20–21.

Herbert, M. 1964. "The Concept and Testing of Brain Damage in Children: A Review." *Journal of Child Psychology and Psychiatry* 5: 197–217.

Herman-Stahl, M., C. Krebs, L. Kroutil, and D. Heller. 2007. "Risk and Protective Factors for Methamphetamine Use and Nonmedical Use of Prescription Stimulants among Young Adults Aged 18 to 25." *Addictive Behaviors* 32: 1003–1015.

Hick, H., J. Kaye, and C. Black. 2004. "Incidence and Prevalence of Drug-Treated Attention Deficit Disorder among Boys in the U.K." *British Journal of General Practitioners* 54 (May): 345–347.

Hickey, K., and L. Lyckholm. 2004. "Child Welfare versus Parental Autonomy: Medical Ethics, the Law, and Faith-Based Healing." *Theoretical Medicine and Bioethics* 25: 265–276.

Hill, D., R. Yeo, R. Campbell, B. Hart, J. Vigil, and W. Brooks. 2003. "Magnetic Resonance Imaging Correlates of Attention-Deficit/Hyperactivity Disorder in Children." *Neuropsychology* 17: 496–506.

Hinshaw, S. 1992. "Externalizing Behavior Problems and Academic Underachievement in Childhood and Adolescence: Causal Relationships and Underlying Mechanisms." *Psychological Bulletin* 111: 127–155.

———. 2002. "Preadolescent Girls with Attention-Deficit/Hyperactivity Disorder: I. Background Characteristics, Comorbidity, Cognitive and Social Functioning, and Parenting Practices." *Journal of Consulting and Clinical Psychology* 70: 1086–1098.

———. 2003. "Impulsivity, Emotion Regulation, and Developmental Psychopathology: Specificity versus Generality of Linkages." *Annals of the New York Academy of Sciences* 149 (December): 149–159.

———. 2007. "Moderators and Mediators of Treatment Outcome for Youth with ADHD: Understanding for Whom and How Interventions Work." *Journal of Pediatric Psychology* 32 (July): 664–675.

Hinshaw, S., and D. Cicchetti. 2000. "Stigma and Mental Disorders: Conceptions of Illness, Public Attitudes, Personal Disclosure, and Social Policy." *Development and Psychopathology* 12: 555–598.

Hinshaw, S., and S. Melnick. 1995. "Peer Relationships in Boys with Attention-Deficit Hyperactivity Disorder with and without Comorbid Aggression." *Development and Psychopathology* 7: 627–647.

Hoagwood, K. 2002. "Making the Translation from Research to Its Application: The *Je Ne Sais Pas* of Evidence-Based Practices." *Clinical Psychology: Science and Practice* 9 (June): 210–213.

Hoagwood, K., K. Kelleher, M. Feil, and D. Comer. 2000. "Treatment Services for Children with ADHD: A National Perspective." *Journal of the American Academy of Child and Adolescent Psychiatry* 39 (February): 198–206.

Hocutt, A., J. McKinney, and M. Montague. 1993. "Issues in the Education of Students with Attention Deficit Disorder: Introduction to the Special Issue." *Exceptional Children* 60 (October–November): 103–107.

Hohman, L. 1922. "Post Encephalitic Behavior Disorders in Children." *Johns Hopkins Hospital Bulletin* 33: 372–375.

Horwitz, A. 2002. *Creating Mental Illness*. Chicago: University of Chicago Press.

Hoza, B., S. Mrug, A. Gerdes, S. Hinshaw, W. Bukowski, J. Gold, et al. 2005. "What Aspects of Peer Relationships Are Impaired in Children with Attention-Deficit/Hyperactivity Disorder?" *Journal of Consulting and Clinical Psychology* 73: 411–423.

Hubbard, J., and A. Newcomb. 1991. "Initial Dyadic Peer Interaction of Attention Deficit-Hyperactivity Disorder and Normal Boys." *Journal of Abnormal Child Psychology* 19: 179–195.

Hunter, J. 1992. *Culture Wars: The Struggle to Define America*. New York: Basic Books.

Hyler, S., J. Williams, and R. Spitzer. 1982. "Reliability in the DSM-III Field Trials." *Archives of General Psychiatry* 39: 1275–1278.

Hynd, G., K. Hern, E. Novey, D. Eliopulos, R. Marshall, J. Gonzalez, et al. 1993. "Attention-Deficit Hyperactivity Disorder and Asymmetry of the Caudate Nucleus." *Journal of Child Neurology* 8: 339–347.

Hynd, G., M. Semrud-Clikeman, A. Lorys, E. Novey, and D. Eliopulos. 1990. "Brain Morphology in Developmental Dyslexia and Attention Deficit Disorder/Hyperactivity." *Archives of Neurology* 47: 919–926.

Iglehart, J. 1996. "Health Policy Report: Managed Care and Mental Health." *New England Journal of Medicine* 335 (July 4): 131–135.

Irwin, P., and R. Conroy-Hughes. 1981. "EPSDT Impact on Health Status." *Health Care Financing Review* 2 (Spring): 25–39.

Jablensky, A. 2005. "Categories, Dimensions and Prototypes: Critical Issues for Psychiatric Classification." *Psychopathology* 38 (July–August): 201–205.

Jellinek, M., and B. Nurcombe. 1993. "Two Wrongs Don't Make a Right: Managed Care, Mental Health, and the Marketplace." *Journal of the American Medicine Association* 270 (October 13): 1737–1738.

Jensen, P., et al. 2007. "3-Year Follow-Up of the NIMH MTA Study." *Journal of the American Academy of Child and Adolescent Psychiatry* 46: 989–1002.

Jensen, P., S. Hinshaw, H. Kraemer, N. Lenora, J. Newcorn, H. Abikoff, et al. 2001. "ADHD Comorbidity Findings from the MTA Study: Comparing Comorbid Subgroups." *Journal of the American Academy of Child and Adolescent Psychiatry* 40: 147–158.

Jensen, P., L. Kettle, M. Roper, M. Sloan, M. Dulcan, C. Hoven, et al. 1999. "Are Stimulants Overprescribed? Treatment of ADHD in Four U.S. Communities." *Journal of the American Academy of Child and Adolescent Psychiatry* 38 (July): 797–804.

Jensen, P., D. Martin, and D. Cantwell. 1997. "Comorbidity in ADHD: Implications for Research, Practice, and DSM-V." *Journal of the American Academy of Child and Adolescent Psychiatry* 36: 1065–1079.

Jensen, P., D. Mrazek, P. Knapp, L. Steinberg, C. Pfeffer, J. Schowalter, et al. 1997. "Evolution and Revolution in Child Psychiatry: ADHD as a Disorder of Adaptation." *Journal of the American Academy of Child and Adolescent Psychiatry* 36 (December): 1672–1681.

Johnson, T. 1997. "Evaluating the Hyperactive Child in Your Office: Is It ADHD?" *American Family Physician* 56 (July): 155–160, 168–170.

Johnston, L., P. O'Malley, J. Bachman, and J. Schulenberg. 2005. *Monitoring the Future National Survey Results on Drug Use, 1975–2004.* Vol. 1, *Secondary School Students.* NIH Publication No. 05–5727. Bethesda, MD: National Institute on Drug Abuse, 2005.

Joint Commission on Mental Health of Children. 1970. *Crisis in Child Mental Health: Challenge for the 1970s.* New Yorker: Harper and Row.

Judd, L. 1998. "NIMH during the Tenure of Director Lewis L. Judd, M.D. (1987–1990): The Decade of the Brain and the Four National Research Plans." *American Journal of Psychiatry* 155 (September): 25–31.

Kadison, R. 2005. "Getting an Edge—Use of Stimulants and Antidepressants in College." *New England Journal of Medicine* 353: 1089–1091.

Kahn, E., and L. Cohen. 1934. "Organic Drivenness: A Brain Stem Syndrome and an Experience with Case Reports." *New England Journal of Medicine* 210: 748–756.

Kaloyanides, K., S. McCabe, J. Cranford, and C. Teter. 2007. "Prevalence of Illicit Use and Abuse of Prescription Stimulants, Alcohol, and Other Drugs among College Students: Relationship with Age at Initiation of Prescription Stimulants." *Pharmacotherapy* 27 (May): 666–674.

Katusic, S., W. Barbaresi, R. Colligan, A. Weaver, C. Leibson, and S. Jacobsen. 2005. "Psychostimulant Treatment and Risk for Substance Abuse among Young Adults with a History of Attention-Deficit/Hyperactivity Disorder: A Population-Based, Birth Cohort Study." *Journal of Child and Adolescent Psychopharmacology* 15: 764–776.

Katzmann, R. 1986. *Institutional Disability: The Saga of Transportation Policy for the Disabled*. Washington, DC: Brookings Institution Press.

Kelleher, K., G. Childs, R. Wasserman, T. McInerny, P. Nutting, and W. Gardner. 1998. "Insurance Status and Recognition of Psychosocial Problems: A Report from PROS and ASPN." *Archives of Pediatric and Adolescent Medicine* 151: 1109–1115.

Kelleher, K., T. McInerny, W. Gardner, G. Childs, and R. Wasserman. 2000. "Increasing Identification of Psychosocial Problems: 1979–1996." *Pediatrics* 105 (June): 1313–1321.

Kelleher, K., and S. Scholle. 1995. "Children with Chronic Medical Conditions II: Managed Care Opportunities and Threats." *Ambulatory Child Health* 1: 139–146.

Kelleher, K., S. Scholle, H. Feldman, and D. Nace. 1999. "A Fork in the Road: Decision Time for Behavioral Pediatrics." *Journal of Developmental Behavioral Pediatrics* 20: 181–186.

Kelleher, K., and M. Wolraich. 1996. "Diagnosing Psychosocial Problems." *Pediatrics* 97: 899–901.

Kelly, J. 2000. "Children's Adjustment in Conflicted Marriage and Divorce: A Decade Review of Research." *Journal of the American Academy of Child and Adolescent Psychiatry* 39 (August): 963–973.

Kemp, E. 1981. "Aiding the Disabled: No Pity, Please." *New York Times*, September 3, A19.

Kendall, J., M. Leo, N. Perrin, and D. Hatton. 2005. "Modeling ADHD Child and Family Relationships." *Western Journal of Nursing Research* 27: 500–518.

Kendell, R. 1975. *The Role of Diagnosis in Psychiatry*. Oxford: Blackwell Scientific Publications.

Kessler, R. 2002. "The Categorical versus Dimensional Assessment Controversy in the Sociology of Mental Illness." *Journal of Health and Social Behavior* 43 (June): 171–188.

Kessler, R., L. Adler, R. Barkley, J. Biederman, C. Conners, O. Demler, et al. 2006. "The Prevalence and Correlates of Adult ADHD in the United States: Results from the National Comorbidity Survey Replication." *American Journal of Psychiatry* 163: 716–723.

Kessler, R., L. Adler, R. Barkley, J. Biederman, C. Conners, S. Faraone, et al. 2005. "Patterns and Predictors of Attention-Deficit/Hyperactivity Disorder Persistence into Adulthood: Results from the National Comorbidity Survey Replication." *Biological Psychiatry* 57: 1442–1451.

Kiesler, C., and C. Simpkins. 1991. "Changes in Psychiatric Inpatient Treatment of Children and Youth in General Hospitals: 1980–1985." *Hospital Community Psychiatry* 42 (June): 601–604.

Kiesler, C., C. Simpkins, and T. Morton. 1989. "The Psychiatric Inpatient Treatment of Children and Youth in General Hospitals." *American Journal of Community Psychology* 17 (December): 821–830.

Kimmel, M. 2006. "A War against Boys?" *Dissent* 53 (Fall): 65–70.

Kindlon, D., and M. Thompson. 1999. *Raising Cain: Protecting the Emotional Lives of Boys.* New York: Ballantine Books.

Kirk, S., and H. Kutchins. 1992. *The Selling of DSM: The Rhetoric of Science in Psychiatry.* New York: Aldine Transaction.

Kirmayer, L., and A. Young. 1999. "Culture and Context in the Evolutionary Concept of Mental Disorder." *Journal of Abnormal Psychology* 108 (August): 446–452.

Kitagawa, E. 1981. "New Life-Styles: Marriage Patterns, Living Arrangements, and Fertility Outside of Marriage." *The Annals of the American Academy of Political and Social Science* 453: 1–27.

Klein, R. 2002. "Alcohol, Stimulants, Nicotine, and Other Drugs in ADHD." In *Attention Deficit Hyperactivity Disorder: State of the Science; Best Practices*, ed. P. Jensen and J. Cooper, 16-1–16-17. Kingston, NJ: Civic Research Institute.

Klein, R., H. Abikoff, L. Hechtman, and G. Weiss. 2004. "Design and Rationale of Controlled Study of Long-Term Methylphenidate and Multimodal Psychosocial Treatment in Children with ADHD." *Journal of the American Academy of Child and Adolescent Psychiatry* 43: 792–801.

Kleinman, A. 2004. "Culture and Depression." *New England Journal of Medicine* 351 (September 2): 951–953.

Knitzer, J. 1982. *Unclaimed Children: The Failure of Public Responsibility to Children and Adolescents in Need of Mental Health Services.* Washington, DC: Children's Defense Fund.

Knopik, V., E. Sparrow, P. Madden, K. Bucholz, J. Hudziak, W. Reich, et al. 2005. "Contributions of Parental Alcoholism, Prenatal Substance Exposure, and Genetic Transmission to Child ADHD Risk: A Female Twin Study." *Psychological Medicine* 35: 625–635.

Koch, K. 2000. "Special Education: Do Students with Disabilities Get the Help They Need?" *CQ Researcher* 10 (November 10): 911.

Kohn, A. 1989. "Suffer the Restless Children." *Atlantic Monthly* 264 (November): 90–98.

Kolata, G. 1990. "Researchers Say Brain Abnormality May Help to Explain Hyperactivity." *New York Times*, November 15, B18.

Kollins, S., L. Greenhill, J. Swanson, S. Wigal, H. Abikoff, J. McCracken, et al. 2006. "Rationale, Design, and Methods of the Preschool ADHD Treatment

Study (PATS)." *Journal of the American Academy of Child and Adolescent Psychiatry* 45: 1275–1283.

Kollins, S., E. MacDonald, and C. Rush. 2001. "Assessing the Abuse Potential of Methylphenidate in Nonhuman and Human Subjects: A Review." *Pharmacology, Biochemistry, and Behavior* 68: 611–627.

Komoroski, A. 2001. "Stimulant Drug Therapy for Hyperactive Children: Adjudicating Disputes between Parents and Educators." *Boston Public Interest Law Journal* 11 (Fall): 100–101.

Kopp, C., and J. Krakow. 1983. "The Developmentalist and the Study of Biological Risk: A View of the Past with an Eye to the Future." *Child Development* 54 (October): 1086–1108.

Kowatch, R., and M. Delbello. 2006. "Pediatric Bipolar Disorder: Emerging Diagnostic and Treatment Approaches." *Child and Adolescent Psychiatric Clinics of North America* 15 (January): 73–108.

Kraepelin, E. 1913. *Lectures on Clinical Psychiatry*. New York: William Wood.

Kramer, P. 1993. *Listening to Prozac*. New York: Viking Press.

Kroll, J. 1979. "Philosophical Foundations of French and U.S. Nosology." *American Journal of Psychiatry* 136: 1135–1138.

Kronebusch, K. 2001. "Medicaid for Children: Federal Mandates, Welfare Reform, and Policy Backsliding." *Health Affairs* 20 (January–February): 97–111.

Kroutil, L., D. Van Brunt, M. Herman-Stahl, D. Heller, R. Bray, and M. Penne. 2006. "Nonmedical Use of Prescription Stimulants in the United States." *Drug and Alcohol Dependence* 84: 135–143.

Kuhlthau, K., J. Perrin, S. Ettner, T. McLaughlin, and S. Gortmaker. 1998. "High-Expenditure Children with Supplemental Security Income." *Pediatrics* 102 (September): 610–615.

Kuntsi, J., G. McLoughlin, and P. Asherson. 2006. "Attention Deficit Hyperactivity Disorder." *Neuromolecular Medicine* 8: 461–484.

Kuther, T. 2003. "Medical Decision-Making and Minors: Issues of Consent and Assent." *Adolescence* 38 (Summer): 343–358.

Kwasman, A., B. Tinsley, and H. Lepper. 1995. "Pediatricians' Knowledge and Attitudes Concerning Diagnosis and Treatment of Attention Deficit and Hyperactivity Disorders: A National Survey Approach." *Archives of Pediatric and Adolescent Medicine* 149 (November): 1211–1216.

Ladd, E. 1970. "Pills for Classroom Peace?" *Saturday Review*, November 21, 66–68, 81–83.

Lahey, B., B. Applegate, K. McBurnett, J. Biederman, L. Greenhill, G. Hynd, et al. 1994. "DSM-IV Field Trials for Attention Deficit/Hyperactivity Disorder in Children and Adolescents." *American Journal of Psychiatry* 151: 1673–1685.

Lahey, B., R. Loeber, M. Stouthammer-Loeber, M. Christ, S. Green. M. Russo, et al. 1990. "Comparison of DSM-III and DSM-III-R Diagnoses for Prepubertal Children: Changes in Prevalence and Validity." *Journal of the American Academy of Child and Adolescent Psychiatry* 29 (July): 620–626.

Lahey, B., W. Pelham, J. Loney, S. Lee, and E. Willcutt. 2005. "Instability of the DSM-IV Subtypes of ADHD from Preschool through Elementary School." *Archives of General Psychiatry* 62 (August): 896–902.

Lakoff, A. 2000. "Adaptive Will: The Evolution of Attention Deficit Disorder." *Journal of the History of the Behavioral Sciences* 36 (Spring): 146–169.

Lambert, N. 2002. "Stimulant Treatment as a Risk Factor for Nicotine Use and Substance Abuse." In *Attention Deficit Hyperactivity Disorder: State of the Science; Best Practices*, ed. P. Jensen and J. Cooper, 18-1–18-24. Kingston, NJ: Civic Research Institute.

Lane, C. 2006. "How Shyness Became an Illness: A Brief History of Social Phobia." *Common Knowledge* 12: 388–409.

Laufer, M. 1975. "In Osler's Day It was Syphilis." In *Explorations in Child Psychiatry*, ed. E. Anthony. New York: Plenum Press.

———. 1980. "Which Adolescents Must Be Helped and by Whom?" *Journal of Adolescence* 3 (December): 265–272.

Laufer, M., E. Denhoff, and G. Solomons. 1957. "Hyperkinetic Impulse Disorder in Children's Behavior Problems." *Psychosomatic Medicine* 19 (January–February): 38–49.

Lear, J. 2007. "Health at School: A Hidden Health Care System Emerges from the Shadows." *Health Affairs* 26 (March–April): 409–419.

Lehmann, H. 1989. "The Introduction of Chlorpromazine to North America." *Psychiatric Journal of the University of Ottawa* 14: 263–265.

Lehmann, H., and G. Hanrahan. 1954. "New Inhibiting Agent for Psychomotor Excitement and Manic States." *Archives of Neurology and Psychiatry* 71: 227–237.

Lenz, C. 2005. "Prescribing a Legislative Response: Educators, Physicians, and Psychotropic Medication for Children." *Journal of Contemporary Health Law and Policy* 22 (Fall): 72–106.

Leslie, D., R. Rosenheck, and S. Horwitz. 2001. "Patterns of Mental Health and Utilization and Costs among Children in a Privately Insured Population." *Health Services Research* 36 (April): 115–118.

Leslie, L., D. Plemmons, A. Monn, and L. Palinkas. 2007. "Investigating ADHD Treatment Trajectories: Listening to Families' Stories about Medication Use." *Journal of Development and Behavioral Pediatrics* 28 (June): 179–188.

Levy, F., and D. Hay. 2001. *Attention, Genes, and ADHD.* Philadelphia: Brunner-Routledge.

Levy, F., D. Hay, M. McStephen, C. Wood, and I. Waldman. 1997. "Attention-Deficit Hyperactivity Disorder: A Category or a Continuum? Genetic Analysis of a Large-Scale Twin Study." *Journal of the American Academy of Child and Adolescent Psychiatry* 36: 737–744.

Lewin, T. 1987. "Drug Makers Fighting Back against Advance of Generics." *New York Times*, July 28, A1.

Lewis, J. 1989. "Are Adolescents Being Hospitalized Unnecessarily? The Current Use of Hospitalization in Psychiatric Treatment." *Journal of Child and Adolescent Psychiatric Mental Health Nursing* 2 (October–December): 134–138.

Lipman, R. 1974. "NIMH-PRB Support of Research in Minimal Brain Dysfunction in Children." In *Clinical Use of Stimulant Drugs in Children*, ed. C. Conners, 203–213. Amsterdam: Excerpta Medica.

Liu, C., A. Robin, S. Brenner, and J. Eastman. 1991. "Social Acceptability of Methylphenidate and Behavior Modification fort Treating Attention Deficit Hyperactivity Disorder." *Pediatrics* 88 (September): 560–565.

Livingston, K. 1998. "Ritalin: Miracle Drug or Cop-Out." *Public Interest* 127 (Spring): 3–18.

Lloyd, J., S. Forness, and K. Kavale. 1998. "Some Methods Are More Effective than Others." *Intervention in School and Clinic* 33: 195–200.

Lock, J., and G. Strauss. 1994. "Psychiatric Hospitalization of Adolescents for Conduct Disorder." *Hospital and Community Psychiatry* 45 (September): 925–928.

Loeber, R., S. Green, B. Lahey, M. Christ, and P. Frick. 1992. "Developmental Sequences in the Age of Onset of Disruptive Child Behaviors." *Journal of Child and Family Studies* 1: 21–41.

Loney, J., J. Kramer, and H. Salisbury. 2002. "Medicated vs. Unmedicated ADHD Children—Involvement with Legal and Illegal Drugs." In *Attention Deficit Hyperactivity Disorder: State of the Science; Best Practices*, ed. P. Jensen and J. Cooper, 17-1–17-16. Kingston, NJ: Civic Research Institute.

Longmore, P. 1995. "Medical Decision Making and People with Disabilities: A Clash of Cultures." *Journal of Law, Medicine, and Ethics* 23: 82–87.

Lopez, F. 2006. "ADHD: New Pharmacological Treatments on the Horizon." *Journal of Developmental Behavioral Pediatrics* 27 (October): 410–416.

Low, K., and A. Gendaszek. 2002. "Illicit Use of Psychostimulants among College Students: A Preliminary Study." *Psychology, Health and Medicine* 7: 283–287.

Luhrmann, T. 2001. *Of Two Minds: The Growing Disorder in American Psychiatry*. New York: Vintage.

Lyons, J. 2004. *Redressing the Emperor: Improving Our Children's Mental Health System*. Westport, CT: Praeger, 2004.

Madow, L. 1976. "The Retreat from a Psychiatry of People." *Journal of the American Academy of Psychoanalysis* 4: 131–135.

Malacrida, C. 2002. "Alternative Therapies and Attention Deficit Disorder: Discourses of Maternal Responsibility and Risk." *Gender and Society* 16 (June): 366–385.

———. 2004. "Medicalization, Ambivalence, and Social Control: Mothers' Descriptions of Educators and ADD/ADHD." *Health* 8: 61–80.

Mallett, C. 2006. "Behaviorally-Based Disorders: The Historical Social Construction of Youths' Most Prevalent Psychiatric Diagnoses." *History of Psychiatry* 17: 437–460.

Mannuzza, S., R. Klein, A. Bessler, P. Malloy, and M. LaPadula. 1993. "Adult Outcome of Hyperactive Boys: Educational Achievement, Occupational Rank, and Psychiatric Status." *Archives of General Psychiatry* 50: 565–576.

———. 1998. "Adult Psychiatric Status of Hyperactive Boys Grown Up." *American Journal of Psychiatry* 155: 493–498.

Mannuzza, S., R. Klein, N. Bonagura, P. Malloy, T. Giampino, and K. Addalli. 1991. "Hyperactive Boys Almost Grown Up: V. Replication of Psychiatric Status." *Archives of General Psychiatry* 48: 77–83.

Mantel, B. 2005. "No Child Left Behind: Is the Law Improving Student Performance?" *CQ Researcher* 15, no. 20 (May 27): 469–492.

Mark, T., R. Coffey, E. King, H. Harwood, D. McKusick, J. Genuardi, et al. 2000. "Spending on Mental Health and Substance Abuse Treatment, 1987–1997." *Health Affairs* 19 (July–August): 113–115.

Markowitz, S., and A. Cuellar. 2007. "Antidepressants and Youth: Healing or Harmful?" *Social Science and Medicine* 64 (May): 2138–2151.

Marks, A. 1980. "Aspects of Biosocial Screening and Health Maintenance in Adolescents." *Pediatric Clinics of North America* 27 (February): 153–161.

Marks, A., and M. Cohen. 1978. "Health Screening and Assessment of Adolescents." *Pediatric Annals* 7 (September): 596–604.

Marland, H., and M. Gijswijt-Hofstra. 2003. *Cultures of Child Health in Britain and the Netherlands in the Twentieth Century.* New York: Rodopi Press.

Marshall, E. 2000. "Epidemiology: Duke Study Faults Overuse of Stimulants for Children." *Science* 289 (August 4): 721.

Martin, A. and D. Leslie. 2003. "Trends in Psychotropic Medication Costs for Children and Adolescents, 1997–2000." *Archives of Pediatric and Adolescent Medicine* 157 (October): 997–1004.

Mashaw, J., J. Perrin, and V. Reno, eds. 1996. *Restructuring the SSI Disability Program for Children and Adolescents.* Washington, DC: National Academy of Social Insurance.

Mason, M., and J. Gibbs. 1992. "Patterns of Adolescent Psychiatric Hospitalization: Implications for Social Policy." *American Journal of Orthopsychiatry* 62 (July): 447–457.

Mattes, J., L. Boswell, and H. Oliver. 1985. "Methylphenidate Effects on Symptoms of Attention Deficit Disorder in Adults." *Archives of General Psychiatry* 41: 1059–1063.

Mayes, R., and R. Berenson. 2006. *Medicare Prospective Payment and the Shaping of U.S. Health Care.* Baltimore: Johns Hopkins University Press.

Mayes, R., and A. Horwitz. 2005. "DSM-III and the Revolution in the Classification of Mental Illness." *Journal of the History of the Behavioral Sciences* 41 (Summer): 249–267.

Mayes, R., and A. Rafalovich. 2007. "Suffer the Restless Children: The Evolution of ADHD and Pediatric Stimulant Use: 1900–1980." *History of Psychiatry* 18 (December): 435–457.

Mayes, S., S. Calhoun, and E. Crowell. 2000. "Learning Disabilities and ADHD: Overlapping Spectrum Disorders." *Journal of Learning Disabilities* 33 (September–October): 417–424.

Maynard, R. 1970. "Omaha Pupils Given 'Behavior Drugs.'" *Washington Post*, June 29, 1.

McBurnett, K., B. Lahey, and L. Pfiffner. 1993. "Diagnosis of Attention Deficit Disorders in DSM-IV: Scientific Basis and Implications for Education." *Exceptional Children* 60 (October–November): 108–117.

McCabe, S., J. Knight, C. Teter, and H. Wechsler. 2005. "Non-Medical Use of Prescription Stimulants among US College Students: Prevalence and Correlates from a National Survey." *Addiction* 99: 96–106.

McCabe, S., C. Teter, and C. Boyd. 2004. "The Use, Misuse and Diversion of Prescription Stimulants among Middle and High School Students." *Substance Use and Misuse* 39 (June): 1095–1116.

———. 2006. "Medical Use, Illicit Use and Diversion of Prescription Stimulant Medication." *Journal of Psychoactive Drugs* 31: 43–56.

McCann, B., and P. Roy-Byrne. 2004. "Screening and Diagnostic Utility of Self-Report Attention Deficit Hyperactivity Disorder Scales in Adults." *Comprehensive Psychiatry* 45: 175–183.

McCubbin, M., and D. Cohen. 1999. "Empirical, Ethical, and Political Perspectives on the Use of Methylphenidate." *Ethical Human Sciences and Services* 1 (Spring): 81–101.

McDaniel, K. 1986. "Pharmacologic Treatment of Psychiatric and Neurodevelopmental Disorders in Children and Adolescents." *Clinical Pediatrics* 25 (February): 65–71.

McDonald, S. 1994. "An Ethical Dilemma: Risk versus Responsibility." *Journal of Psychosocial Nursing in Mental Health Services* 32 (January): 19–25.

McKusick, D., T. Mark, E. King, R. Coffey, and J. Genuardi. 2002. "Trends in Mental Health Insurance Benefits and Out-of-Pocket Spending." *Journal of Mental Health Policy and Economics* 5 (June): 71–78.

McLean, A. 1995. "Empowerment and the Psychiatric Consumer/Ex-Patient Movement in the United States: Contradictions, Crisis and Change." *Social Science and Medicine* 40 (April): 1053–1071.

McLean, B. 2001. "A Bitter Pill: Prozac Made Eli Lilly." *Fortune* 144 (August 13): 118–119.

McLeod, J., D. Fettes, P. Jensen, B. Pescosolido, and J. Martin. 2007. "Public Knowledge, Beliefs, and Treatment Preferences Concerning Attention-Deficit Hyperactivity Disorder." *Psychiatric Services* 58 (May): 626–631.

Mechanic, D. 1998. "Emerging Trends in Mental Health Policy and Practice." *Health Affairs* 17 (November–December): 91–92.

———. 1998. *Mental Health and Social Policy.* 4th ed. New York: Allyn and Bacon.

Melnick, R. 1994. *Between the Lines: Interpreting Welfare Rights.* Washington, DC: Brookings Institution Press.

Merill, R. 1999. "Modernizing the FDA: An Incremental Revolution." *Health Affairs* 18: 96–111.

Michels, R., and P. Marzuk. 1993. "Progress in Psychiatry." *New England Journal of Medicine* 329 (August 19): 552–560, (August 26): 628–638.

Miech, R., A. Caspi, T. Moffitt, B. Wright, and P. Silva. 1999. "Low Socioeconomic Status and Mental Disorders: A Longitudinal Study of Selection and Causation during Young Adulthood." *American Journal of Sociology* 104 (January): 1096–1131.

Mihalik, G., and M. Scherer. 1998. "Fundamental Mechanisms of Managed Behavioral Health." *Journal of Health Care Finance* 24 (Spring): 1–15.

Milberger, S., J. Biederman, S. Faraone, L. Chen, and J. Jones. 1996. "Is Maternal Smoking during Pregnancy a Risk Factor for Attention Deficit Hyperactivity Disorder in Children?" *American Journal of Psychiatry* 153: 1138–1142.

Miller, R. 2003. *Children, Ethics and Modern Medicine*. Bloomington: Indiana University Press.

Millstein, R., T. Wilens, J. Biederman, and T. Spencer. 1997. "Presenting ADHD Symptoms and Subtypes in Clinically Referred Adults with ADHD." *Journal of Attention Disorders* 2: 159–166.

Milne, C. 1999. "Pediatric Research: Coming of Age in the New Millennium." *American Journal of Therapeutics* 6 (September): 263–282.

Minow, M., and R. Weissbourd. 1993. "Social Movements for Children." *Daedalus* 122 (Winter): 1–29.

Mintz, S. 2004. *Huck's Raft: A History of American Childhood*. Cambridge, MA: Belknap Press.

Molina, B. 2007. "Delinquent Behavior and Emerging Substance Use in the MTA at 36 Months: Prevalence, Course, and Treatment Effects." *Journal of the American Academy of Child and Adolescent Psychiatry* 46: 1028–1040.

Molina, B., and W. Pelham, Jr. 2003. "Childhood Predictors of Adolescent Substance Use in a Longitudinal Study of Children with ADHD." *Journal of Abnormal Psychology* 112: 497–507.

Molitch, M., and J. Sullivan. 1937. "The Effect of Benzedrine Sulfate on Children Taking the New Stanford Achievement Test." *American Journal of Orthopsychiatry* 7 (October): 519–522.

Moreno, C., L. Gonzalo, C. Blanco, H. Jiang, A. Schmidt, and M. Olfson. 2007. "National Trends in the Outpatient Diagnosis and Treatment of Bipolar Disorder in Youth." *Archives of General Psychiatry* 64 (September): 1032–1039.

Moreno, C., G. Laje, C. Blanco, H. Jiang, A. Schmidt, and M. Olfson. 2007. "National Trends in the Outpatient Diagnosis and Treatment of Bipolar Disorder in Youth." *Archives of General Psychiatry* 64 (September): 1032–1039.

Morgan, J., D. Robinson, and J. Aldridge. 2002. "Parenting Stress and Externalizing Child Behavior." *Child and Family Social Work* 7 (August): 219–225.

Mossinghoff, G. 1999. "Overview of the Hatch-Waxman Act and Its Impact on the Drug Development Process." *Food and Drug Law Journal* 54: 187–194.

Mrug, S., B. Hoza, and A. Gerdes. 2001. "Children with Attention-Deficit/ Hyperactivity Disorder: Peer Relationships and Peer-Oriented Interventions." In *The Role of Friendship in Psychological Adjustment*, ed. D. W. Nangle and C. A. Erdley, 51–77. San Francisco: Jossey-Bass.

MTA Cooperative Group. 1999. "14-Month Randomized Clinical Trial of Treatment Strategies for Attention Deficit Hyperactivity Disorder." *Archives of General Psychiatry*: 1073–1086.

Mueller, L., and P. Wheeler. 1998. "The Growth in Disability Programs as Seen by SSA Field Office Managers." In *Growth in Disability Benefits*, ed. K. Rupp and D. Stapleton. Kalamazoo, MI: Upjohn.

Muller, U., P. Fletcher, and H. Steinberg. 2006. "The Origin of Pharmacopsychology: Emil Kraepelin's Experiments in Leipzig, Dorpat and Heidelberg (1882–1892)." *Psychopharmacology* 184 (January): 131–138.

Murphy, K., and S. LeVert. 1995. *Out of the Fog: Treatment Options and Coping Strategies for Adult Attention Deficit Disorder*. New York: Hyperion.

Nahata, M. 1994. "More Conflicts of Interest: Review Articles Sponsored by the Pharmaceutical Industry." *Journal of the American Medical Association* 272, no. 16 (October 26): 1253–1254.

———. 1999. "Inadequate Pharmacotherapeutic Data for Drugs Used in Children: What Can Be Done?" *Pediatric Drugs* 1: 245–249.

Needleman, H., A. Schell, D. Bellinger, L. Leviton, and E. Alfred. 1990. "The Long-Term Effects of Exposure to Low Doses of Lead in Childhood: An 11-Year Follow-Up Report." *New England Journal of Medicine* 322: 83–88.

Neufeld, P., and M. Foy. 2006. "Historical Reflections on the Ascendancy of ADHD in North America." *British Journal of Educational Studies.*

Newacheck, P., and W. Taylor. 1992. "Childhood Chronic Illness: Prevalence, Severity, and Impact." *American Journal of Public Health* 82: 364–371.

Newsholme, A. 1935. *Fifty Years in Public Health: A Personal Narrative.* London: Allen and Unwin.

Niederhofer, H., B. Hackenberg, and K. Lazendorfer. 2004. "Family Conflict Tendency and ADHD." *Psychological Reports* 94 (April): 577–580.

Nigg, J. 2001. "Is ADHD a Disinhibitory Disorder?" *Psychological Bulletin* 127: 571–598.

———. 2006. *What Causes ADHD?* New York: Guilford Press.

Nolan, E., K. Gadow, and J. Sprafkin. 2001. "Teacher Reports of DSM-IV ADHD, ODD, and CD Symptoms in Schoolchildren." *Journal of the American Academy of Child and Adolescent Psychiatry* 40: 241–249.

Nolan, J. 1998. *The Therapeutic State.* New York: New York University Press.

O'Brien, R. 2001. *Crippled Justice: The History of Modern Disability Policy in the Workplace.* Chicago: University of Chicago Press.

Office of Child Development and Office of Assistant Secretary for Health and Scientific Affairs, Department of Health, Education, and Welfare. 1971. *Report of the Conference on the Use of Stimulant Drugs in the Treatment of Behaviorally Disturbed Young Children.* Washington, DC, January 11–12.

Okie, S. 2000. "Behavioral Drug Use in Toddlers up Sharply; Research Lacking Effects, Safety." *Washington Post,* February 23, A1.

———. 2006. "ADHD in Adults." *New England Journal of Medicine* 354: 2637–2641.

Olfson, M., C. Blanco, L. Liu, C. Moreno, and G. Laje. 2006. "National Trends in the Outpatient Treatment of Children and Adolescents with Antipsychotic Drugs." *Archives of General Psychiatry* 63: 679–685.

Olfson, M., M. Gameroff, S. Marcus, and P. Jensen. 2003. "National Trends in the Treatment of Attention Deficit Hyperactivity Disorder." *American Journal of Psychiatry* 160 (June): 1071–1077.

Olfson, M., and G. Klerman. 1993. "Trends in the Prescription of Psychotropic Medications: The Role of Physician Specialty." *Medical Care* 31: 559–564.

Olfson, M., S. Marcus, M. Weissman, and P. Jensen. 2002. "National Trends in the Use of Psychotropic Medications by Children." *Journal of the American Academy of Child and Adolescent Psychiatry* 41: 514–521.

Olson, B., P. Rosenbaum, N. Dosa, and N. Roizen. 2005. "Improving Guideline Adherence for the Diagnosis of ADHD in an Ambulatory Pediatric Setting." *Ambulatory Pediatrics* 5 (May–June): 138–142.

Olson, M. 1994. "Political Influence and Regulatory Policy: The 1984 Drug Legislation." *Economic Inquiry* 32: 363–365.

O'Reilly, B. 1994. "Drugmakers under Attack." *Fortune*, July 29, 54–63.

Ouellette, E. 1991. "Legal Issues in the Treatment of Children with Attention Deficit Disorder." *Journal of Child Neurology* 6 (Suppl.): 569–575.

Owens, E., S. Hinshaw, H. Kraemer, L. Arnold, H. Abikoff, D. Cantwell, et al. 2003. "Which Treatment for Whom for ADHD? Moderators of Treatment Response in the MTA." *Journal of Consulting and Clinical Psychology* 71 (June): 540–542.

Palmer, E., and S. Finger. 2001. "An Early Description of ADHD (Inattentive Subtype)." *Child Psychology and Psychiatry Review* 6: 66–73.

Parker, J., and S. Asher. 1987. "Peer Relations and Later Personal Adjustment: Are Low Accepted Children 'At Risk'?" *Psychological Bulletin* 102: 357–389.

Pasnau, R. 1987. "The Remedicalization of American Psychiatry." *Hospital and Community Psychiatry* 38: 145–151.

Pastor, P., and C. Reuben. May 2002. "Attention Deficit Disorder and Learning Disability: United States, 1997–1998." *Vital and Health Statistics*, Series 10, Number 206. Washington, DC: National Center for Health Statistics, 1–12.

Paternite, C., J. Loney, H. Salisbury, and M. Whalen. 1999. "Childhood Inattention-Overactivity, Aggression, and Stimulant Medication History as Predictors of Young Adult Outcomes." *Journal of Child and Adolescent Psychopharmacology* 9: 169–184.

Paul, S., and M. Tohen. 2007. "Conflicts of Interest and the Credibility of Psychiatric Research." *World Psychiatry* 6 (February): 33–34.

Pear, R. 2000. "Effort on Mood Drugs for Young Is Backed; Doctors, Teachers, and Business Endorse White House Plan." *New York Times*, March 21, A18.

Pelham, W. 1999. "The NIMH Multimodal Treatment Study for Attention-Deficit Hyperactivity Disorder: Just Say Yes to Drugs Alone?" *Canadian Journal of Psychiatry* 44: 981–990.

Pelham, W., and M. Bender. 1982. "Peer Relationships in Hyperactive Children." *Advances in Learning and Behavioral Disabilities* 1: 365–436.

Pelham, W., E. Gnagy, L. Burrows-Maclean, A. Williams, G. Fabiano, S. Morrisey, et al. 2001. "Once-a-Day Concerta Methylphenidate versus Three-Times-Daily Methylphenidate in Laboratory and Natural Settings." *Pediatrics* 107: 1417–1418.

Pelham, W., E. Gnagy, A. Greiner, B. Hoza, S. Hinshaw, J. Swanson, et al. 2000. "Behavioral versus Behavioral and Pharmacological Treatment in ADHD Children Attending a Summer Treatment Program." *Journal of Abnormal Child Psychology* 28: 507–525.

Pelham, W., and B. Hoza. 1996. "Intensive Treatment: A Summer Treatment Program for Children with ADHD." In *Psychosocial Treatments for Child* and Adolescent Disorders: Empirically Based Strategies for Clinical Practice, ed. E. D. Hibbs and P. S. Jensen, 311–340. Washington, DC: American Psychological Association.

Pelham, W., T. Wheeler, and A. Chronis. 1998. "Empirically Supported Psychosocial Treatments for Attention Deficit Hyperactivity Disorder." *Journal of Clinical Child Psychology* 27: 190–205.

Pellegrini, A., and M. Horvat. 1995. "A Developmental Contextualist Critique of Attention Deficit Hyperactivity Disorder." *Educational Researcher* 24 (January–February): 13–19.

Perils, R., C. Perils, Y. Wu, C. Hwang, M. Joseph, and A. Nierenberg. 2005. "Industry Sponsorship and Financial Conflict of Interest in the Reporting of Clinical Trials in Psychiatry." *American Journal of Psychiatry* 162, no. 10 (October): 1957–1960.

Perrin, J. 2002. "Health Services Research for Children with Disabilities." *Milbank Quarterly* 80: 303–324.

Perrin, J., K. Kuhlthau, T. McLaughlin, S. Ettner, and S. Gortmaker. 1999. "Changing Patterns of Conditions among Children Receiving Supplemental Security Income Disability Benefits." *Archives of Pediatric and Adolescent Medicine* 153 (January): 80–84.

Perring, C. 1997. "Medicating Children: The Case of Ritalin." *Bioethics* 11 (July): 228–240.

Pfeiffer, D. 1993. "Overview of the Disability Movement: History, Legislative Record, and Political Implications." *Policy Studies Journal* 21 (December): 724–734.

Pfiffner, L., and R. Barkley. 2006. "Treatment of ADHD in School Settings." In *Attention-Deficit Hyperactivity Disorder: A Handbook for Diagnosis and Treatment*. 2nd ed., by R. Barkley, 458–490. New York: Guilford Press.

Phillips, C. 2006. "Medicine Goes to School: Teachers as Sickness Brokers for ADHD." *PloS Medicine* 3 (April): 434.

Pincus, H., T. Tanielian, S. Marcus, M. Olfson, D. Zarin, J. Thompson, et al. 1998. "Prescribing Trends in Psychotropic Medications: Primary Care, Psychiatry, and Other Medical Specialties." *Journal of the American Medical Association* 279 (February 18): 526–531.

Pipher, M. 1995. *Reviving Ophelia: Saving the Selves of Adolescent Girls*. New York: Ballantine.

Plessen, K., R. Bansal, H. Zhu, R. Whiteman, J. Amat, G. Quackenbush, et al. 2006. "Hippocampus and Amygdala Morphology in Attention-Deficit/ Hyperactivity Disorder." *Archives of General Psychiatry* 63: 795–807.

Pliszka, S. 2000. "Patterns of Psychiatric Comorbidity with Attention Deficit/Hyperactivity Disorder." *Child Adolescent Psychiatric Clinics of North America* 9: 525–540.

Polanczyk, G., M. de Lima, B. Horta, J. Biederman, and L. Rohde. 2007. "The Worldwide Prevalence of ADHD: A Systematic Review and Metaregression Analysis." *American Journal of Psychiatry* 164 (June): 942–948.

Pollack, W. 1998. *Real Boys: Rescuing Our Sons from the Myths of Boyhood*. New York: Random House.

Pollard, M. 1990. "Managed Care and a Changing Pharmaceutical Industry." *Health Affairs* 9: 55–65.

Pope, A., and K. Bierman. 1999. "Predicting Adolescent Peer Problems and Antisocial Activities: The Relative Roles of Aggression and Dysregulation." *Developmental Psychology* 35: 335–346.

Pope, A., K. Bierman, and G. Mumma. 1989. "Relations between Hyperactive and Aggressive Behavior and Peer Relations at Three Elementary Grade Levels." *Journal of Abnormal Child Psychology* 17: 253–267.

Porter, N. 2001. "Who Decides What's Best for Your Child?" *Pennsylvania Lawyer* 23 (January–February): 16–17.

Pottick, K., D. McAlpine, and R. Andelman. 2000. "Changing Patterns of Psychiatric Inpatient Care for Children and Adolescents in General Hospitals, 1988–1995." *American Journal of Psychiatry* 157 (August): 1267–1273.

Poulin, C. 2007. "From Attention-Deficit/Hyperactivity Disorder to Medical Stimulant Use to the Diversion of Prescribed Stimulants to Non-Medical Stimulant Use: Connecting the Dots." *Addiction* 102 (May): 740–751.

Poulsen, R. 1992. "Some Current Factors Influencing the Prescribing and Use of Psychiatric Drugs." *Public Health Reports* 107 (January–February): 47–53.

Power, T., T. Costigan, S. Leff, R. Eiraldi, and S. Landau. 2001. "Assessing ADHD across Settings: Contributions of Behavioral Assessment to Categorical Decision-Making." *Journal of Clinical Child Psychology* 30 (September): 399–412.

Price, T., E. Simonoff, P. Asherson, S. Curran, J. Kuntsi, I. Waldman, et al. 2005. "Continuity and Change in Preschool ADHD Symptoms: Longitudinal Genetic Analysis with Contrast Effects." *Behavior Genetics* 35: 121–132.

Prince, J., T. Wilens, T. Spencer, and J. Biederman. 2006. "Pharmacotherapy of ADHD in Adults." In *Attention-Deficit Hyperactivity Disorder: A Handbook for Diagnosis and Treatment*. 3rd ed., ed. R. Barkley. New York: Guilford Press.

Pumariega, A., and E. Rothe. 2003. "Cultural Considerations in Child and Adolescent Psychiatric Emergencies and Crises." *Child and Adolescent Psychiatric Clinics of North America* 12 (October): 723–744.

Quay, H. 1997. "Inhibition and Attention Deficit Hyperactivity Disorder." *Journal of Abnormal Child Psychology* 25: 7–13.

Quist, J., and J. Kennedy. 2001. "Genetics of Childhood Disorders: XXIII. ADHD, Part 7: The Serotonin System." *Journal of the American Academy of Child and Adolescent Psychiatry* 40: 253–256.

Radigan, M., P. Lannon, P. Roohan, and F. Gesten. 2005. "Medication Patterns for Attention-Deficit/Hyperactivity Disorder and Comorbid Psychiatric Conditions in a Low-Income Neighborhood." *Journal of Child and Adolescent Psychopharmacology* 15 (February): 44–56.

Raehtz, T., R. Milewski, and N. Massoud. 1987. "Factors Influencing Prices Offered to Pharmaceutical Purchasing Groups." *American Journal of Hospital Pharmacy* 44 (September): 2073–2076.

Rafalovich, A. 2001. "The Conceptual History of Attention Deficit Hyperactivity Disorder: Idiocy, Imbecility, Encephalitis and the Child Deviant, 1877–1929." *Deviant Behavior: An Interdisciplinary Journal* 22: 93–115.

———. 2005. "Exploring Clinician Uncertainty in the Diagnosis and Treatment of Attention Deficit Hyperactivity Disorder." *Sociology of Health and Illness* 27 (April): 305–323.

Rains, A., and L. Scahill. 2004. "New Long-Acting Stimulants in Children with ADHD." *Journal of Child and Adolescent Psychiatric Nursing* 17 (October–December): 177–179.

Ramey, C. 1974. "Children and Public Policy: A Role for Psychologists." *American Psychologist* 29 (January): 14–18.

Rapin, I. 1964. "Brain Damage in Children." In *Practice of Pediatrics*, ed. J. Brennemann. Hagerstown, MD: Prior.

Rapoport, J., M. Buchsbaum, H. Weingartner, T. Zahn, C. Ludlow, and E. Mikkelsen. 1980. "Dextroamphetamine: The Cognitive and Behavioral Effects in Normal and Hyperactive Boys and Normal Men." *Archives of General Psychiatry* 37 (August): 933–943.

Rapoport, J., M. Buchsbaum, T. Zahn, H. Weingartner, C. Ludlow, and J. Mikkelsen. 1978. "Dextroamphetamine: Cognitive and Behavioral Effects on Normal Prepubertal Boys." *Science* 199: 560–563.

Rappley, M. 2005. "Attention-Deficit Hyperactivity Disorder." *New England Journal of Medicine* 352 (January 13): 165–173.

Rapport, M., S. Scanlan, and C. Denney. 1999. "Attention-Deficit/Hyperactivity Disorder and Scholastic Achievement: A Model of Dual Developmental Pathways." *Journal of Child Psychology and Psychiatry* 40: 1169–1183.

Rascati, J. 1990. "Commentary on Lewin and Sharfstein." *Psychiatry* 53 (May): 125.

Raskin, L., S. Shaywitz, B. Shaywitz, G. Anderson, and D. Cohen. 1984. "Neurochemical Correlates of Attention Deficit Disorder." *Pediatric Clinics of North America* 31: 387–396.

Redick, R., M. Witkin, and R. Manderscheid. 1994. "CMHS Data Highlights On: Availability of Psychiatric Beds, United States, Selected Years, 1970–1990." *Mental Health Statistical Note* (August): 1–7.

Reich, W. 1982. "Psychiatry's Second Coming." *Psychiatry* 41 (August): 189–196.

Reid, R., J. Maag, and S. Vasa. 1993–1994. "Attention Deficit Hyperactivity Disorder as a Disability Category: A Critique." *Exceptional Children* 60 (December–January): 198–214.

Relman, A. 1980. "The New Medical-Industrial Complex." *New England Journal of Medicine* 303: 963–970.

Resnick, R. 2005. "Attention Deficit Hyperactivity Disorder in Teens and Adults: They Don't All Outgrow It." *Journal of Clinical Psychology* 61: 529–533.

Rheinstein, P. 1998. "Overview of the US Food and Drug Administration's Reform Legislation." *Clinical Therapeutics* 20: C4–C11.

Richmond, J. 1970. "Disadvantaged Children: What Have They Compelled Us to Learn?" *Yale Journal of Biology and Medicine* 43 (December): 127–144.

Rissmiller, D., and J. Rissmiller. 2006. "Evolution of the Antipsychiatry Movement into Mental Health Consumerism." *Psychiatric Services* 57 (June): 863–866.

Robison, L., D. Sclar, and T. Skaer. 2005. "Datapoints: Trends in ADHD and Stimulant Use among Adults, 1995–2002." *Psychiatric Services* 56 (December): 1497.

Rodgers, K. 1996. "ADHD Med Reformulated: An Old Drug Reenters Market." *Drug Topics* 140 (March 18): 31–32.

Rogers, J. 1971. "Drug Abuse—Just What the Doctor Ordered?" *Psychology Today*, September, 16–24.

Rogler, L. 1997. "Making Sense of Historical Changes in the Diagnostic and Statistical Manual of Mental Disorders: Five Propositions." *Journal of Health and Social Behavior* 38 (March): 9–20.

Rohde, L., C. Szobot, G. Polanczyk, M. Schmitz, S. Martins, and S. Tramontina. 2005. "Attention-Deficit/Hyperactivity Disorder in a Diverse Culture: Do Research and Clinical Findings Support the Notion of a Cultural Construct for the Disorder?" *Biological Psychiatry* 57 (June): 1436–1441.

Rojas, N., and E. Chan. 2005. "Old and New Controversies in the Alternative Treatment of Attention-Deficit Hyperactivity Disorder." *Mental Retardation and Developmental Disabilities Research Reviews* 11: 116–130.

Rosenbaum, S., and P. Wise. 2007. "Crossing the Medicaid-Private Insurance Divide: The Case of EPSDT." *Health Affairs* 26 (March–April): 382–393.

Rosenhan, D. 1973. "On Being Sane in Insane Places." *Science* 179 (January 19): 250–258.

Rosenman, S. 2006. "Reconsidering the Attention Deficit Paradigm." *Australasian Psychiatry* 14 (June): 127–132.

Ross, D., and S. Ross. 1976. *Hyperactivity: Research, Theory, and Action.* New York: Wiley.

Rothman, D. 1994. "The Problem with 'Cosmetic Psychopharmacology.'" *New Republic* (February 14): 37–38.

Rowland, A., D. Umbach, K. Catoe, L. Stallone, S. Long, D. Rabiner, et al. 2001. "Studying the Epidemiology of Attention-Deficit Hyperactivity Disorder: Screening Method and Pilot Results." *Canadian Journal of Psychiatry* 46 (December): 931–940.

Rowntree, B. 1901. *Poverty: A Study of Town Life.* London: Macmillan.

Rubin, K., W. Bukowski, and J. Parker. 1998. "Peer Interactions, Relationships, and Groups." In *Handbook of Child Psychology.* 5th ed., ed. W. Damon. New York: Wiley.

Rushton, J., K. Fant, and S. Clark. 2004. "Use of Practice Guidelines in the Primary Care of Children with Attention-Deficit/Hyperactivity Disorder." *Pediatrics* 114 (July): 23–28.

Rushton, J., B. Felt, and M. Roberts. 2002. "Coding of Pediatric Behavioral and Mental Disorders." *Pediatrics* 110 (July): e8.

Safer, D. 1971. "Drugs for Problem School Children." *Journal of School Health* 41 (November): 491.

———. 1983. "Broader Clinical Considerations in Child Psychopharmacology Practice." *Comprehensive Psychiatry* 24 (November–December): 567–573.

———. 2000. "Are Stimulants Overprescribed for Youths with ADHD?" *Annals of Clinical Psychiatry* 12 (March): 55–62.

Safer, D., and J. Krager. 1988. "A Survey of Medication Treatment for Hyperactive/Inattentive Students." *Journal of the American Medical Association* 260 (October 21): 2256–2258.

———. 1992. "Effect of a Media Blitz and a Threatened Lawsuit on Stimulant Treatment." *Journal of the American Medical Association* 268 (August 26): 1004–1007.

———. 1994. "The Increased Rate of Stimulant Treatment for Hyperactive/Inattentive Students in Secondary Schools." *Pediatrics* 94 (October): 462–464.

Safer, D., J. Zito, and E. Fine. 1996. "Increased Methylphenidate Usage for Attention Deficit Disorder in the 1990s." *Pediatrics* 98: 1084–1088.

Safer, D., J. Zito, and J. Gardner. 2001. "Pemoline Hepatoxicity and Postmarketing Surveillance." *Journal of the American Academy of Child and Adolescent Psychiatry* 40: 622–629.

Safren, M. Otto, S. Sprich, C. Winett, T. Wilens, and J. Biederman. 2005. "Cognitive-Behavioral Therapy for ADHD in Medication-Treated Adults with Continued Symptoms." *Behaviour Research and Therapy* 43: 831–842.

Sameroff, A. 1995. "General Systems Theories and Developmental Psychopathology." In *Developmental Psychopathology*. Vol. 1, *Theory and Methods*, ed. D. Cicchetti and D. Cohen, 659–695. New York: Wiley.

Sandberg, S., and J. Barton. 1996. "Historical Development." In *Hyperactivity Disorders of Childhood*, ed. S. Sandberg. Cambridge: Cambridge University Press.

Sanua, V. 1990. "Leo Kanner (1894–1981): The Man and the Scientist." *Child Psychiatry and Human Development* 21 (Fall): 3–23.

Satel, S. 2005. *One Nation under Therapy: How the Helping Culture Is Eroding Self-Reliance*. New York: St. Martin's Press.

Satterfield, J., D. Cantwell, L. Lesser, and R. Podosin. 1972. "Physiological Studies of the Hyperkinetic Child." *American Journal of Psychiatry* 128 (May): 1418–1424.

Satterfield, J., L. Lesser, R. Saul, and D. Cantwell. 1973. "EEG Aspects in the Diagnosis and Treatment of Minimal Brain Dysfunction." *Annals of the New York Academy of Sciences* 205 (February 28): 274–282.

Savage, T. 1996. "Ethical Issues Surrounding Attention Deficit Hyperactivity Disorder." *Pediatric Nursing* 22 (May–June): 239–243.

Sax, L., and K. Kautz. 2003. "Who First Suggests the Diagnosis of Attention-Deficit/Hyperactivity Disorder?" *Annals of Family Medicine* 1 (September–October): 171–174.

Schachar, R. 1986. "Hyperkinetic Syndrome: Historical Development of the Concept." In *The Overactive Child*, ed. E. Taylor, 19–40. Oxford: Blackwell.

Scheff, T. 1963. "Decision Rules and Types of Errors, and Their Consequences in Medical Diagnosis." *Behavioral Science* 8: 97–107.

———. 1963. "The Role of the Mentally Ill and the Dynamics of Mental Disorder: A Research Framework." *Sociometry* 26: 436–453.

———. 1966. *Being Mentally Ill*. Chicago: Aldine.

————. 1968. "The Societal Reaction to Deviance: Ascriptive Elements in the Psychiatric Screening of Mental Patients in a Midwestern State." In *The Mental Patient*, ed. S. Spitzer and N. Denzin, 276–290. New York: McGraw-Hill.

Schenk, S., and B. Partridge. 1997. "Sensitization and Tolerance in Psychostimulant Self-Administration." *Pharmacology, Biochemistry and Behavior* 57: 543–550.

————. 1999. "Cocaine-Seeking Produced by Experimenter-Administered Drug Injections: Dose-Effect Relationships in Rats." *Psychopharmacology* 147: 285–290.

Schmied, L., H. Steinberg, and E. Sykes. 2006. "Psychopharmacology's Debt to Experimental Psychology." *History of Psychology* 9 (May): 144–157.

Schneider, H., and D. Eisenberg. 2006. "Who Receives a Diagnosis of Attention-Deficit/Hyperactivity Disorder in the United States Elementary School Population?" *Pediatrics* 117 (April): 601–609.

Schrag, P., and D. Divoky. 1975. *The Myth of the Hyperactive Child and Other Means of Child Control*. New York: Pantheon Books.

Schulz, K., J. Newcorn, K. McKay, J. Himelstein, V. Koda, L. Siever, et al. 2001. "Relationship between Central Serotonergic Function and Aggression in Prepubertal Boys: Effect of Age and Attention-Deficit/Hyperactivity Disorder." *Psychiatry Research* 101: 1–10.

Schulz, K., C. Tang, J. Fan, D. Marks, A. Cheung, J. Newcorn, et al. 2005. "Differential Prefrontal Cortex Activation during Inhibitory Control in Adolescents with and without Childhood Attention-Deficit/Hyperactivity Disorder." *Neuropsychology* 19: 390–402.

Scotch, R. 1989. "Politics and Policy in the History of the Disability Rights Movement." *Milbank Quarterly* 67: 380–400.

Sealander, J. 2003. *The Failed Century of the Child: Governing America's Young in the Twentieth Century*. New York: Cambridge University Press.

Segal, H., and H. Yahraes. 1978. "Protecting Children's Mental Health." *Children Today* 7 (September–October): 23–25.

Semrud-Clikeman, M., R. Steingard, P. Filipek, J. Biederman, K. Bekken, and P. Renshaw. 2000. "Using MRI to Examine Brain-Behavior Relationships in Males with Attention Deficit Disorder with Hyperactivity." *Journal of the American Academy of Child and Adolescent Psychiatry* 39: 477–484.

Shader, R., and J. Oesterheld. 2006. "Facts and Public Policy: Should I Keep My Child on ADHD Drugs?" *Journal of Clinical Psychopharmacology* 26 (June): 223–224.

Shapiro, J. 1994. *No Pity: People with Disabilities Forging a New Civil Rights Movement*. New York: Times Books.

Shaw, P., K. Eckstrand, W. Sharp, J. Blumenthal, J. Lerch, D. Greenstein, et al. 2007. "Attention-Deficit/Hyperactivity Disorder Is Characterized by a Delay in Cortical Maturation." *Proceedings of the National Academy of Sciences* 104 (November): 19649–19654.

Shaywitz, S., and B. Shaywitz. 1988. "Increased Medication Use in Attention-Deficit Hyperactivity Disorder: Regressive or Appropriate?" *Journal of the American Medical Association* 260 (October 21): 2270–2273.

Shear, L. 1998. "From Competition to Complementarity: Legal Issues and Their Clinical Implications in Custody." *Child and Adolescent Psychiatric Clinics of North America* 7 (April): vi–viii, 311–334.

Sherer, D. 1991. "The Capacities of Minors to Exercise Voluntariness in Medical Treatment Decisions." *Law and Human Behavior* 15 (August): 431–449.

Sherman, D., W. Iacono, and M. McGue. 1997. "Attention-Deficit Hyperactivity Disorder Dimensions: A Twin Study of Inattention and Impulsivity-Hyperactivity." *Journal of the American Academy of Child and Adolescent Psychiatry* 54: 745–753.

Shore, M., and A. Beigel. 1986. "Sounding Board: The Challenges Posed by Managed Behavioral Health Care." *New England Journal of Medicine* (January 11): 116–118.

Shorter, E. 1997. *A History of Psychiatry: From the Age of the Asylum to the Age of Prozac.* New York: Wiley.

Sieg, K., G. Gaffney, D. Preston, and J. Hellings. 1995. "SPECT Brain Imaging Abnormalities in Attention Deficit Hyperactivity Disorder." *Clinical Nuclear Medicine* 20: 55–60.

Silk, J., S. Nath, L. Siegel, and P. Kendall. 2000. "Conceptualizing Mental Disorders in Children: Where Have We Been and Where Are We Going?" *Development and Psychopathology* 12: 713–735.

Silverman, I., and D. Ragusa. 1992. "Child and Maternal Correlates of Impulse Control in 24-Month Old Children." *Genetic, Social, and General Psychology Monographs* 116: 435–473.

Singh, I. 2002. "Biology in Context: Social and Cultural Perspective on ADHD." *Children and Society* 16: 360–367.

———. 2006. "A Framework for Understanding Trends in ADHD Diagnosis and Stimulant Drug Treatment: School and Schooling as a Case Study." *BioSocieties* 1: 439–452.

———. 2007. "Clinical Implications of Ethical Concepts: Moral Self-Understandings in Children Taking Methylphenidate for ADHD." *Clinical Child Psychology and Psychiatry* 12 (April): 167–182.

———. 2007. "Not Just Naughty: 50 Years of Stimulant Drug Advertising." In *Medicating Modern America: Prescription Drugs in History*, ed. A. Tone and A. Watkins, 134–135. New York: New York University Press.

Skounti, M., A. Philalithis, and E. Galanakis. 2007. "Variations in Prevalence of Attention Deficit Hyperactivity Disorder Worldwide." *European Journal of Pediatrics* 166 (February): 117–123.

Sleator, E., and R. Ullmann. 1981. "Can the Physician Diagnose Hyperactivity in the Office?" *Pediatrics* 67 (January): 13–17.

Smith, M. 1991. *A Social History of the Minor Tranquilizers: The Quest for Small Comfort in the Age of Anxiety.* New York: Haworth Press.

Smith, R. 2005. "Medical Journals Are an Extension of the Marketing Arm of Pharmaceutical Companies." *PloS Medicine* 2, no. 5 (May): 364–366.

Smith, S., and D. Wesson. 1973. *Uppers and Downers*. Englewood Cliffs, NJ: Prentice-Hall.

Sommer, R. 1990. "Family Advocacy and the Mental Health System: The Recent Rise of the Alliance for the Mentally Ill." *Psychiatric Quarterly* 61 (Fall): 205–221.

Sommers, C. 2001. *The War against Boys: How Misguided Feminism Is Harming Our Young Men*. New York: Simon and Schuster.

Sommers, C., and Satel, S. 2005. *One Nation under Therapy: How the Helping Culture Is Eroding Self-Reliance*. New York: St. Martin's Press.

Sparks, J., and B. Duncan. 2004. "The Ethics and Science of Medicating Children." *Ethical Human Psychology and Psychiatry* 6 (Spring): 25–39.

Spencer, T. 2006. "Antidepressant and Specific Norepinephrine Reuptake Inhibitor Treatments." In *Attention-Deficit Hyperactivity Disorder: A Handbook for Diagnosis and Treatment*. 3rd ed., by R. Barkley, 648–657. New York: Guilford Press.

Spencer, T., J. Biederman, and E. Mick. 2007. "Attention-Deficit/Hyperactivity Disorder: Diagnosis, Lifespan, Comorbidities, and Neurobiology." *Ambulatory Pediatrics* 7 (January–February): 73–81.

Spencer, T., J. Biederman, and T. Wilens. 2000. "Pharmacotherapy of Attention Deficit Hyperactivity Disorder." *Psychopharmacology* 9: 77–97.

Spencer, T., J. Biederman, T. Wilens, S. Faraone, J. Prince, K. Gerard, et al. 2001. "Efficacy of a Mixed Amphetamine Salts Compound in Adults with Attention-Deficit/Hyperactivity Disorder." *Archives of General Psychiatry* 58: 775–782.

Spencer, T., J. Biederman, T. Wilens, M. Harding, D. O'Donnell, and S. Griffin. 1996. "Pharmacotherapy of Attention-Deficit Hyperactivity Disorder Across the Life Cycle." *Journal of the American Academy of Child and Adolescent Psychiatry* 35: 409–432.

Spencer, T., T. Wilens, J. Biederman, S. Faraone, J. Ablon, and K. Lapey. 1995. "A Double-Blind, Crossover Comparison of Methylphenidate and Placebo in Adults with Childhood-Onset Attention-Deficit Hyperactivity Disorder." *Archives of General Psychiatry* 52: 434–443.

Sperber, M. 1992. "Short-Sheeting the Psychiatric Bed: State-Level Strategies to Curtail the Unnecessary Hospitalization of Adolescents in For-Profit Mental Health Facilities." *American Journal of Law and Medicine* 18: 251–276.

Spetie, L., and L. Arnold. 2007. "Ethical Issues in Child Psychopharmacology Research and Practice." *Psychopharmacology* 191 (March): 15–26.

Spiegel, A. 2005. "The Dictionary of Disorder: How One Man Revolutionized Psychiatry." *New Yorker*, January 3, 56–63.

Spitzer, R. 1975. "On Pseudoscience in Science, Logic in Remission, and Psychiatric Diagnosis: A Critique of Rosenhan's 'On Being Sane in Insane Places.'" *Journal of Abnormal Psychology* 84 (October): 442–452.

———. 1976. "More on Pseudoscience in Science and the Case for Psychiatric Diagnosis. A Critique of D. L. Rosenhan's 'On Being Sane in Insane Places' and 'The Contestual Nature of Psychiatric Diagnosis.'" *Archives of General Psychiatry* 33 (April): 459–470.

———. 1981. "The Diagnostic Status of Homosexuality in DSM-III: An Insider's Perspective." *American Journal of Psychiatry* 138 (February): 210–215.

Spitzer, R., M. Sheehy, and J. Endicott. 1977. "DSM-III: Guiding Principles." In *Psychiatric Diagnosis*, ed. V. Rakoff, H. Stancer, and H. Kedward. New York: Brunner/Mazel.

Spitzer, R., J. Williams, and A. Skodal. 1980. "DSM-III: The Major Achievements and an Overview." *American Journal of Psychiatry* 137: 151–164.

Sprague, R. 1978. "Principles of Clinical Trials and Social, Ethical and Legal Issues of Drug Use in Children." In *Pediatric Psychopharmacology: The Use of Behavior Modifying Drugs in Children*, ed. J. Werry. New York: Branner-Mazel.

Staton, D. 1991. "Psychiatry's Future: Facing Reality." *Psychiatric Quarterly* 62 (Summer): 165–176.

Steen, P. 1931. "Epidemic Encephalitis." *American Journal of Nursing* 31 (November): 1235–1239.

Stein, M. 2004. "Innovations in Attention-Deficit/Hyperactivity Disorder Pharmacotherapy: Long-Acting Stimulant and Nonstimulant Treatments." *American Journal of Managed Care* 10 (July): S89–S98.

Stein, M., N. Marx, J. Beard, M. Lerner, B. Levin, F. Glascoe, et al. 2004. "ADHD: The Diagnostic Process from Different Perspectives." *Journal of Developmental and Behavioral Pediatrics* 25 (February): 53–58.

Stevens, J., J. Harman, and K. Kelleher. 2004. "Ethnic and Regional Differences in Primary Care Visits for Attention-Deficit Hyperactivity Disorder." *Journal of Developmental and Behavioral Pediatrics* 25 (October): 318–325.

———. 2005. "Race/Ethnicity and Insurance Status as Factors Associated with ADHD Treatment Patterns." *Journal of Child and Adolescent Psychopharmacology* 15 (February): 88–96.

Stewart, M., F. Pitts, A. Craig, and W. Dieruf. 1966. "The Hyperactive Child Syndrome." *American Journal of Orthopsychiatry* 36 (October): 861–867.

Still, G. 1902. "The Goulstonian Lectures on Some Abnormal Psychical Conditions in Children." *Lancet* 1 (April 12): 1008–1012, (April 19): 1079–1082, (April 26): 1163–1167.

Stolberg, S. 2002. "Preschool Meds." *New York Times*, November 17, E58.

Stoller, R., J. Marmor, I. Bieber, R. Gold, C. Socarides, R. Green, et al. 1973. "A Symposium: Should Homosexuality Be in the APA Nomenclature?" *American Journal of Psychiatry* 130 (November): 1207–1216.

Stone, A. 1995. "Psychotherapy and Managed Care: The Bigger Picture." *Harvard Mental Health Letter* 11 (February): 5–7.

Stone, D. 1979. *The Disabled State*. Philadelphia: Temple University Press.

Strauss, A., and L. Lehtinen. 1947. *Psychopathology and Education of the Brain-Injured Child*. New York: Grune and Stratton.

Strauss, A., and H. Werner. 1942. "Disorders of Conceptual Thinking in the Brain-Injured Child." *Journal of Nervous and Mental Disease* 96: 153–172.

———. 1943. "Comparative Psychopathology of the Brain-Injured Child and the Traumatic Brain-Injured Adult." *American Journal of Psychiatry* 99: 835–838.

Strauss, G., M. Chassin, and J. Lock. 1994. "Can Experts Agree When to Hospitalize Adolescents?" *Journal of the American Academy of Child and Adolescent Psychiatry* 34: 418–424.

Strauss, G., J. Yager, and G. Strauss. 1984. "The Cutting Edge in Psychiatry." *American Journal of Psychiatry* 141 (January): 38–43.

Strecker, E., and F. Ebaugh. 1924. "Neuropsychiatric Sequelae of Cerebral Trauma in Children." *Archives of Neurology and Psychiatry* 12: 443–453.

Strother, C. 1973. "Minimal Cerebral Dysfunction: A Historical Overview." *Annals of the New York Academy of Sciences* 205 (February 28): 6–17.

Stroul, B., S. Pires, M. Armstrong, and J. Meyers. 1998. "The Impact of Managed Care on Mental Health Services for Children and Their Families." *Future of the Child* 8 (Summer–Fall): 119–133.

Sturm, R. 2000. "How Does Risk Sharing between Employers and a Managed Behavioral Health Organization Affect Mental Health Care?" *Health Services Research* 35 (October): 761–776.

Swanson, J. 2007. "Secondary Evaluations of MTA 36-Month Outcomes: Propensity Score and Growth Mixture Model Analyses." *Journal of the American Academy of Child and Adolescent Psychiatry* 46: 1003–1014.

Swanson, J., G. Elliott, L. Greenhill, T. Wigal, L. Arnold, B. Vitiello, et al. 2007. "Effects of Stimulant Medication on Growth Rates across 3 Years in the MTA Follow-Up." *Journal of the American Academy of Child and Adolescent Psychiatry* 46: 1015–1027.

Swanson, J., L. Greenhill, T. Wigal, S. Kollins, A. Stehli-Nguyen, M. Davies, et al. 2006. "Stimulant-Related Reductions of Growth Rates in the PATS." *Journal of the American Academy of Child and Adolescent Psychiatry* 45: 1304–1313.

Swanson, J., M. Lerner, and L. Williams. 1995. "More Frequent Diagnosis of Attention-Deficit Hyperactivity Disorder." *New England Journal of Medicine* 333 (October 5): 944.

Swanson, J., K. McBurnett, D. Christian, and T. Wigal. 1995. "Stimulant Medications and the Treatment of Children with ADHD." In *Advances in Clinical Child Psychology*. Vol. 17, ed. T. Ollendick and R. Prinz. New York: Plenum Press.

Swanson, J., K. McBurnett, T. Wigal, L. Pfiffner, M. Lerner, L. Williams, et al. 1993. "Effect of Stimulant Medication on Children with Attention Deficit Disorder: A 'Review of Reviews.'" *Exceptional Children* 60: 154–162.

Swazey, J. 1974. *Chlorpromazine in Psychiatry: A Study of Therapeutic Innovation.* Cambridge, MA: MIT Press.

Szasz, T. 1961. *The Myth of Mental Illness.* New York: Hoeber-Harper.

———. 1963. *Law, Liberty, and Psychiatry.* New York: MacMillan.

———. 1970. *The Manufacture of Madness*. New York: Harper and Row.

Szatmari, P. 1992. "The Epidemiology of Attention-Deficit Hyperactivity Disorders." *Child and Adolescent Psychiatric Clinics of North America* 1: 361–372.

Szatmari, P., D. Offord, and M. Boyle. 1989. "Correlates, Associated Impairments, and Patterns of Service Utilization of Children with Attention Deficit Disorders: Findings from the Ontario Child Health Study." *Journal of Child Psychology and Psychiatry* 30: 205–217.

Tannock, R. 1998. "Attention Deficit Hyperactivity Disorder: Advances in Cognitive, Neurobiological, and Genetic Research." *Journal of Child Psychology and Psychiatry* 39: 65–100.

Taube, C., J. Lave, A. Rupp, H. Goldman, and R. Frank. 1988. "Psychiatry under Prospective Payment: Experience in the First Year." *American Journal of Psychiatry* 145 (February): 210–213.

Taube, C., J. Thompson, B. Burns, P. Widem, and C. Prevost. 1985. "Prospective Payment and Psychiatric Discharges from General Hospitals with and without Psychiatric Units." *Hospital Community Psychiatry* 36 (July): 754–760.

Taylor, E., and J. Rogers. 2005. "Practitioner Review: Early Adversity and Developmental Disorders." *Journal of Child Psychology and Psychiatry* 46 (May): 451–467.

Taylor, W. 1971. "Developmental Theory: Unsolved Problem for Child Psychiatry." *American Journal of Orthopsychiatry* 41 (July): 557–565.

Teter, C., S. McCabe, C. Boyd, and S. Guthrie. 2003. "Illicit Methylphenidate Use in an Undergraduate Student Sample: Prevalence and Risk Factors." *Pharmacotherapy* 23: 609–617.

———. 2005. "Prevalence and Motives for Illicit Use of Prescription Stimulants in an Undergraduate Student Sample." *Journal of American College Health* 53: 253–262.

Thomas, C., P. Conrad, R. Casler, and E. Goodman. 2006. "Trends in the Use of Psychotropic Medications among Adolescents, 1994 to 2001." *Psychiatric Services* 57 (January): 63–69.

Thornton, A., and D. Freedman. 1983. "The Changing American Family." *Population Bulletin* 38 (October): 1–44.

Timimi, S. 2004. "ADHD Is Best Understood as a Cultural Construct." *British Journal of Psychiatry* 184: 8–9.

Tirosh, E., J. Berger, M. Cohen-Ophir, M. Davidovitch, and A. Cohen. 1998. "Learning Disabilities with and without Attention Deficit-Hyperactivity Disorder: Parents' and Teachers' Perspectives." *Journal of Child Neurology* 13 (June): 270–276.

Tomes, N. 2006. "The Patient as a Policy Factor: A Historical Case Study of the Consumer/Survivor Movement in Mental Health." *Health Affairs* 25 (May–June): 720–729.

Tone, A., and E. Watkins, eds. 2007. *Medicating Modern America: Prescription Drugs in History*. New York: New York University Press.

Tredgold, A. 1922. *Mental Deficiency (Amentia)*. 4th ed. New York: William Wood.

U.S. Congress. House. 1990. *Education of the Handicapped Act Amendments of 1990: Report to Accompany H.R. 1013.* 101st Cong., 2nd sess. H. Rept. 101-544.

———. 1990. Committee on Education and Labor. Subcommittee on Select Education. *Hearings on the Reauthorization of the EHA Discretionary Programs.* 101st Cong., 2nd sess., 352–355.

———. 2002. Committee on Government Reform. *Attention Deficit/Hyperactivity Disorder—Are We Over-Medicating Our Children?* 107th Cong., 2nd sess., September 26.

———. 1971. Committee on Ways and Means. *The Social Security Amendments of 1971.* 92nd Cong., 2nd sess. H. Rept. 92-231.

———. 1970. Subcommittee of the Committee on Government Operations. *Federal Involvement in the Use of Behavior Modification Drugs on Grammar School Children on the Right to Privacy Inquiry.* 91st Cong., 2nd sess., September 29.

U.S. Congress. Senate. 1973. Committee on Labor and Public Welfare. Subcommittee on the Handicapped. "Education for All Handicapped Children, 1973–1974." Hearings, 93rd Cong., 1st sess., May 7.

U.S. Department of Education. 2002. *To Assure the Free Appropriate Public Education of All Children with Disabilities.* Washington, DC: Government Printing Office.

U.S. Department of Health and Human Services. 2000. *Mental Health: A Report of the Surgeon General.* Washington, DC: Government Printing Office.

U.S. General Accounting Office. September 1994. *Social Security: Rapid Rise in Children on SSI Disability Rolls Follows New Regulations.* GAO/HEHS-94-225. Washington, DC: Government Printing Office.

———. January 27 1995. *Supplemental Security Income: Recent Growth in the Rolls Raises Fundamental Program Concerns.* GAO/T-HEHS-95-67. Washington, DC.

Vaczek, D. 1996. "The Rise of the Generic Drug Industry." *American Druggist* (April): 41–45.

Visser, S., C. Lesesne, and R. Perou. 2007. "National Estimates and Factors Associated with Medication Treatment for Childhood Attention-Deficit/Hyperactivity Disorder." *Pediatrics* 119 (February, Suppl.): S99–S106.

Vitiello, B. 2001. "Psychopharmacology for Young Children: Clinical Needs and Research Opportunities." *Pediatrics* 108 (October): 983–989.

Vitiello, B., S. Zuvekas, and G. Norquist. 2006. "National Estimates of Antidepressant Medication Use among U.S. Children." *Journal of the American Academy of Child and Adolescent Psychiatry* 45: 271–279.

Volkow, N., Y. Ding, J. Fowler, G. Want, J. Logan, J. Gatley, et al. 1995. "Is Methylphenidate Like Cocaine? Studies on Their Pharmacokinetics and Distribution in the Human Brain." *Archives of General Psychiatry* 52: 456–463.

Volkow, N., G. Wang, S. Gatley, J. Fowler, Y. Ding, J. Logan, et al. 1996. "Temporal Relationships between the Pharmacokinetics of Methylphenidate in the

Human Brain and Its Behavioral and Cardiovascular Effects." *Psychopharmacology* 123: 26–33.

Wahlback, K., and C. Adams. 1999. "Beyond Conflicts of Interest: Sponsored Drug Trials Show More Favorable Outcomes." *British Medical Journal* 318, no. 7181 (February 13): 465.

Waldrop, M., R. Bell, B. McLaughlin, and C. Halverson. 1978. "Newborn Minor Physical Anomalies Predict Short Attention Span, Peer Aggression, and Impulsivity at Age 3." *Science* 199 (February 3): 563–565.

Waldrop, M., F. Pederson, and R. Bell. 1968. "Minor Physical Anomalies and Behavior in Preschool Children." *Child Development* 39 (June): 391–400.

Walker, S. 1999. *The Hyperactive Hoax: How to Stop Drugging Your Child and Find Real Medical Help*. New York: St. Martin's Press.

Wallen, J., and H. Pincus. 1988. "Care of Children with Psychiatric Disorders at Community Hospitals." *Hospital and Community Psychiatry* 39 (February): 167–172.

Wallis, C. 1994. "Life in Overdrive." *Time*, July 18, 42.

Wardell, W., M. May, and G. Trimble. 1982. "New Drug Development by U.S. Pharmaceutical Firms." *Clinical Pharmacology and Therapeutics* (October): 407–417.

Ware, N., W. Lachicotte, S. Kirschner, D. Cortes, and B. Good. 2000. "Clinician Experiences of Managed Mental Health Care: A Rereading of the Threat." *Medical Anthropology Quarterly* 14: 3–27.

Warner-Rogers, J., A. Taylor, E. Taylor, and S. Sandberg. 2000. "Inattentive Behavior in Childhood: Epidemiology and Implications for Development." *Journal of Learning Disabilities* 33 (November): 520–536.

Wax, P. 1997. "Analeptic Use in Clinical Toxicology: A Historical Appraisal." *Journal of Toxicology: Clinical Toxicology* 35 (March): 203–209.

Weatherwax, J., and E. Benoit. 1962. "Concrete and Abstract Thinking in Organic and Non-Organic Mentally Retarded Children." In *Readings on the Exceptional Child: Research and Theory*, ed. E. Trapp and P. Himmelstein. New York: Appleton-Century-Crofts.

Weaver, R. 2000. *Ending Welfare as We Know It*. Washington, DC: Brookings Institution Press.

Wechsler, J. 2001. "FDA: A History of Leadership, Partnership, and Transformation." *Pharmaceutical Technology* (July): 14–16.

Weiner, B. 1985. "An Overview of Child Custody Laws." *Hospital and Community Psychiatry* 36 (August): 838–843.

Weiner, J., A. Lyles, D. Steinwachs, and K. Hall. 1991. "Impact of Managed Care on Prescription Use." *Health Affairs* 10 (Spring): 140–154.

Weiss, M., L. Hechtman, and G. Weiss. 1989. *ADHD in Adulthood: A Guide to Current Theory, Diagnosis, and Treatment*. Baltimore: Johns Hopkins University Press.

Weiss, N. 1977. "Mother, the Invention of Necessity: Dr. Benjamin Spock's Baby and Child Care." *American Quarterly* 29: 519–546.

Weithorn, L. 1988. "Mental Hospitalization of Troublesome Youth: An Analysis of Skyrocketing Admission Rates." *Stanford Law Review* 40 (February): 773–838.

Welke, R. 1999. "Litigation Involving Ritalin and the Hyperactive Child." *Detroit College Law Review* (Spring): 125–176.

Wells, K. 1995. "Parent Management Training." In *Conduct Disorders in Children and Adolescents*, ed. G. Sholevar, 213–236. Washington, DC: American Psychiatric Association.

Wells, K., W. Pelham, Jr., R. Kotkin, B. Hoza, H. Abikoff, A. Abramowitz, et al. 2000. "Psychosocial Treatment Strategies in the MTA Study: Rationale, Methods, and Critical Issues in Design and Implementation." *Journal of Abnormal Child Psychology* 28: 483–505.

Wender, P. 1995. *Attention-Deficit Hyperactivity in Adults.* New York: Oxford University Press.

———. 2000. *ADHD: Attention-Deficit Hyperactivity Disorder in Children and Adults.* New York: Oxford University Press.

Wender, P., and F. Reimherr. 1990. "Buproprion Treatment of Attention Deficit Hyperactivity Disorder in Adults." *American Journal of Psychiatry* 147: 1018–1020.

Wender, P., F. Reimherr, D. Wood, and M. Ward. 1995. "A Controlled Study of Methylphenidate in the Treatment of Attention Deficit Disorder, Residual Type, in Adults." *American Journal of Psychiatry* 142: 547–552.

Werry, J. 1978. *Pediatric Psychopharmacology: The Use of Behavior Modifying Drugs in Children.* New York: Brunner/Mazel, Publishers.

Whalen, C., and B. Henker. 1992. "The Social Profile of Attention-Deficit Hyperactivity Disorder: Five Fundamental Facets." *Child and Adolescent Psychiatric Clinics of North America* 1: 395–410.

Whalen, C., B. Henker, L. Jamner, S. Ishikawa, J. Floro, R. Swindle, et al. 2006. "Toward Mapping Daily Challenges of Living with ADHD: Maternal and Child Perspectives Using Electronic Devices." *Journal of Abnormal Child Psychology* 34: 15–30.

Whalen, C., L. Jamner, B. Henker, R. Delfino, and J. Lozano. 2002. "The ADHD Spectrum and Everyday Life: Experience Sampling of Adolescent Moods, Activities, Smoking, and Drinking." *Child Development* 73 (January–February): 209–227.

Whittaker, A., R. Van Rossem, J. Feldman, I. Schonfeld, J. Pinto-Martin, C. Torre, et al. 1997. "Psychiatric Outcomes in Low-Birth-Weight Children at Age 6 Years: Relation to Neonatal Cranial Ultrasound Abnormalities." *Archives of General Psychiatry* 54: 847–856.

Widiger, T., and D. Samuel. 2005. "Diagnostic Categories or Dimensions? A Question for the Diagnostic and Statistical Manual of Mental Disorders—Fifth Edition." *Journal of Abnormal Psychology* 114 (November): 494–504.

Wigal, T., L. Greenhill, S. Chuang, J. McGough, B. Vitiello, A. Skrobala, et al. 2006. "Safety and Tolerability of Methylphenidate in Preschool Children with ADHD." *Journal of the American Academy of Child and Adolescent Psychiatry* 45: 1294–1303.

Wilens, T., J. Biederman, S. Brown, et al. 2002. "Psychiatric Comorbidity and Functioning in Clinically Referred Preschool Children and School-Age Youth with ADHD." *Journal of the American Academy of Child and Adolescent Psychiatry* 41: 262–268.

Wilens, T., J. Biederman, J. Prince, et al. 1996. "Six-Week, Double-Blind, Placebo-Controlled Study of Desipramine for Adult Attention Deficit Hyperactivity Disorder." *American Journal of Psychiatry* 153: 1147–1153.

Wilens, T., S. Faraone, J. Biederman, and S. Gunawardene. 2003. "Attention-Deficit/Hyperactivity Disorder Beget Later Substance Abuse? A Meta-Analytic Review of the Literature." *Pediatrics* 111: 179–185.

Wilens, T., M. Gignac, A. Swezey, M. Monuteaux, and J. Biederman. 2006. "Characteristics of Adolescents and Young Adults with ADHD Who Divert or Misuse Their Prescribed Medications." *Journal of the American Academy of Child and Adolescent Psychiatry* 45: 408–414.

Wilens, T., and T. Spencer. 2000. "The Stimulants Re-visited." *Child and Adolescent Psychiatric Clinics of North America* 9: 573–603.

Wilens, T., T. Spencer, and J. Biederman. 1998. "Pharmacotherapy of Adult ADHD." In *Attention-Deficit Hyperactivity Disorder: A Handbook for Diagnosis and Treatment.* 2nd ed., by R. Barkley, 592–606. New York: Guilford Press.

Williams, J., K. Klinepeter, G. Palmes, A. Pulley, and J. Foy. 2004. "Diagnosis and Treatment of Behavioral Health Disorders in Pediatric Practice." *Pediatrics* 114 (September): 601–606.

Willis, T., and I. Lovaas. 1977. "A Behavioral Approach to Treating Hyperactive Children: The Parent's Role." In *Learning Disabilities and Related Disorders*, ed. J. Millichap, 119–140. Chicago: Year Book Medical.

Wilson, J.T. 1999. "An Update on the Therapeutic Orphan." *Pediatrics* 104: 585–590.

Wilson, M. 1993. "DSM-III and the Transformation of American Psychiatry: A History." *American Journal of Psychiatry* 150 (March): 399–410.

Wolraich. M. 1999. "Attention Deficit Hyperactivity Disorder: The Most Studied and Yet the Most Controversial Diagnosis." *Mental Retardation and Developmental Disabilities Research Reviews* 5: 163–168.

Wolraich, M., L. Greenhill, W. Pelham, J. Swanson, T. Wilens, D. Palumbo, et al. 2001. "Randomized, Controlled Trial of OROS Methylphenidate Once a Day in Children with Attention-Deficit/Hyperactivity Disorder." *Pediatrics* 108: 883–892.

Wood, D., F. Reimherr, P. Wender, et al. 1976. "Diagnosis and Treatment of Minimal Brain Dysfunction in Adults." *Archives of General Psychiatry* 33: 1453–1460.

Woodward, B., and B. Weiser. 1994. "Costs Soar for Children's Disability Program: How 26 Words Cost the Taxpayers Billions in New Entitlement Payments." *Washington Post*, February 4, A1.

Wortis, J. 1986. "Adolph Meyer: Some Recollections and Impressions." *British Journal of Psychiatry* 149 (December): 677–681.

Wright, L. 1979. "Health Care Psychology: Prospects for the Well-Being of Children." *American Psychologist* 34 (October): 1001–1006.

Wynia, M., D. Cummins, J. VanGeest, and I. Wilson. 2000. "Physician Manipulation of Reimbursement Rules for Patients: Between a Rock and a Hard Place." *Journal of the American Medical Association* 283 (April 12): 1858–1865.

Yelowitz, A. 1998. "The Impact of Health Care Costs and Medicaid on SSI Participation." In *Growth in Income Entitlement Benefits for Disability: Explanations and Policy Implications*, ed. K. Rupp and D. Stapleton, 109–133. Kalamazoo, MI: Upjohn Institute.

Yost, R., and D. Flowers. 1987. "New Roles for Wholesalers in Hospital Drug Distribution." *Topics in Hospital Pharmacy Management* 7 (August): 84–90.

Young, A. 1995. *The Harmony of Illusions: Inventing Post-Traumatic Stress Disorder*. Princeton, NJ: Princeton University Press.

Young, D. 2006. "FDA Ponders Cardiovascular Risks of ADHD Drugs." *American Journal of Health-Systems Pharmacy* 63 (March 15): 492–494.

Zahn, T., J. Rapoport, and C. Thompson. 1980. "Autonomic and Behavioral Effects of Dextroamphetamine and Placebo in Normal and Hyperactive Prepubertal Boys." *Journal of Abnormal Child Psychology* 8 (June): 145–160.

Zametkin, A., L. Liebenauer, G. Fitzgerald, A. King, D. Minjunas, P. Herscovitch, et al. 1993. "Brain Metabolism in Teenagers with Attention-Deficit Hyperactivity Disorder." *Archives of General Psychiatry* 50: 333–340.

Zametkin, A., T. Nordahl, M. Gross, A. King, W. Semple, J. Rumsey, et al. 1990. "Cerebral Glucose Metabolism in Adults with Hyperactivity of Childhood Onset." *New England Journal of Medicine* 323: 1361–1366.

Zamiska, N. 2004. "Students Turn to Drugs to Ace Admissions Exams." *Wall Street Journal*, November 8, A1.

Zernike, K., and M. Petersen. 2001. "Schools' Backing of Behavior Drugs Comes under Fire; Legislatures Set Limits." *New York Times*, August 19, 1.

Zipkin, D., and M. Steinman. 2005. "Interactions between Pharmaceutical Representatives and Doctors in Training." *Journal of General Internal Medicine* 20 (August): 777–786.

Zito, J., and H. Koplewicz. 2007. "The Pharmaceutical Industry, Academic Medicine and the FDA." *Journal of Child and Adolescent Psychopharmacology* 17: 275–278.

Zito, J., D. Safer, S. dosReis, J. Gardner, M. Boles, and F. Lynch. 2000. "Trends in the Prescribing of Psychotropic Medications to Preschoolers." *Journal of the American Medical Association* 283: 1025–1030.

Zito, J., D. Safer, S. dosReis, J. Gardner, L. Magder, K. Soeken, et al. 2003. "Psychotropic Practice Patterns for Youth: A 10-Year Perspective." *Archives of Pediatric and Adolescent Medicine* 157: 17–25.

Zito, J., D. Safer, S. dosReis, L. Magder, J. Gardner, and D. Zarin. 1999. "Psychotherapeutic Medication Patterns for Youths with Attention-Deficit/Hyperactivity Disorder." *Archives of Pediatrics and Adolescent Medicine* 153 (December): 1257–1265.

Zito, J., D. Safer, S. dosReis, L. Magder, and M. Riddle. 1997. "Methylphenidate Patterns among Medicaid Youths." *Psychopharmacology Bulletin* 33: 143–147.

Zuvekas, S. 2001. "Trends in Mental Health Services Use and Spending." *Health Affairs* 20 (March–April): 214–224.

———. 2005. "Prescription Drugs and the Changing Patterns of Treatment for Mental Disorders, 1996–2001." *Health Affairs* 24 (January–February): 195–205.

Zuvekas, S., B. Vitiello, and G. Norquist. 2006. "Recent Trends in Stimulant Medication Use among U.S. Children." *American Journal of Psychiatry* 163 (May): 579–585.

# Index

Ablechild, 161, 163

Academic performance: stimulants and, 4–5, 8, 9, 12, 160–164, 170, 207; ADHD impact on, 16, 17, 18, 19, 23, 166–169; peer rejection and, 24–25, 202; combined treatments and, 40, 41–42; special education for, 97, 100, 105–112, 117, 121–123; modification of standards, 124–125, 132; educators' role, 159, 164–166, 168, 169, 170, 281n130

Accommodations: for disabled individuals, 96, 97, 101, 102, 104, 169; special education reform and, 108, 111, 112, 124, 132, 133–134, 269n115

ADD. *See* Attention deficit disorder (ADD)

ADHD. *See* Attention deficit/hyper-activity disorder (ADHD)

Adjustment disorders, 25–26, 32, 54, 79

Adolescents, ADHD in: inpatient mental health services for, 8, 60, 63, 73, 78, 84–87; prevalence, 19–20; peer rejection outcomes, 24–25; DSM-III focus on, 79–84, 194; drug abuse and stimulant use, 147–148, 187–193; illicit stimulant use, 175–180, 185

Ad-pscyh units, 85, 87

Adults/adulthood, ADHD in: stimulant therapy for, 2, 10, 148, 196–198, 208; prevalence, 19, 194; peer rejection outcomes, 24–25; tranquilizers for, 58, 59, 244n112; identity related to,

103–105; disabilities with, 115, 118–119; research on, 145, 196–198; illicit stimulant use by, 177–180; substance use correlation, 192–193; diagnostic criteria, 194–196, 210

Adverse reactions, to stimulants, 34, 158–159, 212

Advocacy/advocates: for mental health, 2–3, 8, 93, 97, 101–102, 133, 141; research applications, 12–13, 67, 78; for ADHD prevention, 22, 66–67; for inpatient services, 84–87; antipoverty, 97–99, 112–114, 115–116, 120–123, 127, 137–138; for disability reform, 99–105, 115; for special education, 105–112; opposing stimulant therapy, 143–144, 159, 161–164, 165, 166; for stimulant therapy, 146–147

African Americans, diagnostic trends in, 109, 283n168

"Age-appropriate" standards, for functional assessment, 117

Age, off-label psychotropics use and, 151–152, 156, 171

Age of onset, in ADHD diagnosis, 17–18, 19, 194, 291n24

Aggressive behavior, in ADHD, 23–24, 150

Aid to Families with Dependent Children (AFDC), 121–122, 135

Alcohol abuse: ADHD associated with, 30–31, 176; stimulants and, 180, 182, 183, 185, 187, 189, 191

Alerting, in ADHD, 26